THE COMPLETE
ILLUSTRATED
GUIDE TO

CHINESE MEDICINE

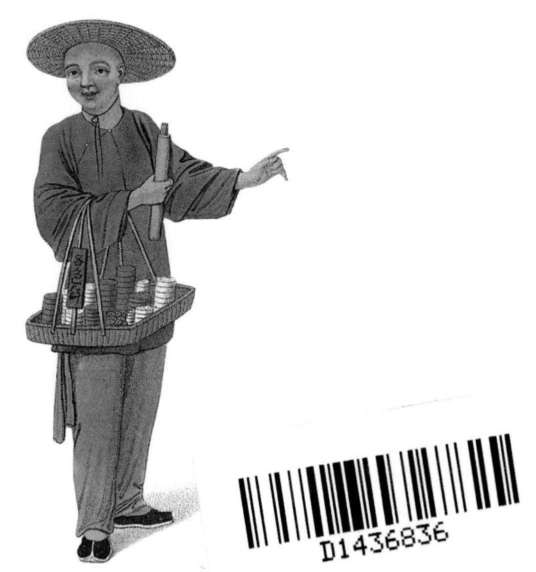

D1436836

ABERDEENSHIRE
LIBRARIES

WITHDRAWN
FROM LIBRARY

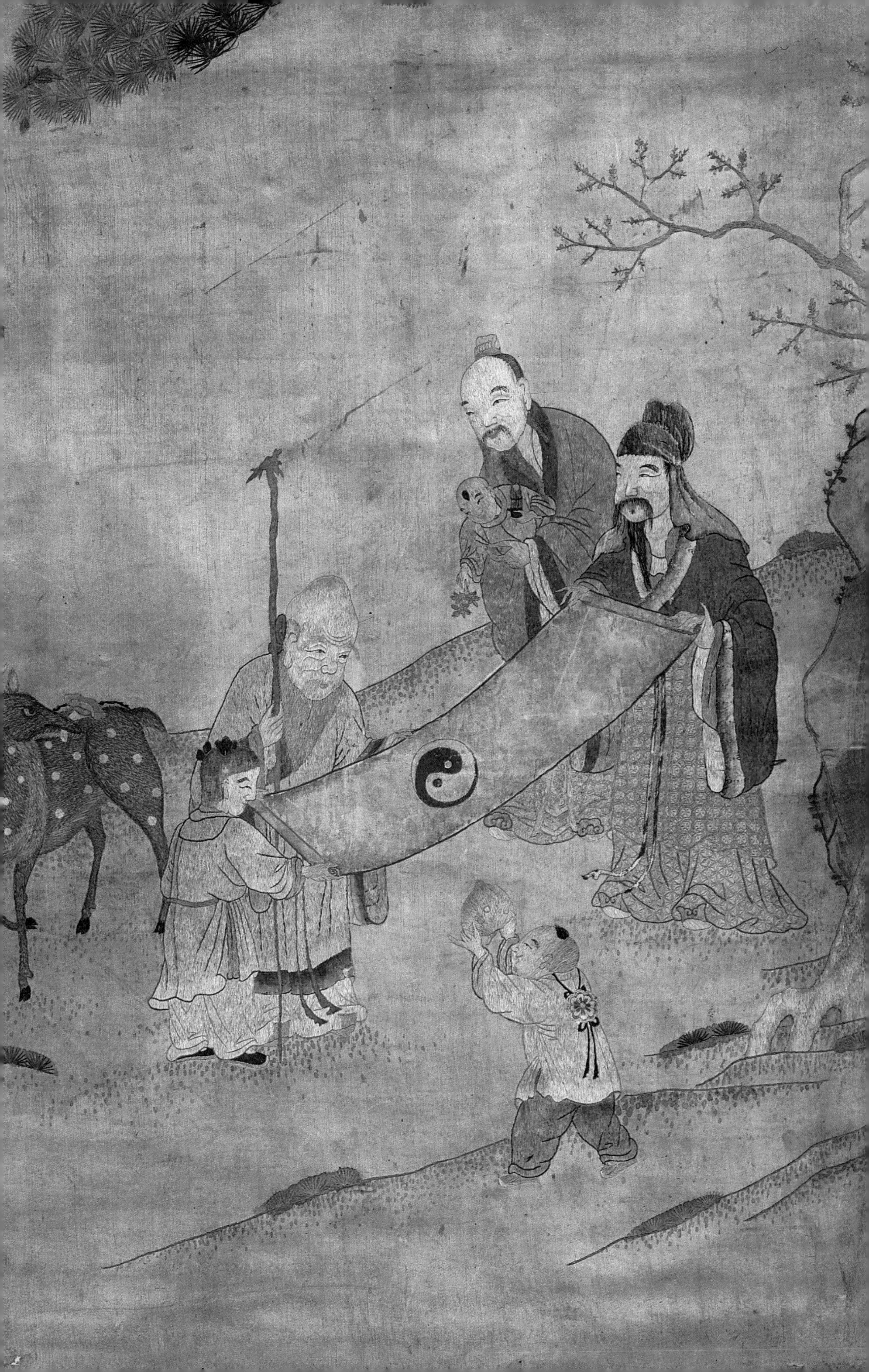

THE COMPLETE ILLUSTRATED GUIDE TO CHINESE MEDICINE

A Comprehensive System for Health and Fitness

TOM WILLIAMS PH.D.

FOREWORD BY
DR. HAN LIPING

ELEMENT

Shaftesbury, Dorset • Rockport, Massachusetts • Brisbane, Queensland

© Element Books 1996
Text © Tom Williams 1996

Williams, Tom

The complete illustrated guide to

615.
85

1461988

First published in Great Britain in 1996 by
ELEMENT BOOKS LIMITED
Shaftesbury, Dorset SP7 8BP

Published in the USA in 1996 by
ELEMENT BOOKS, INC.
PO Box 830, Rockport, MA 01966

Published in Australia in 1996 by
ELEMENT BOOKS LIMITED
for JACARANDA WILEY LIMITED
33 Park Road, Milton, Brisbane 4064

All rights reserved.
No part of this book may be reproduced or utilized in any form or by any means, electronic or mechanical, without prior permission in writing from the Publisher.

NOTE FROM THE PUBLISHER
Any information given in this book is not intended to be taken as a replacement for medical advice. Any person with a condition requiring medical attention should consult a qualified practitioner or therapist.

The moral right of the author has been asserted.

Designed and created for Element Books by
THE BRIDGEWATER BOOK COMPANY

Art director: **Peter Bridgewater**
Designer: **Kevin Knight**
Layout/Page makeup: **Ed White**
Managing editor: **Anne Townley**
Editor: **Margaret Crowther**
Picture research: **Vanessa Fletcher**
Three-dimensional models: **Mark Jamieson**
Studio photography: **Guy Ryecart and Silvio Dokov**
Illustrators: **Lorraine Harrison, Andrew Kulman**

Printed and bound in Great Britain by
Butler & Tanner Ltd, Frome, Somerset

British Library Cataloguing in Publication
data available

Library of Congress Cataloging in Publication
data available

ISBN 1-85230-881-8 Hardback
ISBN 1-85230-904-0 Paperback

ACKNOWLEDGMENTS

The publishers wish to thank the following for the use of pictures:

Archive für Kunst und Geschichte: p.130
e.t. archive: pp.2, 15T, 83, 227
S & R Greenhill: p.162
The Hutchison Library: pp.10B, 15R, 25M, 33T, 81, 188, 189, 213
The Image Bank: pp.12/13, 24B, 41, 44, 77, 78, 82T, 101, 210, 212
Images Colour Library: pp.11, 13, 14B, 41 inset, 49, 79B, 208, 228T, 229 both
The Mansell Collection: pp.14T, 167, 180/181
The Royal Collection © Her Majesty Queen Elizabeth II: p.36
The Science Photo Library: pp.33B, 76, 79L, 92, 125, 163
Trustees of The Wellcome Institute: pp.131, 235, 244

Special thanks go to:

Caroline Dorling and Flint House, Lewes, East Sussex, for help and advice in the preparation of this book
Keith Wright for help with the photography of acupuncture and acupressure
Tom Aitken / Rebecca Carver / Ian Clegg / Judith Cox
Nina Downey / Carly Evans / Julia Holden / Simon Holden
Janice Jones / Pippa Losh / Chloe McCausland
Clare Packman / Emma Ridley / Sally-Ann Russell
Sarah Stanley / Stephen Sparshatt / Tony Wiles
Robin Yarnton
for help with the photography
AcuMedic Ltd, London
The Clinic of Chinese Acupuncture, Brighton, East Sussex
Mayway (UK) Company Ltd, London
for help with properties

AUTHOR'S ACKNOWLEDGMENTS

I would like to express my ongoing thanks to Han Liping, Charlie Buck and Mike Burgess for their knowledge and support in the whole field of Chinese medicine.

Caroline Myss, as ever, ensures that I never accept second best from myself – thank you again.

Finally a thank you to all the readers of the initial paperback version of my book on Chinese medicine who have taken the time and trouble to write to me. Your encouragement is most welcome.

I would like to dedicate this book to my mother, Mary Williams, who died before she was able to see the final version. Thank you for your patience and understanding.

TITLE PAGE

This 17th-century Chinese painting depicts a family studying the Yin and Yang symbol, which represents the opposing and complementary principles that govern the universe and the human body alike.

CONTENTS

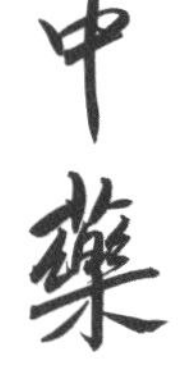

FOREWORD

BY DR. HAN LIPING

TO SOME *Western readers, aspects of Chinese medicine may seem somewhat exotic or strange, but I believe that this excellent book will shed light on matters that at first seem mysterious. Chinese medicine is based on a profound philosophy and also on a particularly rich empirical tradition.*

A doctor trained in traditional Chinese medicine will use four methods (looking, listening, asking, palpation) to gain information in order to make a diagnosis. Such information is of direct assistance in diagnosis, which defines the treatment; for example, if the diagnosis is "Wind-Heat invasion," then the treatment will be to expel Wind-Heat. Therefore, it is vital to get the correct diagnosis.

As well as a sophisticated analytical framework, Chinese medicine is soundly based on empirical observation. Some of the earliest extant Chinese texts refer to the use of medicinal herbs or to the effect of nutrition on health. The book Huang Di Nei Jing *("the Yellow Emperor's Classic of Internal Medicine"), dating to the third century* B.C. *but containing much older material, shows how advanced practical medical knowledge was, even in ancient times; by 200* B.C., *the* Shang Han Lun *("Discussion of Cold Diseases") lists more than a hundred extracts from herbal, mineral, and animal sources and discusses their therapeutic properties. As another example, a Tang dynasty physician, Sun Simiao, discovered the cause of both goiter and berberi; he prescribed extracts of lamb and deer thyroid for the former, and specific herbs and animal products for the latter. There is a general understanding in the West*

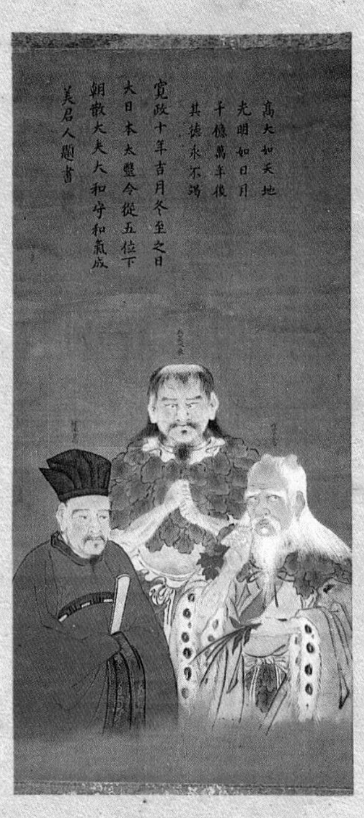

ABOVE
Three influential figures in Chinese medicine: Huang Ti, Fu Hsi, and Chi'en Nung.

that orthodox Western medicine is good at treating acute illness, while Chinese medicine is good at treating chronic illness. With the increasing use of Chinese medicine in the West; it is beginning to be realized that Chinese medicine can be useful in acute as well as chronic conditions. For example, in ancient China physicians used herbs to treat appendicitis, heavy bleeding, high fevers, and many other acute illnesses.

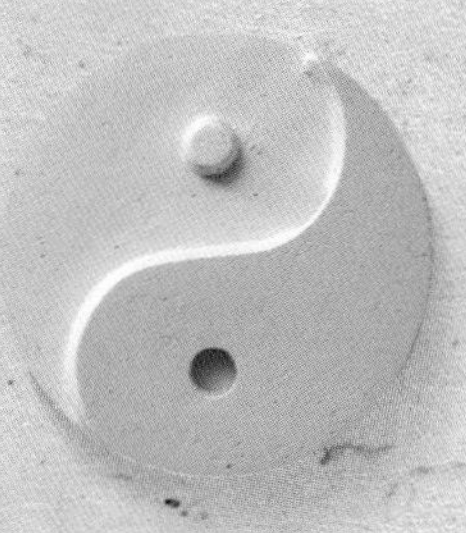

ABOVE
Yin and Yang contain each other.

Finally, it has given me great satisfaction to see that Chinese medicine is equally effective when used in the West, or in some cases even better than in China! I have been delighted to observe that thousands of patients, of all nationalities, respond well to Chinese herbs, acupuncture, and other forms of treatment.

I am sure that this authoritative guide to the many facets of Chinese medicine will provide Western readers with a more informed understanding of this extraordinary heritage. Readers should become familiar with our concepts of the nature of the body, and of health and disease; further, they can begin to understand what kind of therapies may be appropriate for certain conditions, and why medical practitioners may prescribe as they do. Last but not least, the ultimate responsibility for our health devolves upon each of us as individuals: how we eat, sleep, work, and take exercise. By absorbing simple guidance on how to live in harmony with nature, and in particular with human nature, we can hopefully implement our own programs for good health.

DR. HAN LIPING

Dr. Han Liping grew up in China. She graduated from the Beijing College of Traditional Chinese Medicine and worked as a physician for many years in the China Academy of Traditional Chinese Medicine, Beijing. In 1989 she took up residence in England and became director of the teaching clinic of the Northern College of Acupuncture, Bradford, England and a tutor for their Chinese herbal medicine course. She is also in private practice.

HOW TO USE THIS BOOK

THIS BOOK provides a complete guide to every aspect of Chinese medicine as it is practiced today – particularly in the West. It is not meant to be a self-help or self-treatment manual but aims to give, in comprehensive, fully illustrated form, information about the concepts and principles of the Chinese system of medicine and how they are put into practice. Anyone who is considering seeking the advice of a practitioner of Chinese medicine will gain from the book a clear idea of what is involved in diagnosis and the various forms of treatment. Armed with an understanding of the philosophy and practice of Chinese medicine, you will be able to decide whether it is for you, and you will know what to expect from it.

As well as covering every aspect of Chinese medicine and focusing attention on the most important ideas behind it, the book gives detailed descriptions of some of the therapeutic exercises that are beneficial to everyone as a means of developing good health. Finally, for those wishing to study aspects of the subject in more detail, there are lists of useful addresses and further reading.

Authentic Chinese calligraphy is used throughout.

THE MERIDIANS

THE TWELVE REGULAR CHANNELS

PART I

Information is summed up in simple tables and boxes.

Theories are made clear by diagrams or photography.

In Chinese medicine, the parts of the body are seen in a highly conceptual way as parts of the whole energy system. This is represented by a label on a snooker ball.

PART II

key concepts highlighted

The area to be treated is highlighted on an image of the human figure.

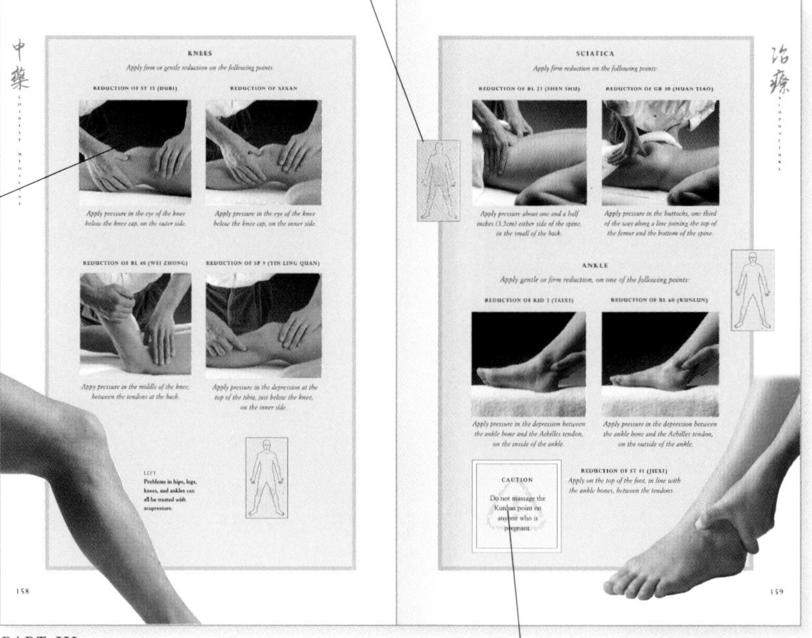

PART III

Step-by-step guide to safe home acupressure techniques for common medical problems. Each step is clearly described and illustrated.

Caution boxes draw attention to situations where care should be taken and to warn of any possible danger.

Straightforward text describes the many concepts of Chinese medicine that are difficult for the Western mind to grasp.

Throughout the book, when Western terms are used to denote a concept of Chinese medicine, a capital letter is used. "Blood" will be spelled with a capital "B" when the word is being used in the Chinese medicine sense. When the word is spelled "blood" the word is being used in the normal Western sense.

The first part of the book covers the theories of Chinese medicine, which has developed from ancient traditions in the light of practical but deeply philosphical observation of the natural world and our place in it as human beings.

The second part of the book explains how a condition is diagnosed by a practitioner of Chinese medicine. Diagnosis is based on a complex but well-defined philosophy of nature in all its aspects and the physician ends up with a descriptive picture of the person and the illness as a whole.

Case studies enable the reader to see in a real-life context how a diagnosis is made.

LUNGS

WHAT IS GOING ON WITH JOHN?

WHAT MIGHT HAVE CAUSED JOHN'S PROBLEM?

WHAT CAN CHINESE MEDICINE DO TO HELP JOHN?

OTHER LUNG PATTERNS

The third part of the book concerns treatment. Many factors help to decide on the most appropriate form of treatment, which is designed to fit the full description of the patient's state. Although the two main modes of treatment, herbalism and acupuncture (known as "modalities"), are often practiced separately, the principle is always the same – to promote dynamic equilibrium and to dispel the disharmony of the illness.

MOXABUSTION

DIRECT MOXABUSTION

INDIRECT MOXABUSTION

PART III

Ingredients used in Chinese medicine, specially prepared and photographed for the book.

Instruments and equipment discussed in the text are clearly illustrated

Photographs of professional techniques in action

INTRODUCTION

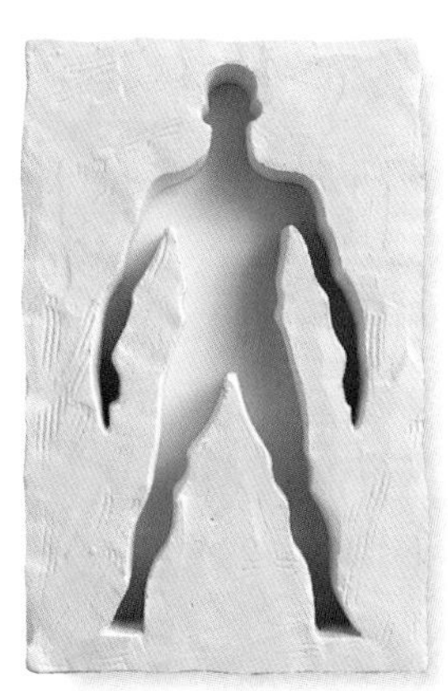

ABOVE
Chinese medicine views the body as a microcosm of the universe.

CHINESE MEDICINE is a system of diagnosis and healthcare approaches that has evolved over the last 3,000 years. The Chinese approach to understanding the human body is unique. It is based on the holistic concept of the universe outlined in the spiritual insights of Daoism, and it has produced a highly sophisticated set of practices designed to cure illness and to maintain health and well-being.

These practices include acupuncture, herbal remedies, diet, meditation, and both static and moving exercises; although they appear very different in approach, they all share the same underlying sets of assumptions about the nature of the human body and its place in the universe.

The last twenty years or so have seen a dramatic increase in the popularity of a whole range of therapies that have their origins well outside the accepted boundaries of Western scientific thought. The derivatives of Chinese medicine – particularly acupuncture, herbal remedies, and Qigong exercises – have been among the most notable, and they now enjoy a growing respect, not only from patients who have experienced their benefits at first hand but also from the medical fraternity in the West, who were initially extremely skeptical.

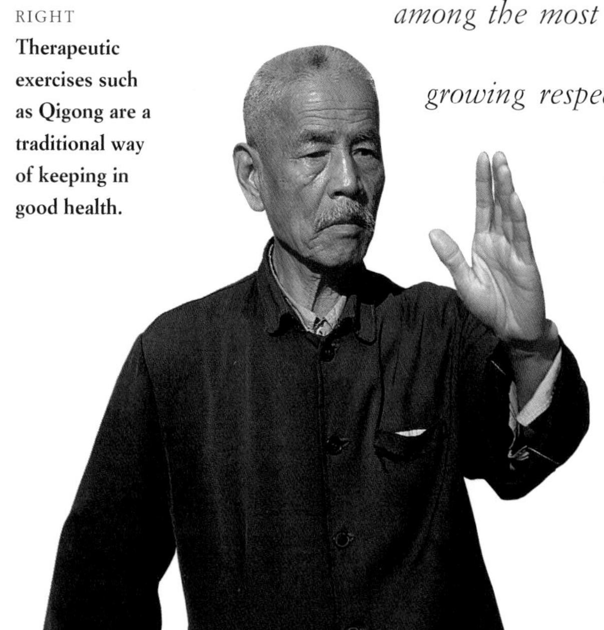

RIGHT
Therapeutic exercises such as Qigong are a traditional way of keeping in good health.

Despite the therapeutic benefits, however, it is likely that patients will, at some point in the process, ask themselves the question "How does this work?"

It is only common sense to wonder why the insertion of fine needles into a variety of points in the body – often bearing no obvious relationship to the actual problem – can have such a dramatic effect. Any patient wrestling with the problem of trying to consume a herbal mixture that would do justice to the witches in Macbeth *must, at times, question what is going on.*

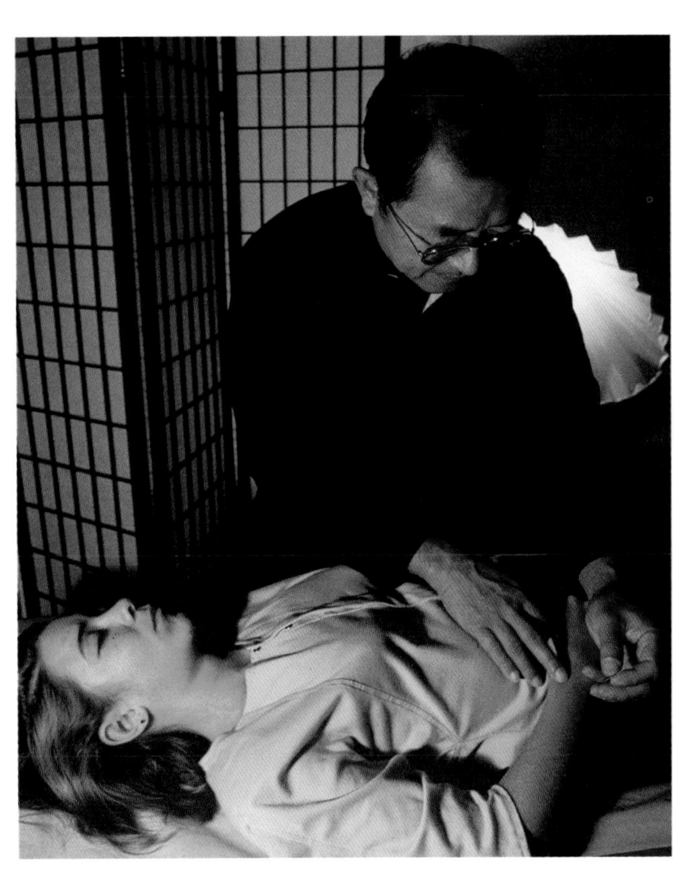

ABOVE
Acupuncture – fine needles inserted in carefully determined points – is a standard treatment.

Many hundreds of practitioners who experience for themselves the benefits of Chinese "Soft Exercises" – Taiji, Qigong, and so on – find themselves wondering how these therapies differ from Western-oriented aerobic exercise. Yet, in all cases, the proof is there in terms of symptomatic relief and improved health and well-being. Often a more balanced view of life in general is a result of practicing these therapies.

So, what is this body of knowledge that is having such an impact throughout the Western world? How does it differ from the systems we have grown up with? What does it have to offer us ? This book aims to provide the answers.

THE WHOLE VIEW

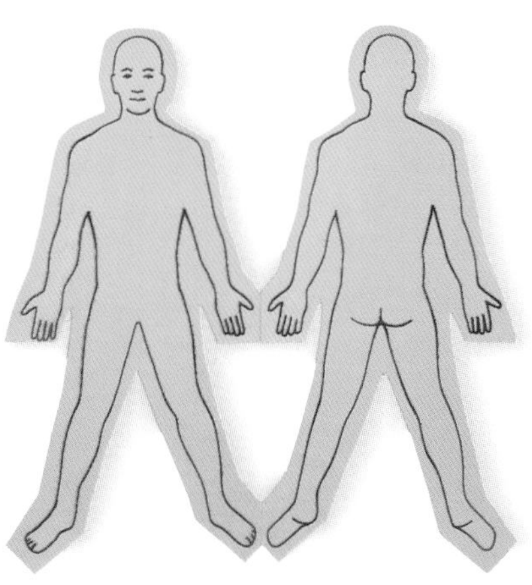

ABOVE
A holistic view looks at the person as a whole.

TO UNDERSTAND any system of healing it is necessary to understand the cultural context within which it developed. Culture articulates the philosophy and the worldview that together define the way the system operates. The healer, the patient, and the techniques used in medicine are intimately tied up with the view that the culture takes of life. The Western scientific worldview is based on a reductionist ideology – that is, it seeks to understand a system by breaking it down into its constituent parts. This has meant that the science and practice of medicine are essentially reductionist too. Analytical specificity is emphasized, and holism – the view that approaches the person as a "whole" being, comprising body, mind, and spirit – is underplayed. This analytical emphasis has brought many marvelous insights to the treatment of disease, but it still lacks the overview that ties all aspects of the human condition together. Chinese medicine has the potential to help redress this balance. The worldview that underpins the principles and practices of Chinese medicine is based on the Daoist understanding of a universe where everything is interdependent and mutually interactive. Nothing is excluded; nothing is analyzed or interpreted without reference to the whole. When it comes to medical theory and practice, this view requires a set of assumptions and parameters quite different from those operating in Western medicine. As human beings we exist as an integral part of an energetic – energy-filled – universe. Within this universe our mind, body, and spirit are merely different manifestations of the same life force and consequently cannot be considered separately.

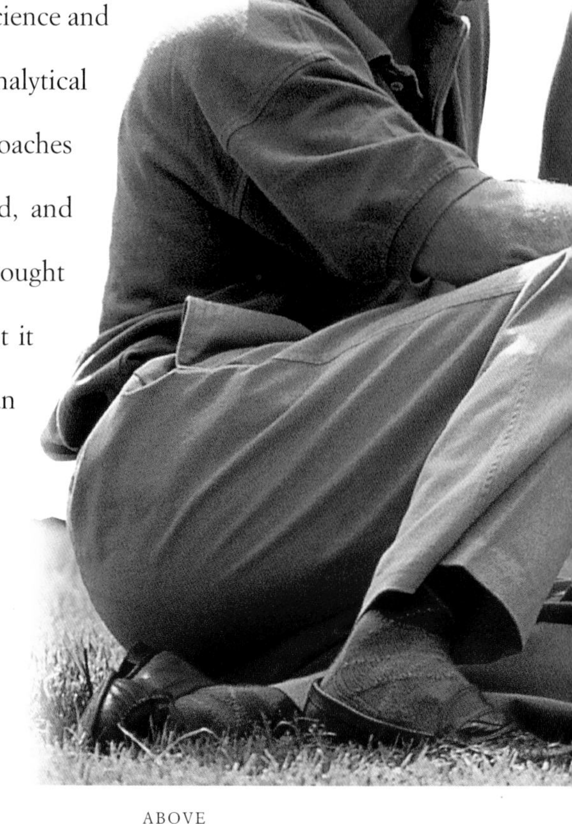

ABOVE
Body, mind, and spirit are seen as one. Qi is the vital force of energy within the body and the universe.

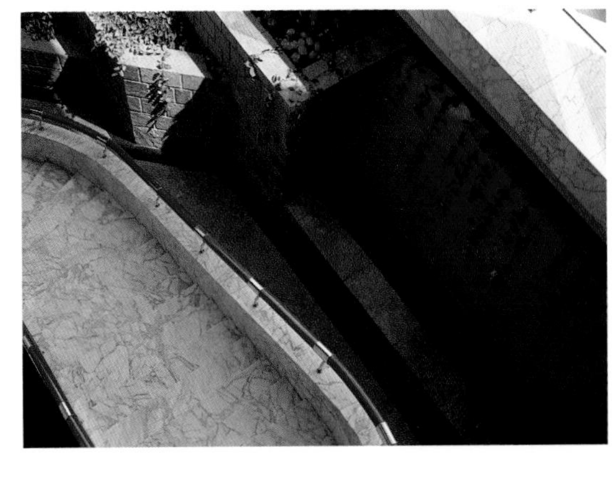

ABOVE
The art of Feng Shui teaches how to adapt the environment to achieve balanced energy flow.

Thus, practitioners of Chinese medicine define their patients' difficulties in terms that naturally emerge from the Daoist philosophical traditions. The diagnosis will place the signs and symptoms into an interdependent tapestry where physical symptoms, emotional reactions, and spiritual beliefs are set alongside social and environmental factors in order to understand how the energy dynamics of the individual lead to health or disharmony.

The treatments used in Chinese medicine are also energetic interventions that seek to reestablish harmony and equilibrium for each individual within his or her unique environment. Thus, whether the practitioner uses acupuncture, prescribes herbal remedies, suggests Qigong exercises, recommends meditation practices, or, indeed, proposes a Feng Shui reading to balance the energetics of the patient's environment at work or at home, there is an overarching commonality of purpose that will see these interventions as mutually interdependent and reinforcing.

The principles of Chinese medicine do not have to await the arrival of illness. Indeed, to understand these principles and to apply them in daily life is as much a part of the Chinese system of health as are the treatment specialisms applied. Thus, prevention and cure are not simply good practices in operation – there is no other way that such a system could operate.

LEFT
Needles are used to stimulate energy flow and restore balance.

HISTORICAL OVERVIEW

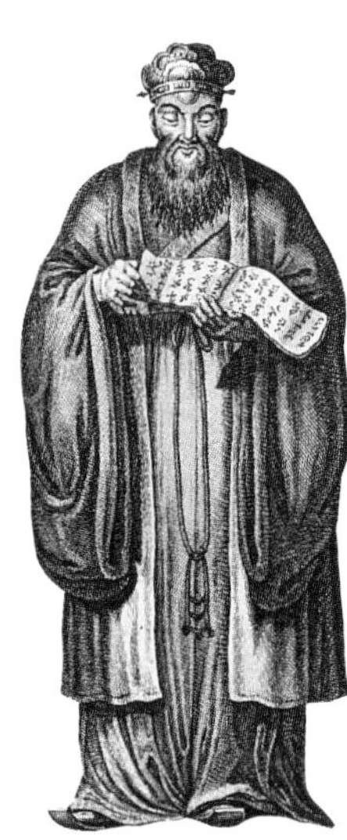

ABOVE
Confucius (551–479 B.C.) had a formidable influence on Chinese thought.

IT IS worth looking briefly at the growth and development of Chinese medicine over the centuries in order to provide a contextual backdrop for the discussions in this book.

There is evidence dating back to the Shang Dynasty (*c.* 1000 B.C.) of a relatively sophisticated approach to medical problems. Archeological digs have unearthed early types of acupuncture needles, and observations on medical conditions have been found inscribed on bones dating back to this time.

In keeping with the Chinese emphasis on the balancing and governing forces of nature, it seems likely that medical practices developed through the observation of the natural world. Many of the graceful postures in Taiji and Qigong stem from the observation of animal behavior. For example, the movements of wild geese form the basis of Dayan Qigong, which relates these movements to the acupuncture points and the energy body. There is clear evidence of a Shamanic culture existing in early Asian civilization, and many Shamanic practices are believed to lie at the foundation of Chinese medicine. By the sixth century B.C., the link between the Shaman and the medical practitioner was clear. Confucius is quoted as having said that "a man without persistence will never make a good Shaman or a good physician."

BELOW
The Shamanistic dragon head is still a vital symbol, believed to affect energy flow.

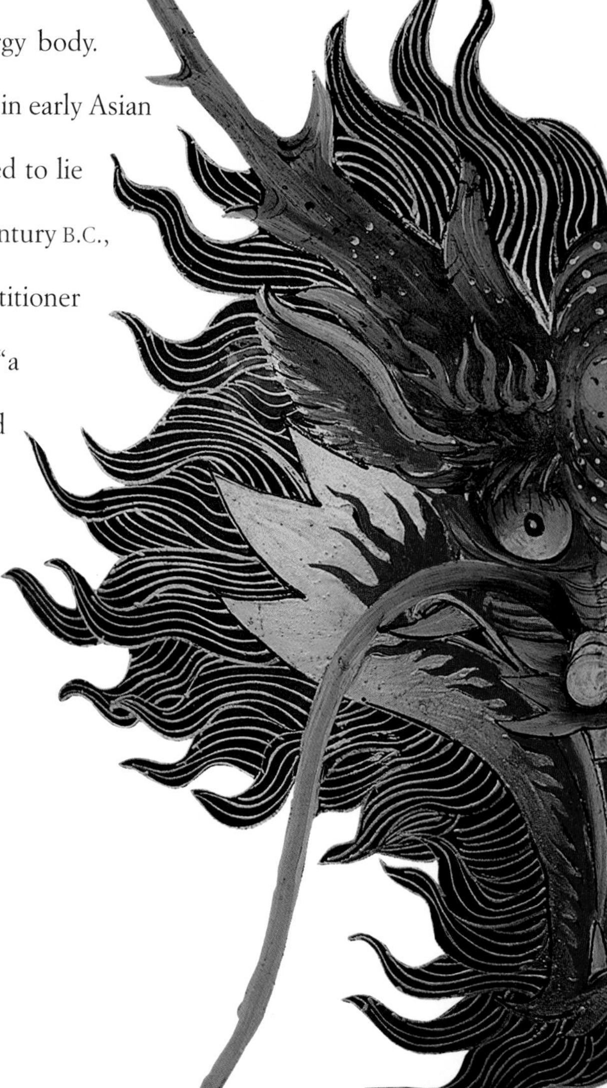

The practice of both acupuncture and massage developed in an empirical manner through the observation of the effects they produced on certain parts of the body and on specific internal ailments. Early acupuncture was carried out using sharpened bone fragments before other tools were developed.

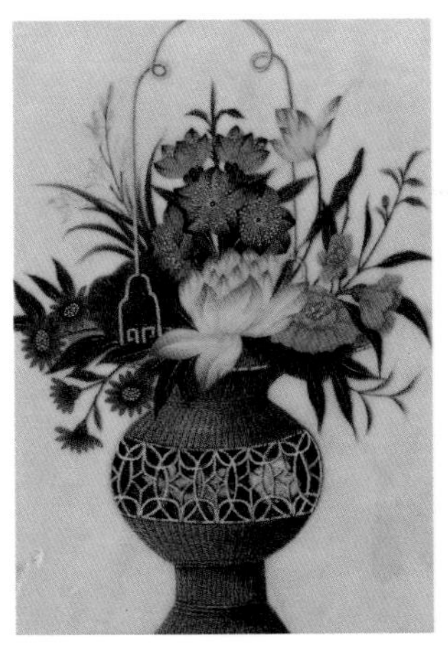

ABOVE
This 19th-century Chinese watercolor expresses perfect harmony and balance.

By the first century A.D. the first and most important classic text of Chinese medicine had been completed. This work, known as the *Inner Classic* and probably compiled over several centuries by various authors, takes the form of a dialogue between the legendary Yellow Emperor and his minister Qi Bo on the topic of medicine. Over the following centuries, these basics were expanded, and specific works emerged on acupuncture and on herbal remedies. Right into the twentieth century much of the practice of Chinese medicine reflected the traditions that had developed over the course of the preceding 3,000 years.

By then, however, Western culture was also making an impact in China. The initial response was for the more traditional theories based on Yin and Yang and the Five Elements to withdraw under the weight of Western scientific determinism. By the time the communists took power in China in 1949, there was a real dilemma regarding how best to deal with the apparent dichotomy between Western-based medical practices and those followed by traditional Chinese practitioners.

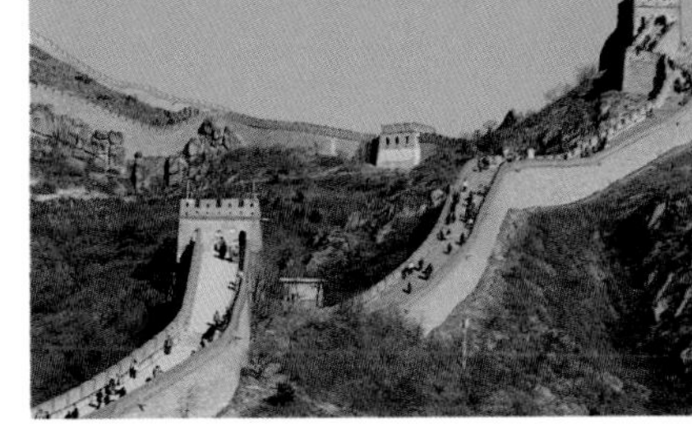

ABOVE
The Great Wall of China: a potent symbol of Eastern culture.

By 1954, the government officially recognized traditional practitioners as representing a "medical legacy of the motherland" and thus began a parallel development of Western and Chinese medical practices. Texts from major teaching centers in China have been translated, and efforts have been made to make the principles of Chinese medicine accessible to the Western reader.

THE FUTURE

將來

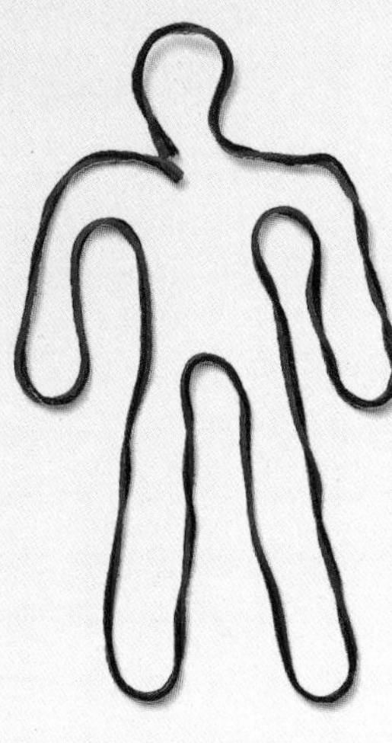

ABOVE
Chinese medicine has a role to play in the West.

CLEARLY IT is necessary to step back into the past to understand where Chinese medicine has come from and to understand how it links with ancient philosophical thinking; but this book aims to help people understand Chinese medicine and its holistic approach in today's Western industrialized society, and to suggest the place that it can rightly occupy in the developing medicine and healthcare of the 21st century.

Patients will more and more come to expect that, when they put themselves in the hands of a professional healthcare worker, whether it is a Western-trained doctor or a practitioner of Chinese medicine, they will be offered an explanation about what is being done and why. This is as it should be, and this book aims to equip patients with a basic understanding of the principles of Chinese medicine so that they will not feel confused when talking with their Chinese medical practitioner.

The herbs and drugs, the acupuncture needles, and surgeon's scalpels of Chinese and Western medicine may seem diametrically opposed, yet Chinese and Western practitioners are increasingly ready to acknowledge the strength of each other's approaches.

EAST

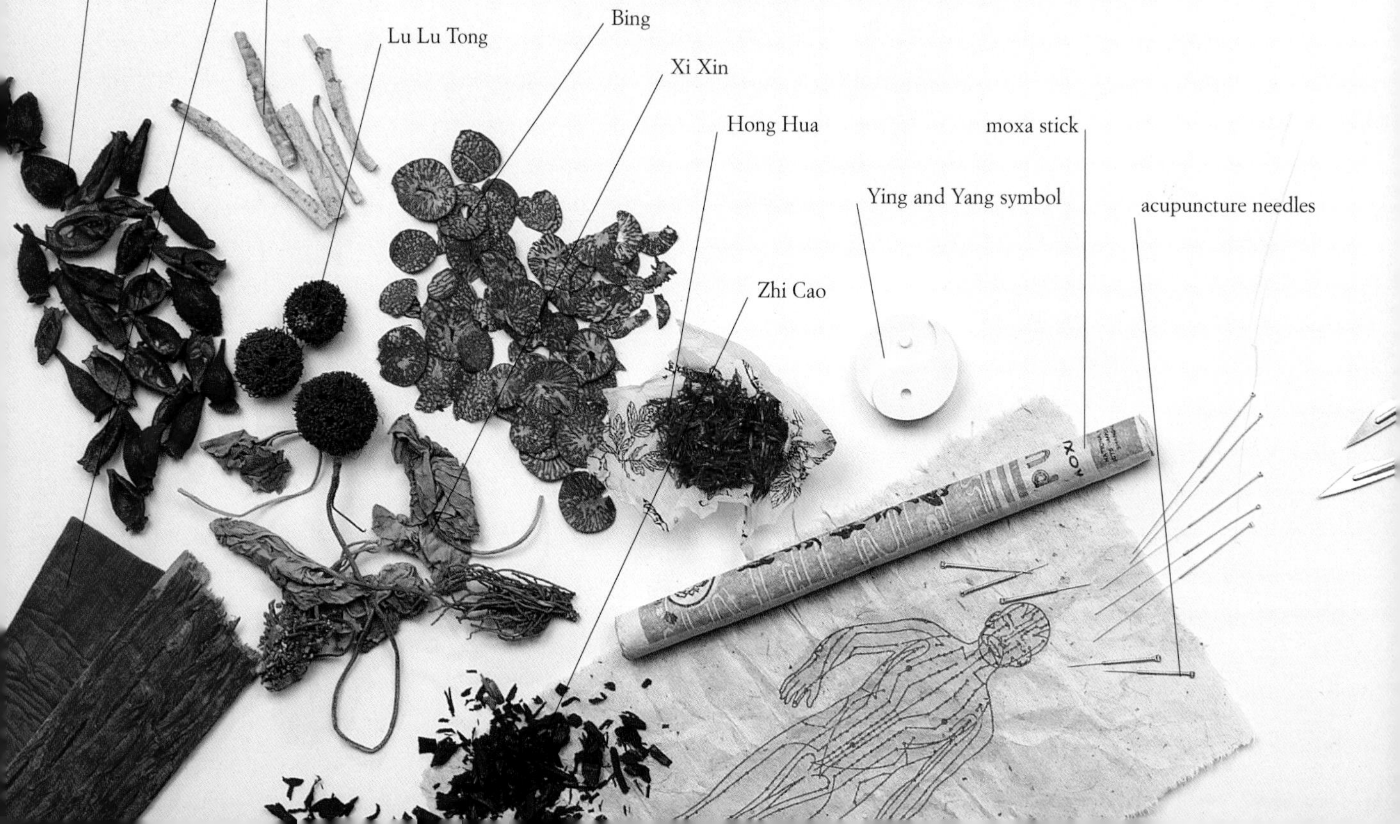

Huang Bai
Jin Ying
Tai Zi Shen
Lu Lu Tong
Bing
Xi Xin
Hong Hua
moxa stick
Ying and Yang symbol
acupuncture needles
Zhi Cao

This is a fascinating and enthralling journey. You will be asked to view your world from a very different perspective, but once you get used to the new landscape the view can be breathtaking and the rewards second to none. Read on and enjoy!

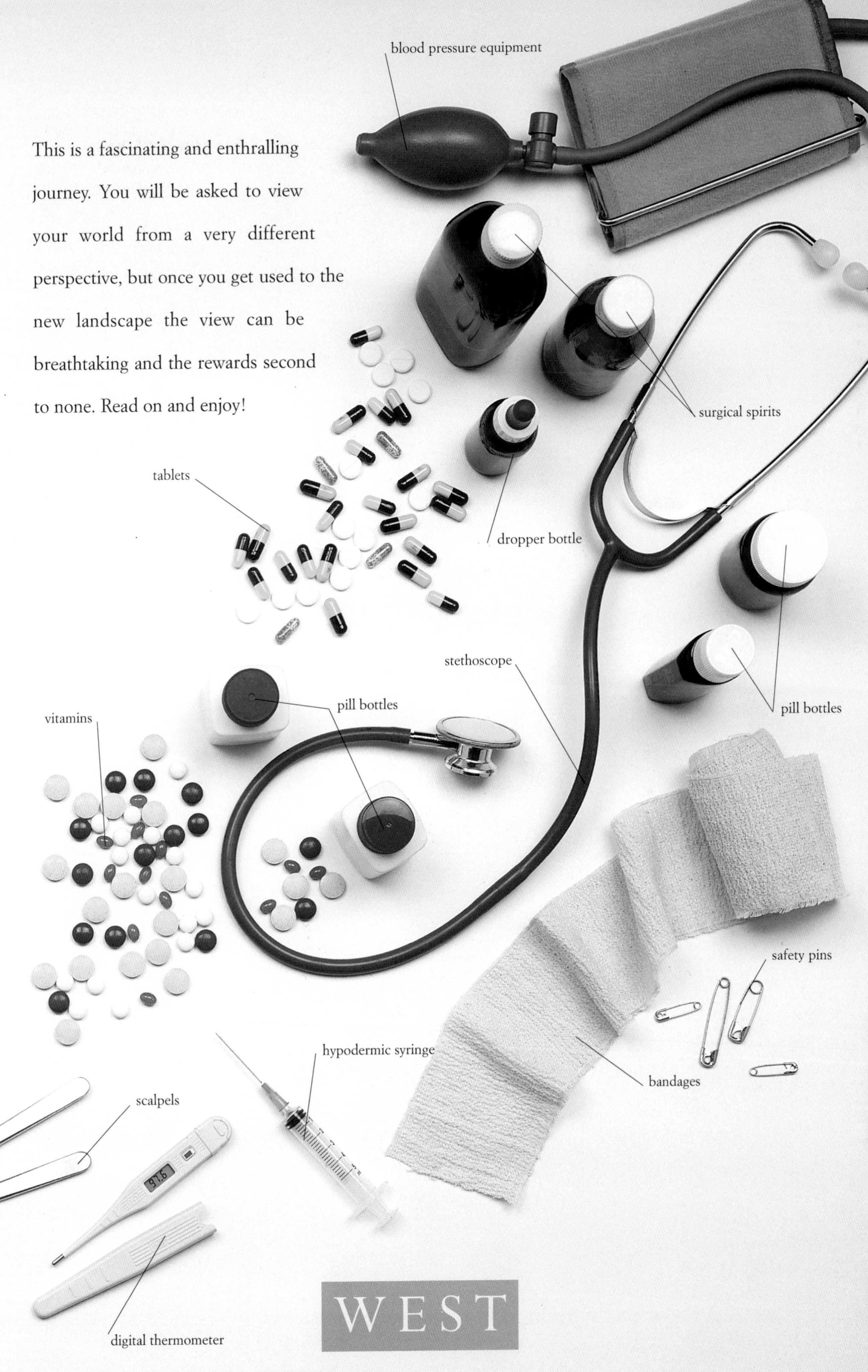

WEST

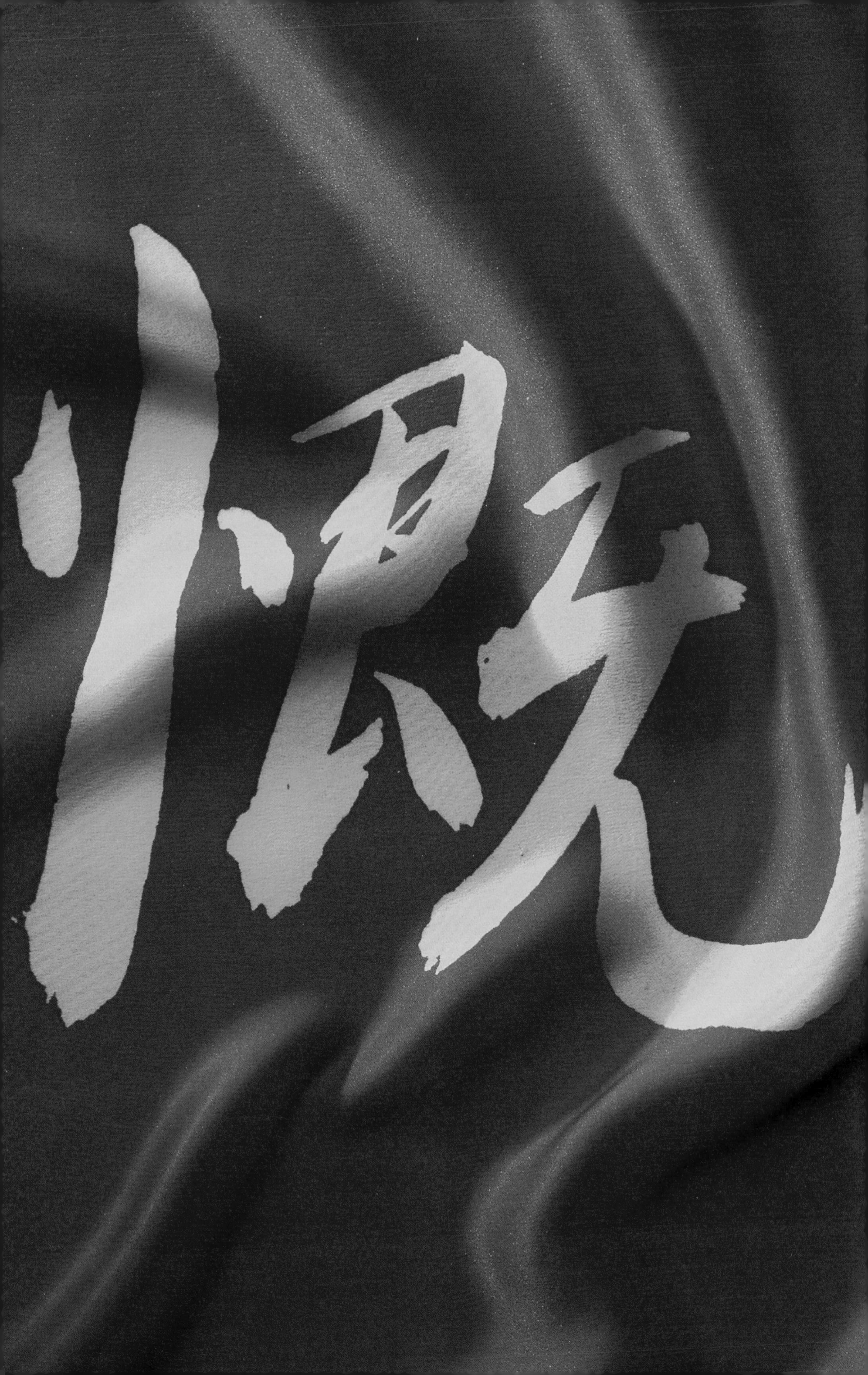
慨

THE IDEAS BEHIND CHINESE MEDICINE

✦ ✦ ✦ ✦ ✦

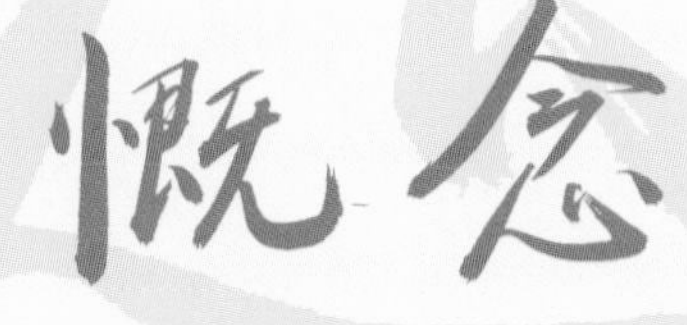

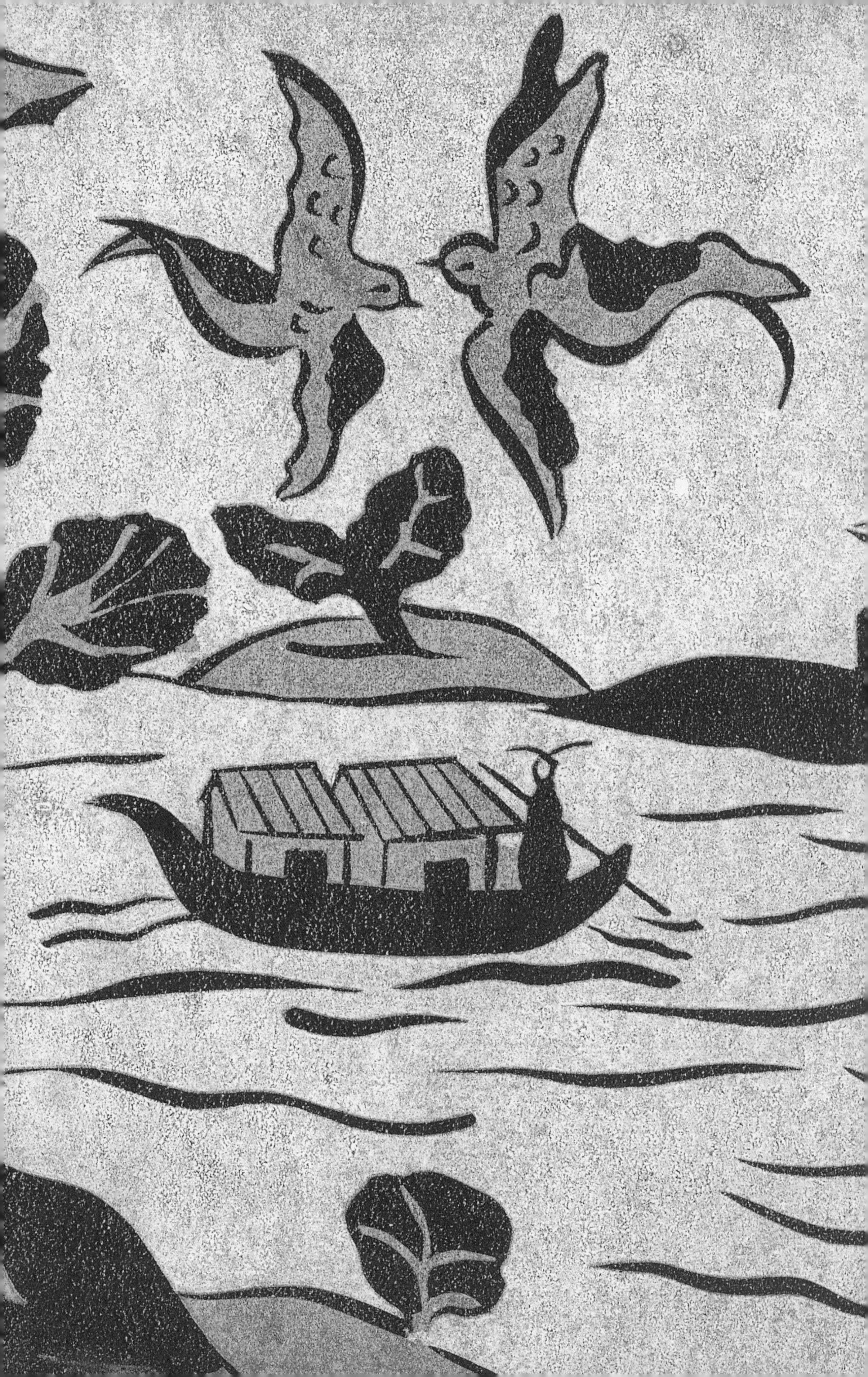

THE BASIC PRINCIPLES

WHEN WE think of medical practices in the West, we make the valid assumption that the skills of the doctor are founded on scientific research regarding how the body works and what mechanisms can go wrong in the course of illness. Thus, the practice of medicine, as the patient experiences it, is based on a firm foundation of scientific principle.

It is important to understand that the subtlety and complexities of Chinese medicine are based on equally firm philosophies and principles that, while differing dramatically from those in the West, are nonetheless rigorous and valid. To understand what Chinese medicine is all about, it is important first to explore this different frame of reference. Without an understanding of its precepts, the system the Chinese use to explain health and sickness in terms of the body's harmonies and disharmonies will seem like mumbo-jumbo designed to confuse rather than to enlighten. In this chapter, we will explore the key concepts of YIN AND YANG *and the* FIVE ELEMENTS.

YIN AND YANG

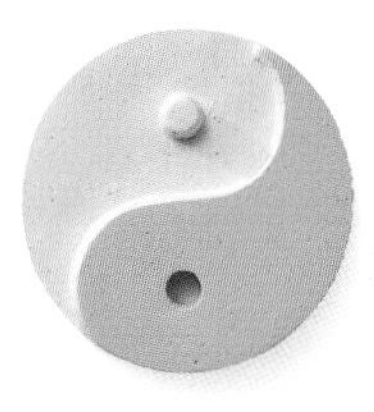

ABOVE
The symbol for Yin and Yang shows them intertwined.

THE CONCEPT of Yin and Yang is fundamental to an understanding of Chinese medicine. The ideas behind Yin and Yang developed from observing the physical world.

It was observed that nature appears to group into pairs of mutually dependent opposites, each giving meaning to the other. Thus, for example, the concept of "night" has no meaning without the concept of "day," the concept of "up" has no meaning without a concept of "down," and so on. The implications of this apparently straightforward observation lead us in a direction quite at odds with the Aristotelian logic that underpins Western scientific thought. To take a simple example: in Western thought a circle is a circle and it is not a square. Measurement and properties define it as a circle. However, from the Chinese perspective of Yin and Yang, a circle contains within it the potential of a square, and vice versa, and thus dichotomies are avoided.

In Chinese thought, the emphasis is on process rather than on structure – a topic that will be revisited time and again in the course of our discussions – and it is important to understand the concept that Yin and Yang are essentially descriptors of the dynamic interactions that underpin all aspects of the universe. Thus, Yin and Yang should not be seen as "things" in the Western sense, but as a key to the system of thinking about the world.

陰
陽

ABOVE
The Chinese characters for Yin (top) and Yang (below).

The Chinese characters for Yin and Yang give a sense of this. The character for Yin translates literally as the "dark side of the mountain" and represents such qualities as cold, stillness, passiveness, darkness, within, and potential. The character for Yang translates literally as the "bright side of the mountain" and represents such qualities as warmth, activity, light, outside, and expression.

OPPOSITE
Chinese philosophy, which underlies Chinese medicine, developed from observation of the world of nature.

BELOW
Dark and cold, bright and warm, Yin (below) and Yang (right) can be seen as complementary aspects of the whole.

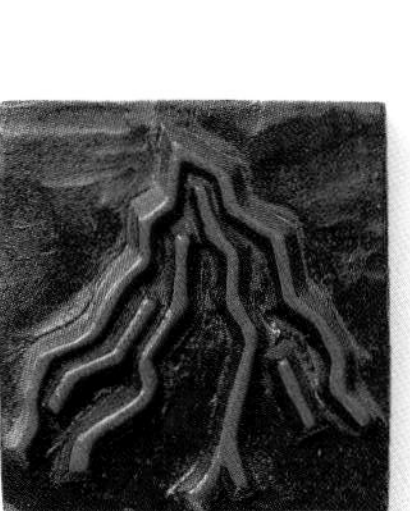

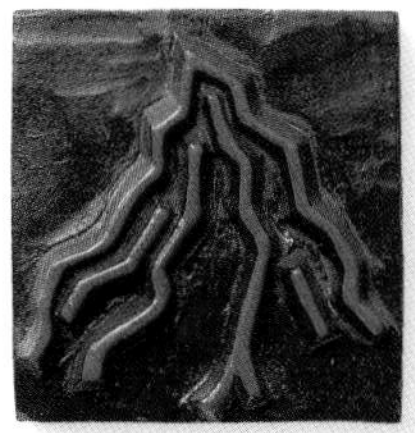

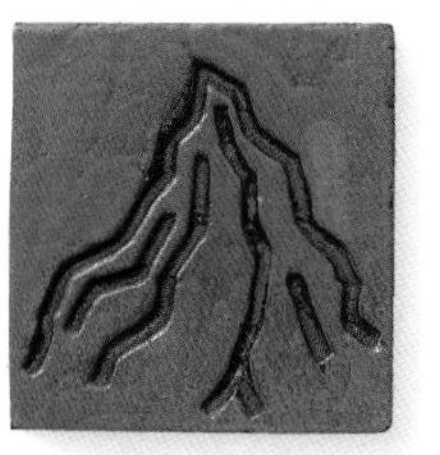

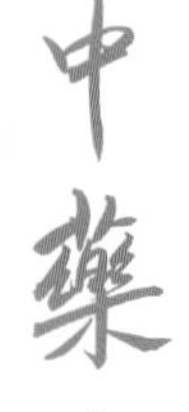

YIN AND YANG ASPECTS

IT WOULD be true to say that, according to the Chinese view, everything has physical existence exactly because everything manifests both Yin and Yang qualities. The relative emphasis of Yin and Yang will vary, but both aspects are always present. In viewing the organs of the body, for example, the Chinese system emphasizes the two qualities. The Liver is considered to be principally a Yin organ since it is quite solid, but it also has the function of promoting the flow of Qi or energy, so to that extent it has a Yang quality. The Stomach, on the other hand, is hollow and moves food through it, so is thus considered to be primarily Yang. However, the Stomach also has a storing aspect that will represent the Yin function. Nevertheless, all these aspects of Yin and Yang are fundamentally interdependent in their relationship.

SUBDIVISIONS OF YIN AND YANG

IN THEORY all Yin and Yang can be infinitely subdivided into aspects that are themselves Yin and Yang. Steam, for example, would be considered a Yang quality of water, whereas ice would be considered a Yin quality. However, both steam and ice can be seen in terms of water molecules that themselves have Yin particles – protons and neutrons – in relation to Yang particles – electrons. No doubt if we delved further into quantum physics we would see further aspects of Yin and Yang appearing. In Chinese medicine, the front of the body is considered Yin in relation to the back, which is Yang, but the upper part of the front – the chest – would be seen as Yang in relation to the lower part of the front – the abdomen.

TYPES OF IMBALANCE BETWEEN YIN AND YANG

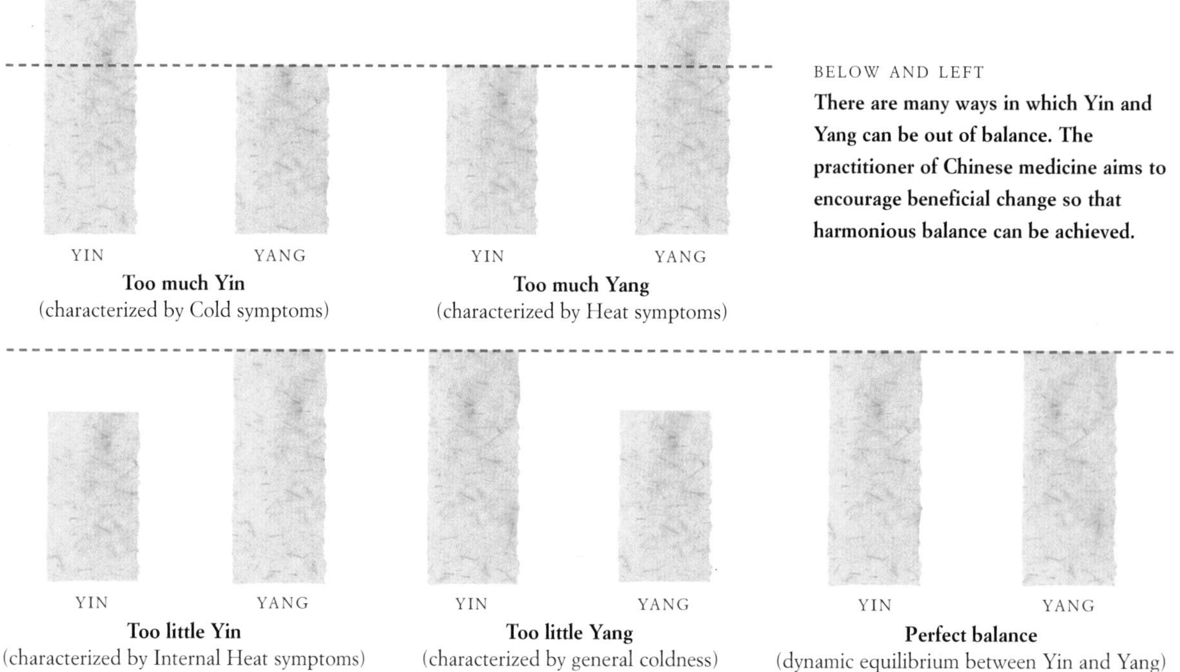

BELOW AND LEFT
There are many ways in which Yin and Yang can be out of balance. The practitioner of Chinese medicine aims to encourage beneficial change so that harmonious balance can be achieved.

YIN AND YANG INTERACTION

THE INTERPENDENCE of Yin and Yang points to the dynamic interaction between the two. Change is at the root of all things, and it manifests itself as Yang transforming into Yin and vice versa. If the Yin and Yang aspects are prevented from achieving balance through this mutual transformation process, the consequences may be catastrophic since, ultimately, balance will forcibly be achieved.

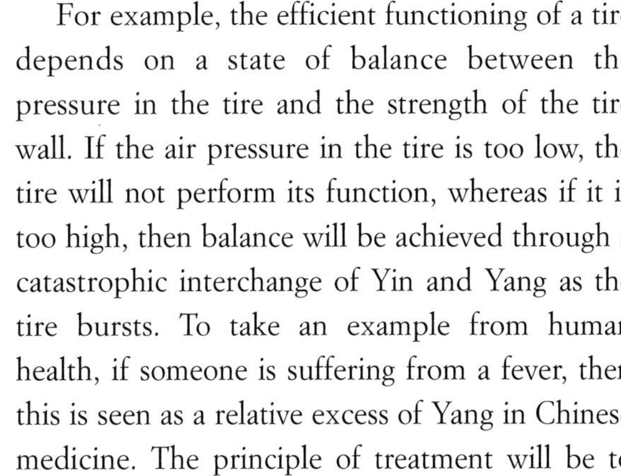

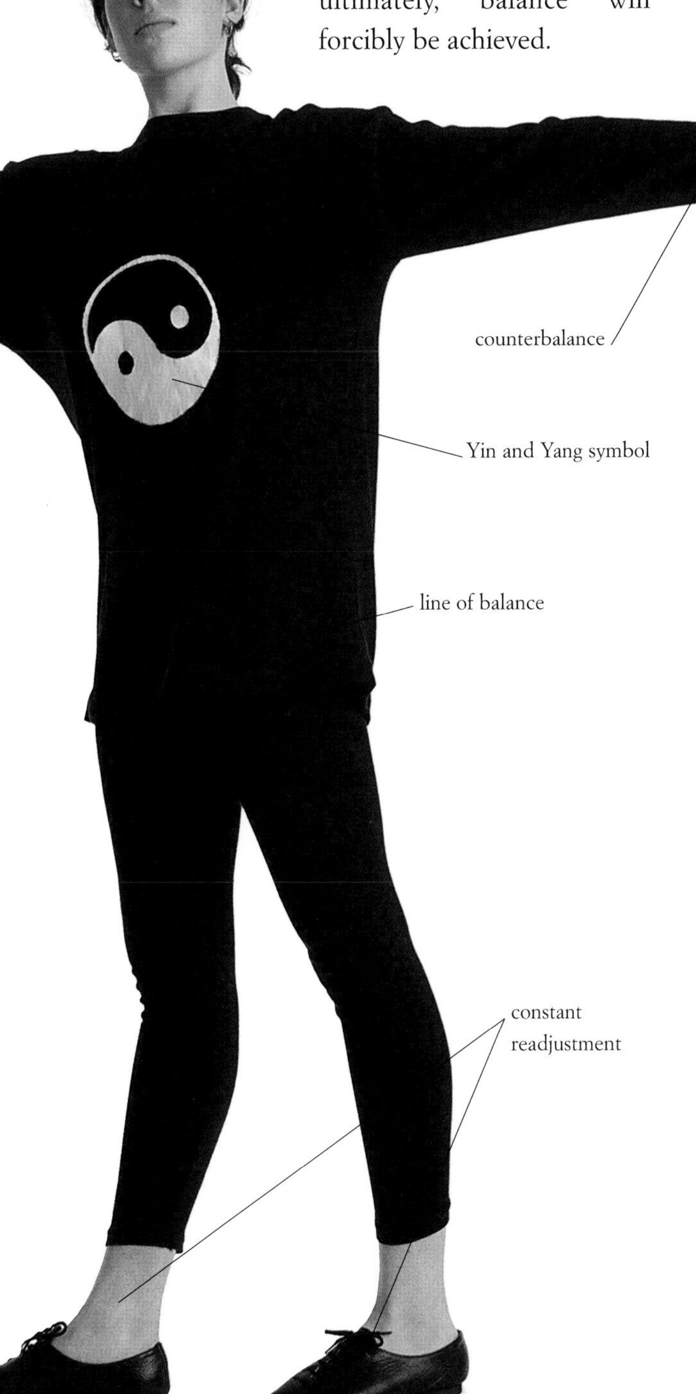

For example, the efficient functioning of a tire depends on a state of balance between the pressure in the tire and the strength of the tire wall. If the air pressure in the tire is too low, the tire will not perform its function, whereas if it is too high, then balance will be achieved through a catastrophic interchange of Yin and Yang as the tire bursts. To take an example from human health, if someone is suffering from a fever, then this is seen as a relative excess of Yang in Chinese medicine. The principle of treatment will be to allow the transformation of the excess Yang into Yin in order to re-establish a state of equilibrium and also of biological homeostasis. By this means the fever would break and the temperature would begin to return to normal – Yang transforming into Yin. It is interesting to note that the early manifestation of a fever is likely to be seen as a relative excess of Yin, with chills and Cold signs. As the condition develops, then the Yin transforms into Yang and the fever develops.

Chinese medicine views the body in terms of Yin and Yang aspects. A dynamic balance between these Yin and Yang aspects of the body is characterized by a healthy state, and, by implication, an unhealthy state is indicative of some imbalance between the Yin and Yang of the body.

Essentially, all disharmonies can be reduced to a pattern of imbalance of Yin and Yang (see opposite). These patterns will be discussed later in greater detail, but at present they serve to illustrate the importance of Yin and Yang in understanding body processes.

LEFT
Balance is just as vital within the human being as it is in the universe. This involves constantly readjusting energy forces.

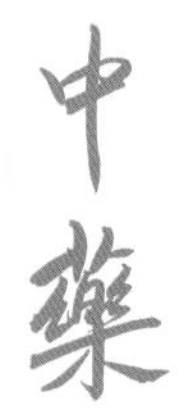

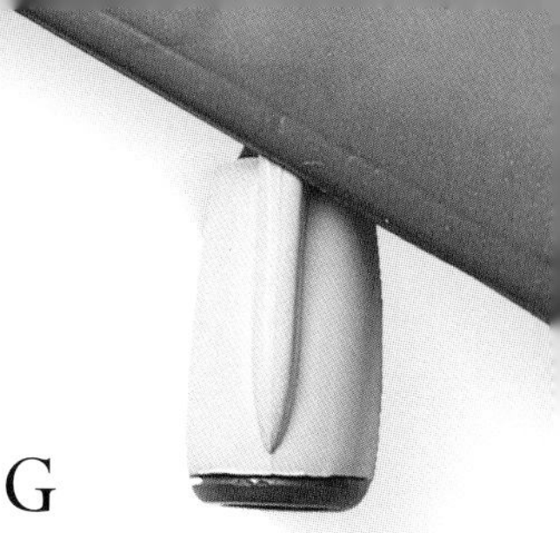

C H I N E S E M E D I C I N E

UNDERSTANDING YIN AND YANG

THE OBJECT of this exercise – which you should not take too seriously – is to see if you have grasped the concept of Yin and Yang, which is so central to Chinese philosophy in general and to Chinese medicine in particular.

Below, there is a list of twenty-five objects, situations, ideas, and so on. For each one in turn, first decide whether it represents something that is predominantly Yin or predominantly Yang. Second, for each one, suggest how it might be changed so that it represents the other quality. If you think the original is basically Yin, think how it would have to change to become basically Yang, and vice versa. An example illustrates the process.

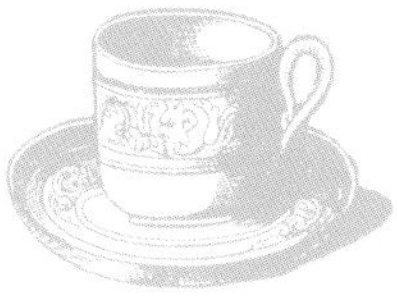

ABOVE
As hot tea cools, Yang changes to Yin.

For example, a cup of hot tea is predominantly Yang in nature. Leave it to cool to room temperature for half an hour and it would become predominantly Yin.

Remember, in every situation Yin and Yang coexist; it is just that there is a relative balance toward one or the other. Also, Yin and Yang contain each other and are continually interacting, and in the process one will transform into the other. Ultimately, there are no absolute right or wrong answers in this exercise.

Compare your answers to mine in the Answers box, but don't feel you necessarily have to agree with my analysis all the time.

✶ *1. a rowdy school classroom*

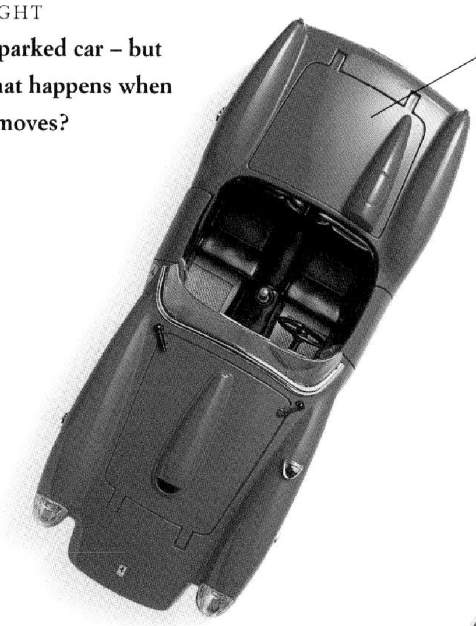

✶ *2. a parked car*

✶ *3. a block of ice*

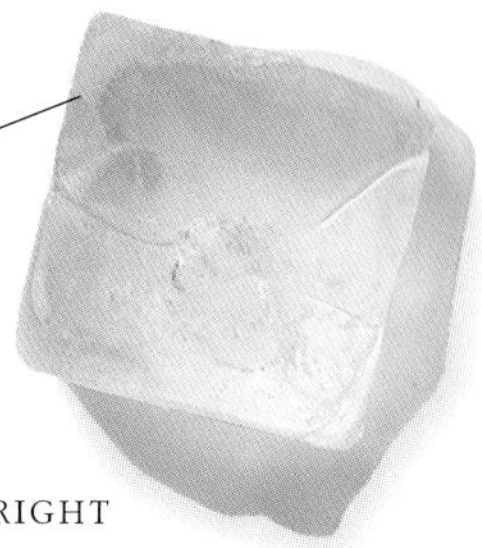

✶ *4. a migraine headache*

✶ *5. an incomplete jigsaw puzzle*

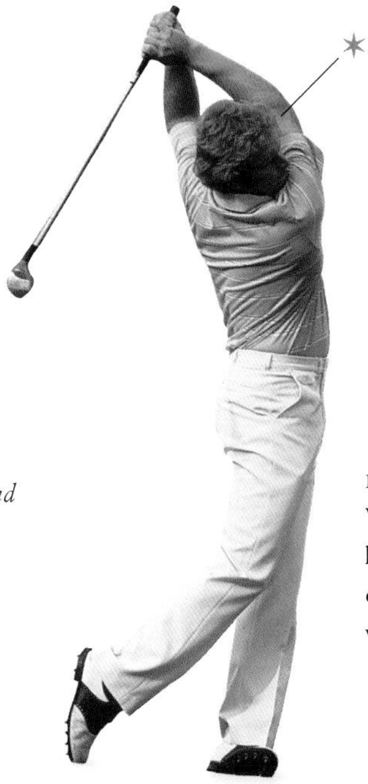

✶ *6. a golfer taking a shot*

✶ *7. a bout of diarrhea*

✶ *8. an ice-cream cone*

✶ *9. a politician delivering a speech*

✶ *10. a hard-boiled egg*

✶ *11. a piano sonata being played*

✶ *12. a CD of a rock band*

✶ *13. a raw egg*

✶ *14. a baby with colic*

RIGHT
A parked car – but what happens when it moves?

RIGHT
A block of ice – but what if it melts?

LEFT
When the golfer has driven the ball down the fairway, what happens next?

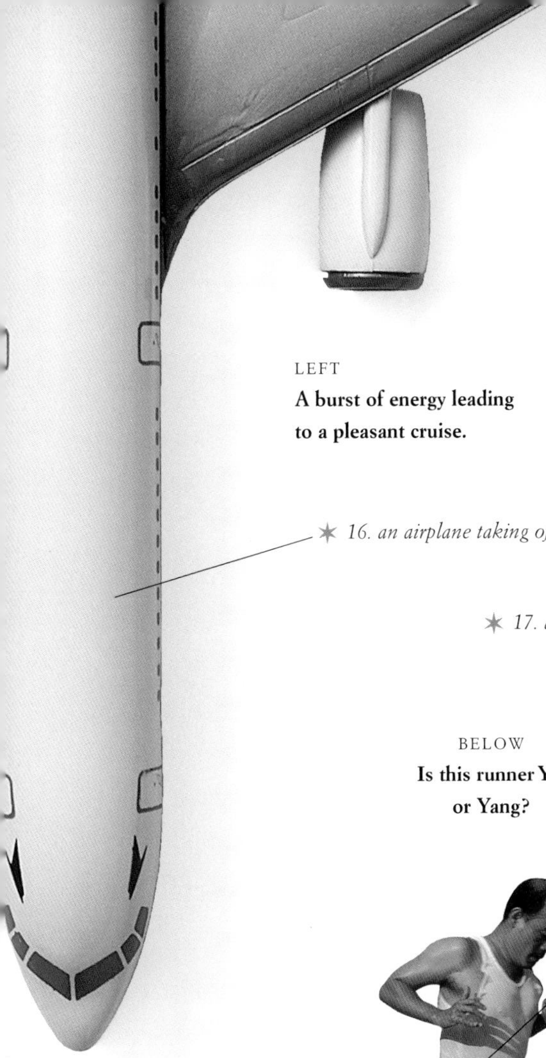

LEFT
A burst of energy leading to a pleasant cruise.

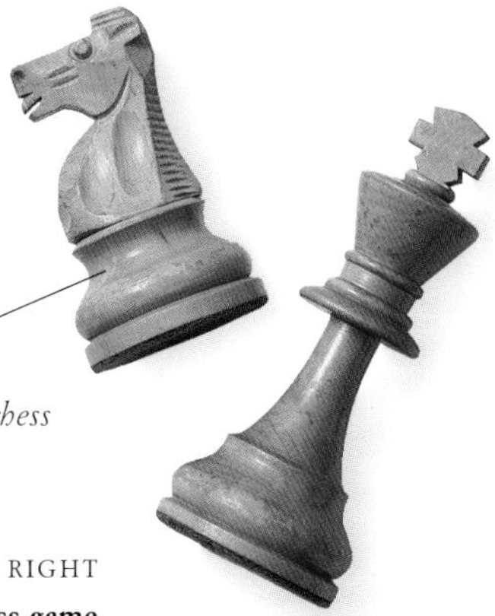

✶ *15. a game of chess*

RIGHT
A chess game involves quiet deliberation.

✶ *16. an airplane taking off*

✶ *17. a car that has run out of fuel*

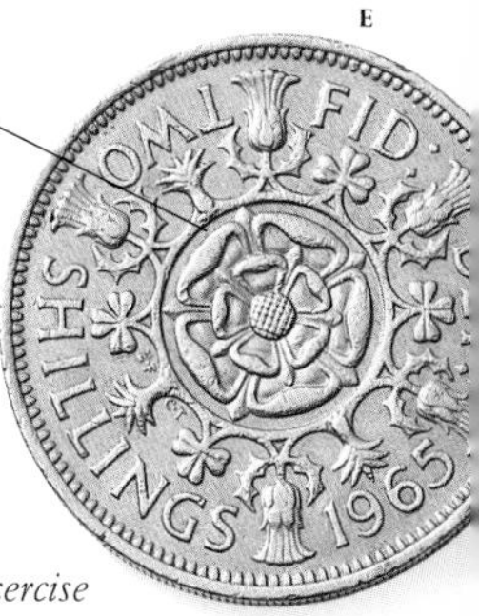

BELOW
Money – a means of exchange with no value of its own.

✶ *18. a hot summer's day*

BELOW
Is this runner Yin or Yang?

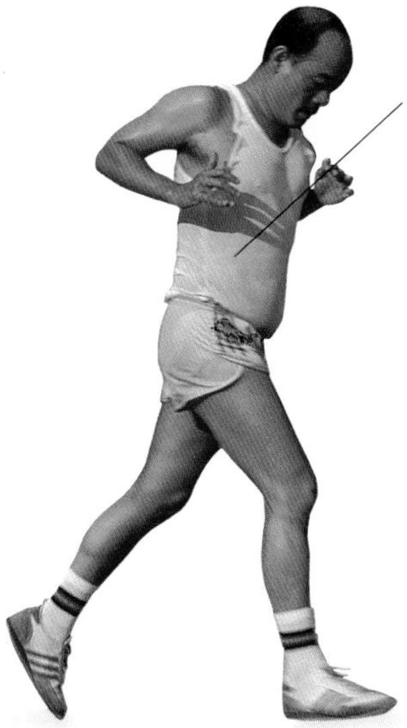

✶ *19. a coin*

✶ *20. a yawn*

✶ *21. someone doing Taiji exercise*

✶ *22. a runner finishing a marathon*

✶ *23. your thought processes now*

✶ *24. a video of an aerobics exercise*

✶ *25. a book*

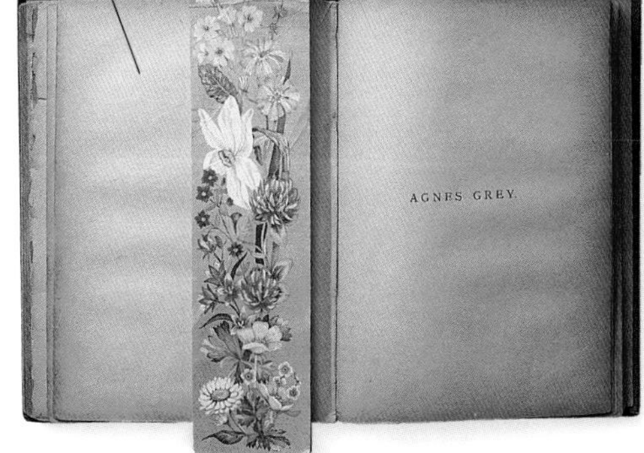

ABOVE
An open book. Has it the same Yin/Yang value when it's closed?

THE ANSWERS

In these answers, we list the number, followed by whether the situation is Yin or Yang, followed by the suggested change.

1. a rowdy school classroom	Yang	*Teachers sets the class work.*
2. a parked car	Yin	*Get in and drive off.*
3. a block of ice	Yin	*Heat it and melt it.*
4. a migraine headache	Yang	*Take an analgesic.*
5. an incomplete jigsaw puzzle	Yin	*Complete the puzzle.*
6. a golfer taking a shot	Yang	*He takes a rest.*
7. a bout of diarrhea	Yang	*Take appropriate medication.*
8. an ice-cream cone	Yin	*lick the ice-cream.*
9. a politician delivering a speech	Yang	*Politician stops talking.*
10. a hard-boiled egg	Yin	*Roll it down the hill.*
11. a piano sonata being played	Yang	*Stop playing the piano.*
12. a CD of a rock band	Yin	*Play it.*
13. a raw egg	Yin	*Boil it.*
14. a baby with colic	Yang	*Settle baby with feed.*
15. a game of chess	Yin	*Start playing.*
16. an airplane taking off	Yang	*Airplane in cruise flight.*
17. a car that has run out of fuel	Yin	*Fill it up and start the engine.*
18. a hot summer's day	Yang	*Summer night.*
19. a coin	Yin	*Spend it.*
20. a yawn	Yang	*Go to sleep.*
21. someone doing Taiji exercise	Yang	*Static Qigong posture.*
22. a runner finishing a marathon	Yang	*Runner starting a marathon.*
23. your thought processes now	?	*Only you know.*
24. a video of an aerobics exercise	Yin	*Follow the video exercise.*
25. a book	Yin	*Read it.*

THE FIVE ELEMENTS

THE PHILOSOPHICAL origins of Chinese medicine have grown, as we have seen, out of the tenets of Daoism (often written as "Taoism"). The ideas of Daoism are closely based on observation of the natural world and the manner in which it operates. In Chinese medicine, this leads to a metamorphic view of the human body that manifests the Yin and Yang interchanges that are seen in the natural world.

The Chinese observed that everywhere in nature there is dynamic interchange.The seed (Yin) grows into the plant (Yang), which itself dies back into the earth (Yin). This takes place within the changes of the seasons – Winter (Yin) transforms through the Spring into Summer (Yang), which in turn transforms through the Fall into Winter again. The Chinese medical system draws extensively on these metaphors. This is most fully articulated in the system of the "Five Elements" or "Five Phases": water, fire, wood, metal, and earth.

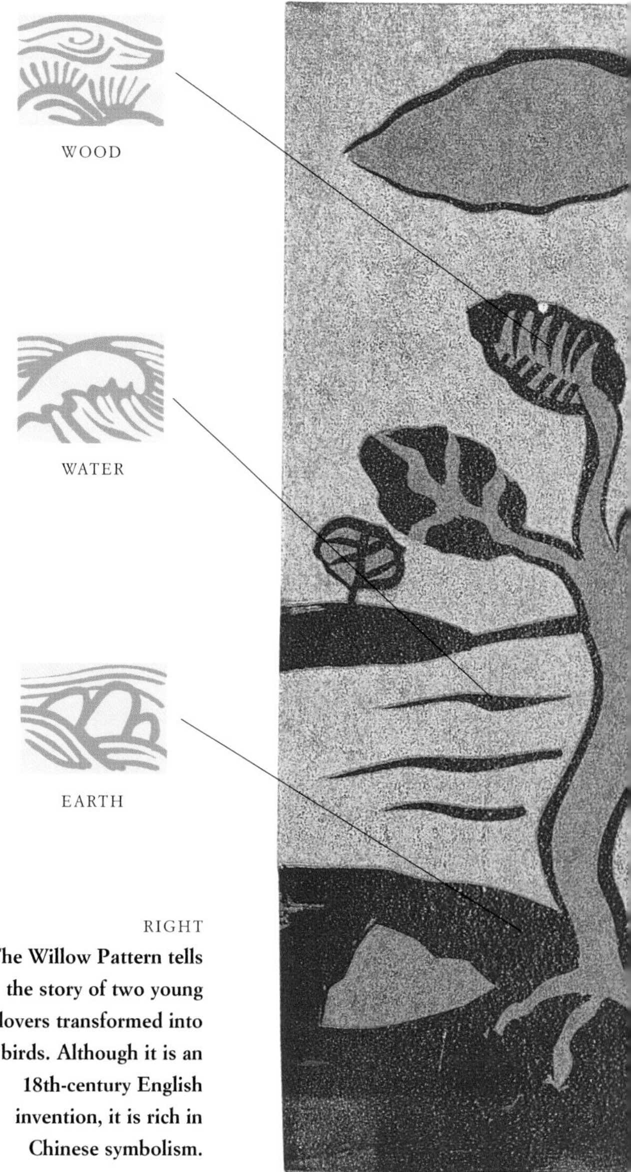

RIGHT
The Willow Pattern tells the story of two young lovers transformed into birds. Although it is an 18th-century English invention, it is rich in Chinese symbolism.

Theories of the Five Elements emerged from an observation of the various groups of dynamic processes, functions, and characteristics observed in the natural world.

WATER	**wet, cool, descending, flowing, yielding**
FIRE	**dry, hot, ascending, moving**
WOOD	**growing, flexible, rooted**
METAL	**cutting, hard, conducting**
EARTH	**productive, fertile, potential for growth**

The characteristics described here are merely exemplars of how the elements can be seen, but the important feature is that they will all contain both Yin and Yang aspects, thus reflecting the underlying principle of mutually interactive duality, so central to Chinese thought.

Each Element is seen as having a series of correspondences relating both to the natural world and to the human body. Fire, for example, corresponds to Heat and to the Heart. A pattern of interrelationships between the Five Elements is used as a model for the way in which the processes of the body support each other. These are defined mainly through the Sheng and Ke cycles.

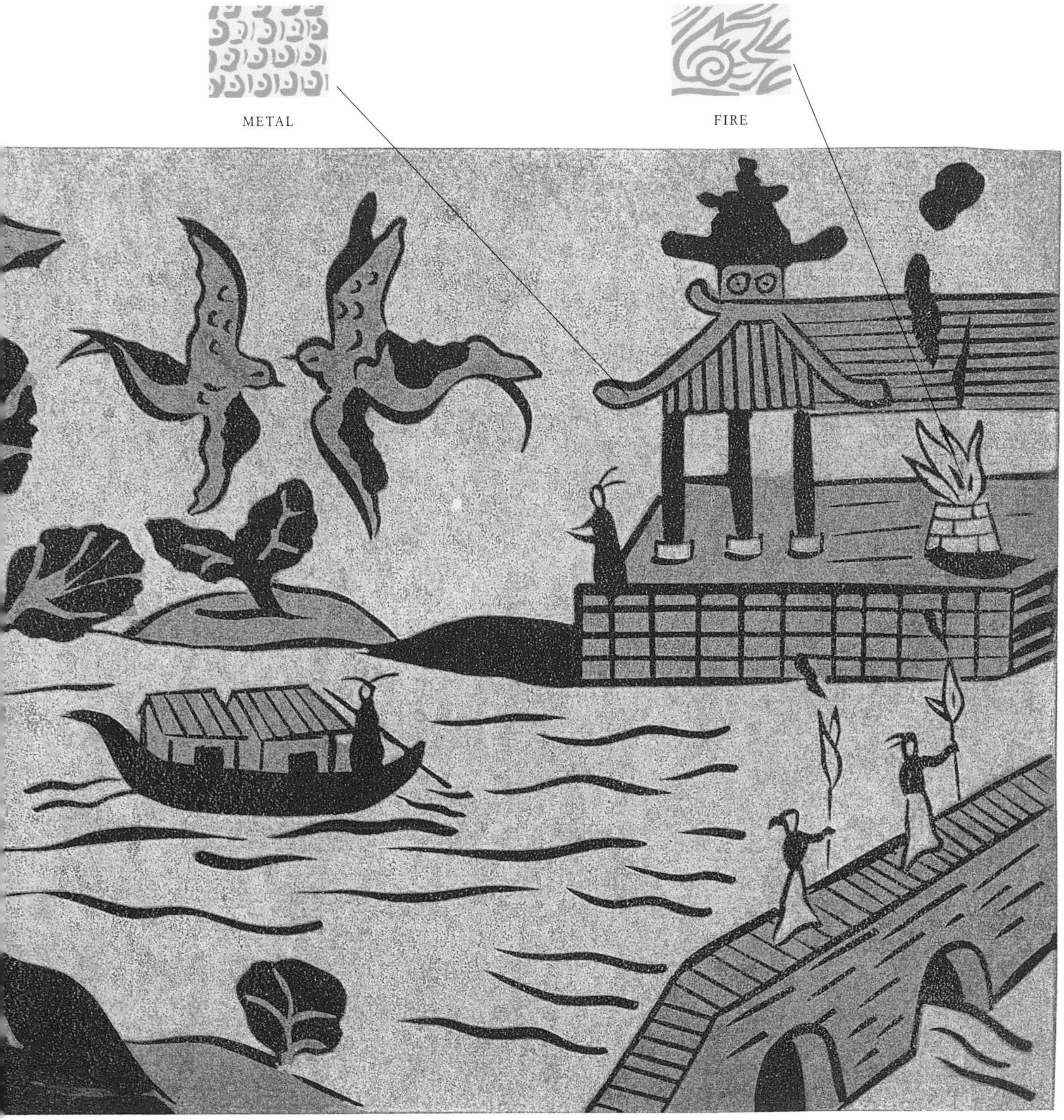

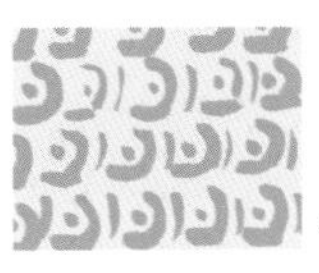
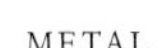

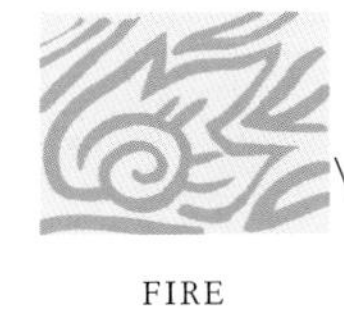

	WOOD	FIRE	EARTH	METAL	WATER
Season	*Spring*	*Summer*	*Late Summer*	*Autumn*	*Winter*
Direction	*East*	*South*	*Center*	*West*	*North*
Climate	*Wind*	*Heat*	*Dampness*	*Dryness*	*Cold*
Color	*Blue/Green*	*Red*	*Yellow*	*White*	*Blue/Black*
Taste	*Sour*	*Bitter*	*Sweet*	*Pungent*	*Salty*
Smell	*Rancid*	*Burnt*	*Fragrant*	*Rotting*	*Putrid*
Yin Organ *(Zang)*	*Liver*	*Heart*	*Spleen*	*Lungs*	*Kidney*
Yang Organ *(Fu)*	*Gall Bladder*	*Small Intestine*	*Stomach*	*Large Intestine*	*Bladder*
Orifice	*Eyes*	*Tongue*	*Mouth*	*Nose*	*Ears*
Tissue	*Tendons*	*Blood Vessels*	*Muscles*	*Skin*	*Bones*
Emotion	*Anger*	*Joy*	*Pensiveness*	*Grief*	*Fear*
Voice	*Shout*	*Laugh*	*Sing*	*Weep*	*Groan*

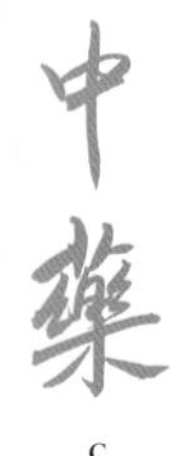

THE SHENG CYCLE

Mutual Production or Promotion

THIS CYCLE represents the manner in which the elements – and by implication the organ systems of the body – support and promote one another: Fire burns to create Earth, Water nourishes the growth of Wood, and so on. When Chinese medicine applies this promotion cycle to the organ system, similar relationships develop: the Heart supports the Spleen, the Spleen supports the Lungs, and so on.

This is sometimes referred to as the "Mother and Son" cycle. For example, the Kidney would be "mother" to her "son," the Liver. An example of this is when the Kidney Yin energy is deficient, which often leads to the deficiency of Liver Yin energy, and the "mother" can be used to treat the "son." If the Lung energy were deficient, this could be treated by toning the Spleen.

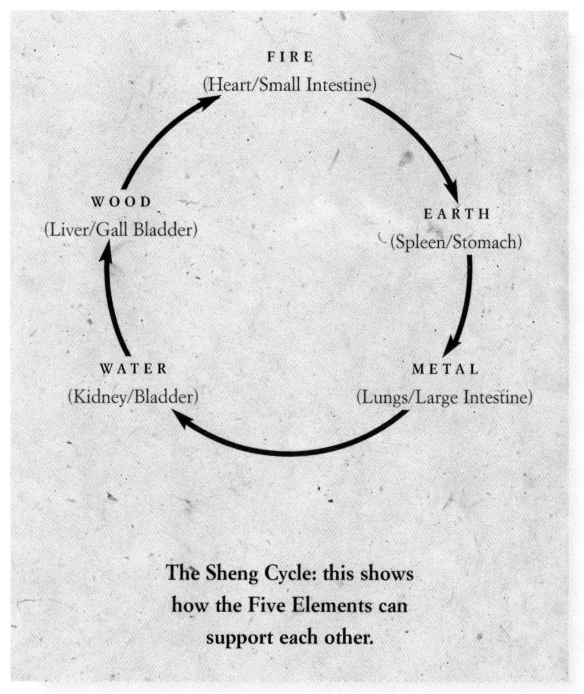

The Sheng Cycle: this shows how the Five Elements can support each other.

THE KE CYCLE

The Cycle of Mutual Control

THIS SET of relationships refers to the manner in which the Elements in the natural world are seen to control each other as part of the process of dynamic equilibrium. Thus Fire will "control" Metal in the sense that Fire will melt Metal, while Water will "control" Fire. In Chinese medicine, the notion of control is seen as part of the process of one organ assisting another. When disharmony occurs, a weak organ may be unable to exert the control and assistance needed by another.

If the Lung energy is weak there may be a tendency for the Liver energy to be uncontrolled and to rise. This may manifest itself in headaches or high blood pressure. If the Spleen is overly damp, it may inhibit the Liver's ability to move energy around the body.

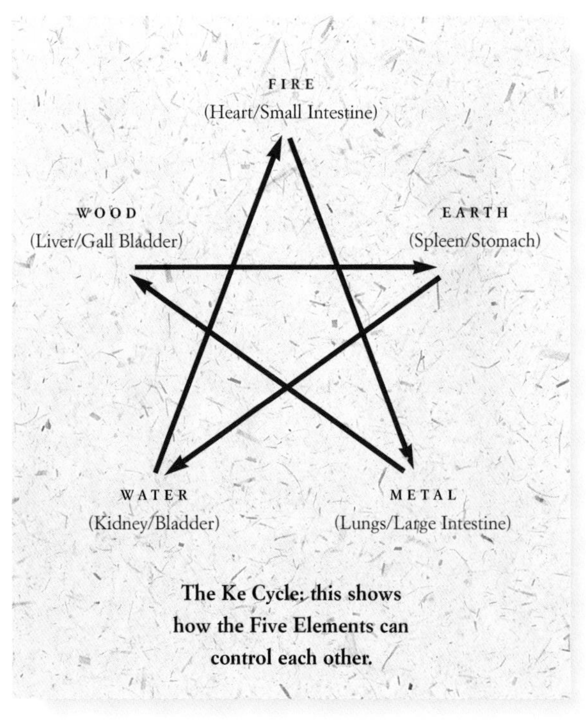

The Ke Cycle: this shows how the Five Elements can control each other.

THE COSMOLOGICAL SEQUENCE

Mirror of the Human Body

THE THIRD sequence that arises from the Five Elements view, and has its roots not only in the Daoist nature view but also in Chinese numerology, is known as the Cosmological Sequence. This sequence places the Water Element at the root and thus at the cycle's most important point.

As the Water Element corresponds to the Kidneys, this points to the importance in Chinese medicine of the Kidneys. They are viewed as the root of the Yin and Yang energy in the body and, by implication, in all the other organs.

The Spleen, which is placed at the center of the Cosmological Sequence, is seen as the origin of Qi in the body and as such the focus of support of all the other organs.

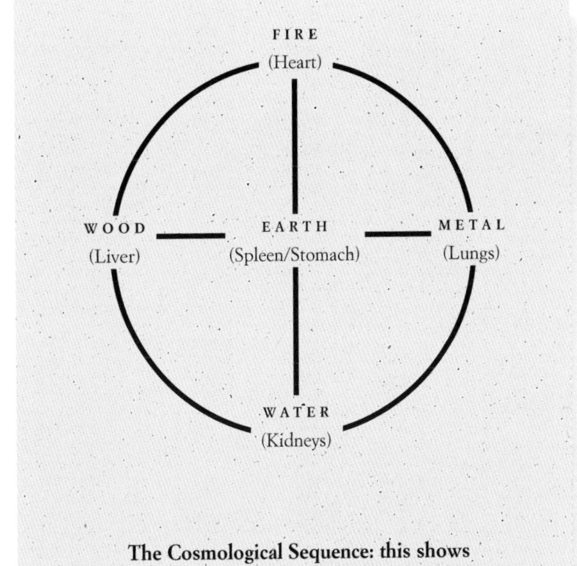

The Cosmological Sequence: this shows how the Five Elements mirror the Chinese view of the human body.

THE FIVE-ELEMENT APPROACH

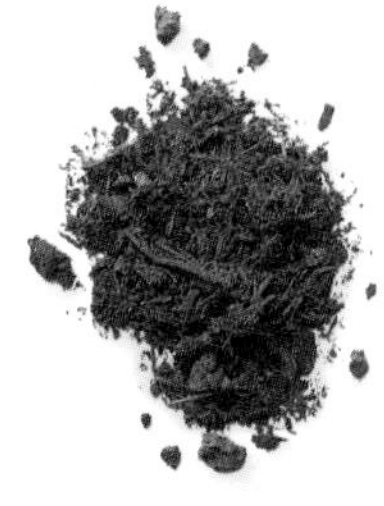

EARTH

THE FIVE-ELEMENTS view is important from the perspective of demonstrating the way in which the Chinese system of medicine has built on the Daoist view of balance, process, and harmony in the natural world. Some practitioners will approach their understanding of a patient's difficulties from the perspective of the Five Elements and determine their interventions according to these principles. Other practitioners will take the basic Yin and Yang perspective and build up their understanding of the patient's difficulties by elaborating on ideas of excess and deficient energy patterns. It is this latter approach – reflecting the more dominant practices in China today – that will form the basis of this book. However, readers interested in finding out more about the Five Element approach may care to explore some of the references given in the bibliography to extend their knowledge of the subject.

WOOD

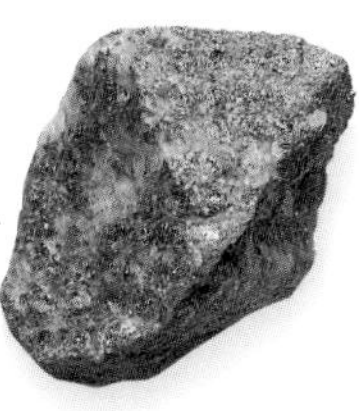

METAL

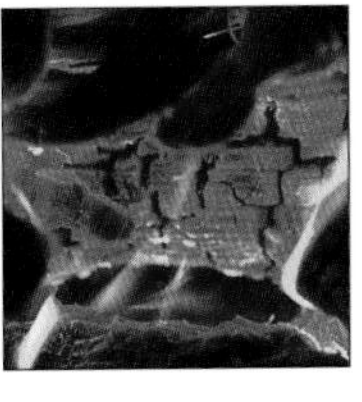

FIRE

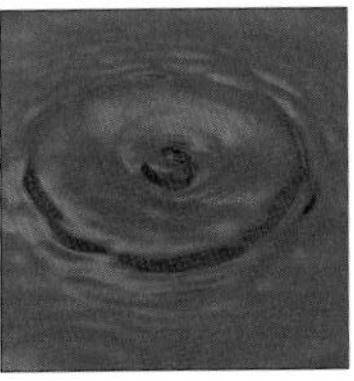

WATER

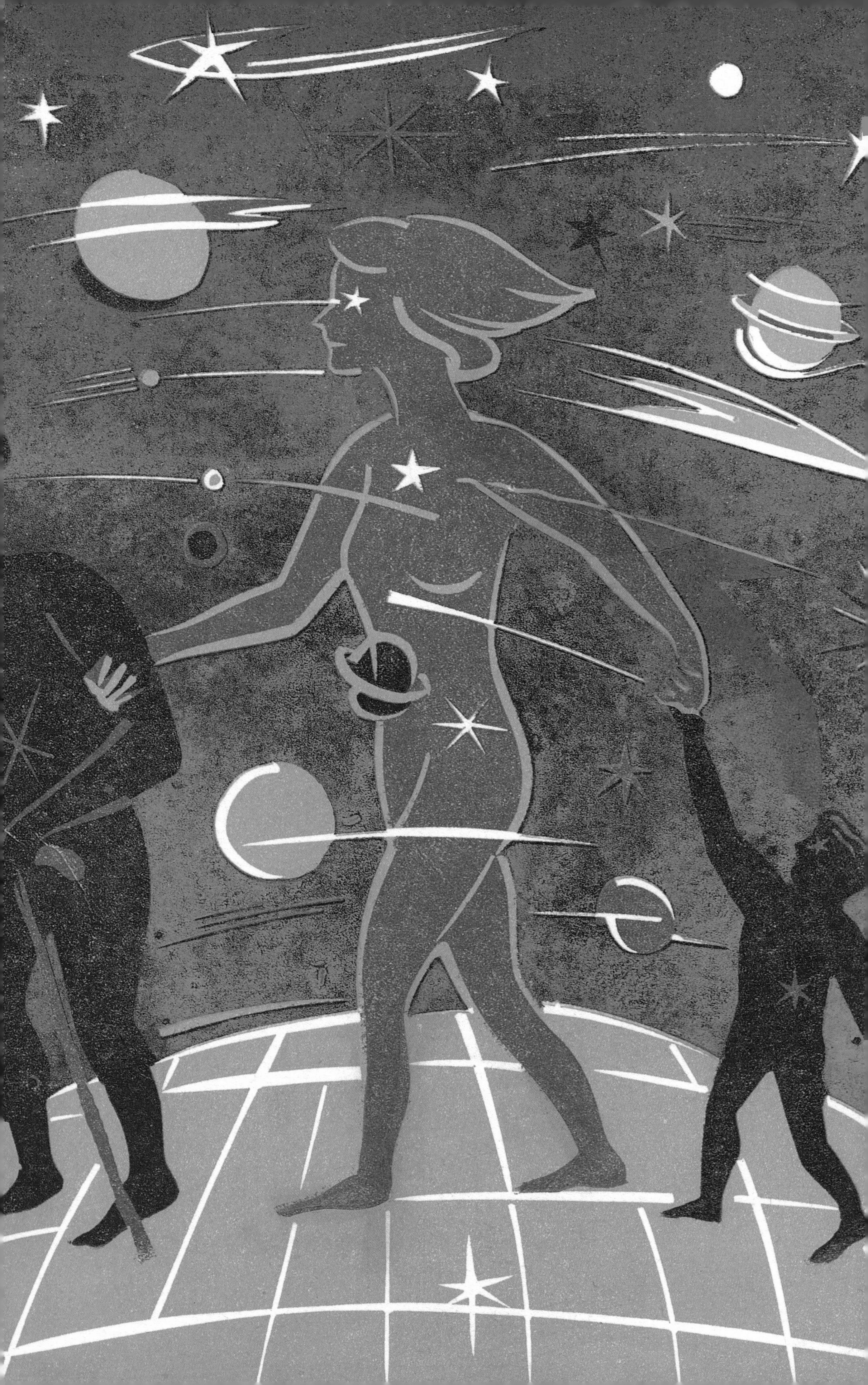

THE BASIC SUBSTANCES

As we have noted, the conventional Western view of the human body emphasizes the physical structures and components that interact in a very subtle and complex manner. Anatomy and physiology map these structures from the largest – bones, muscles, skin, and so on – to the smallest – cells and their components. This structural map forms the basis of the model of cause and effect that dominates Western medical practice.

The Chinese model is very different. Here, we consider components of process rather than of structure. The human body is seen first and foremost as an energy system in which various substances interact to create the whole physical organism. These basic substances, which range from the material to the immaterial, are Qi, Jing, Blood, Body Fluids, and Shen.

Although we will be looking at each in turn, it is important always to remember that none of them can be considered as separate from the rest and that in the Chinese model there is a continuous dynamic interaction between them.

For each of the basic substances in turn we will consider the following:

✦ *ORIGIN* ✦ *TYPES* ✦ *FUNCTIONS* ✦ *DISHARMONIES.*

QI

氣

ABOVE
The Chinese character for Qi.

THERE IS nothing more fundamental to Chinese medicine than understanding the concept of Qi (pronounced: "Chee"; often written as Chi). Qi has variously been translated as "energy," "vital energy," or "life force"; however, it is impossible to capture the concept fully in one English word or phrase. Everything in the universe is composed of Qi, yet it is seen neither as some fundamental particle or substance nor as mere energy. Ted Kaptchuk is a well-respected Western practitioner of Chinese medicine who has written extensively for Western audiences. Perhaps one could say that he captures best the essence of Qi when he describes it as "matter on the verge of becoming energy, or energy at the point of materializing." As the Chinese say, "When Qi gathers, so the physical body is formed; when Qi disperses, so the body dies."

Ultimately, it is probably wise not to debate endlessly what Qi is; rather, it is best to try to understand Qi by being aware of what it does.

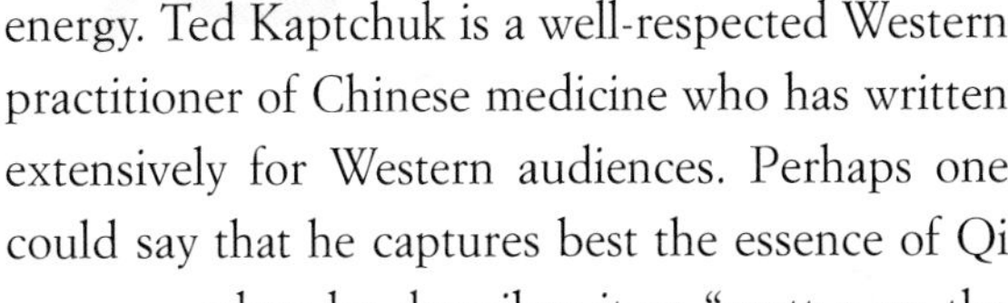

OPPOSITE
Energy (Qi) flows through the universe and through its microcosm – the human body.

LEFT
This depiction of the pulmonic acu-tract (c. 1624) shows 22 acu-points in the body's energy-flow system. (The right side mirrors the left.)

ORIGIN AND TYPES OF QI

WE BEGIN with Original Qi (Yuan Qi), also known as Prenatal or Before Heaven Qi, which is inherited from our parents at conception.

This is augmented by Postnatal or After Heaven Qi, which is derived from the Qi in the world we live in. There are two main sources of Postnatal Qi – food and air. Gu Qi is derived from the food we eat, and the main organ associated with this process is the Spleen. Kong Qi is derived from the air that we breathe, and the main organ associated with this process is the Lung.

Gu Qi and Kong Qi mix together to form Gathering Qi (Zong Qi), sometimes known as Qi of the Chest.

Finally, the Zong Qi is catalyzed by the action of the Yuan Qi to form Normal or Upright Qi (Zheng Qi), which becomes the Qi that circulates through the channels and organs of the body. Since Zheng Qi flows around the body, several functions are based on it, as we now see.

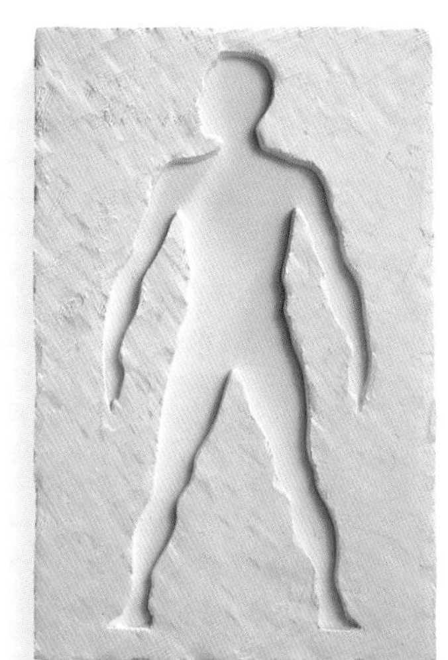

ABOVE

We are born with inherited Qi and this acts upon Qi from the food we eat and the air we breathe.

Zheng Qi forms the basis of Nutritive Qi (Ying Qi), which is essential in the process of nourishing all the tissues of the body. It also forms the basis of Defensive Qi (Wei Qi), which circulates on the outside of the body and protects it from the external factors that might give rise to disharmony and illness.

When the Zheng Qi flows through each of the various internal organs of the body, the Qi functions with respect to the characteristics of that organ. Thus, for example, the activity of Liver Qi will be different from that of Lung Qi, but they are both manifestations of Zheng Qi. This is called Organ Qi (Zangfu Zhi Qi). Similarly, when Zheng Qi flows through the channels or meridians of the body it is called Meridian Qi (Jing Luo Zhi Qi).

TYPES OF QI AND THEIR ORIGINS

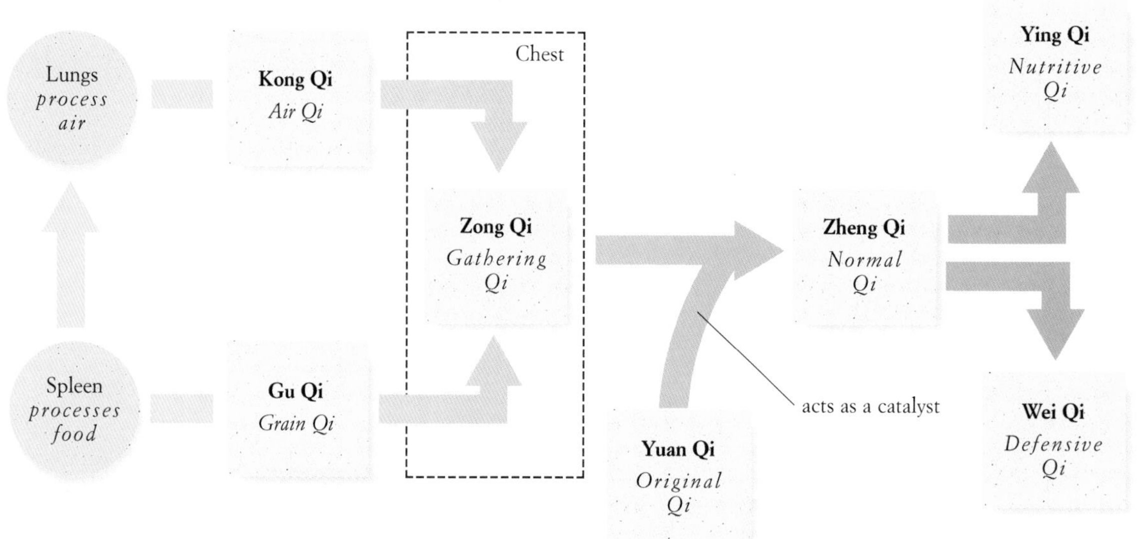

ABOVE

The diagram shows the process whereby food-derived Qi (Gu Qi), processed by the Spleen, and air-derived Qi (Kong Qi), processed by the Lungs, are acted upon by original Qi (Yuan Qi) to nourish the body and form its defensive system.

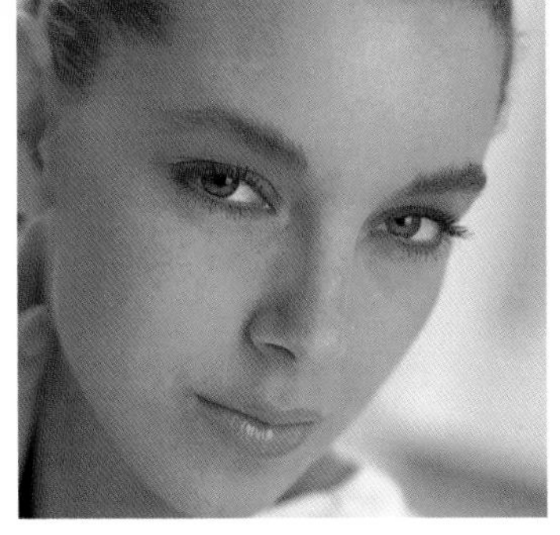

ABOVE
When Qi is in harmony, health and well-being result.

FUNCTIONS OF QI

THERE ARE five main functions of Qi in the body.

1. Source of Body Activity and Movement

Every aspect of movement in the body, both voluntary and involuntary, is a manifestation of the flow of Qi. Qi is constantly ascending, descending, entering, and leaving the body, and health and well-being are dependent on this continuous dynamic activity.

2. Warming the Body

The maintenance of normal body temperature is a function of the warming action of Qi.

3. Source of Protection for the Body

Wei Qi is responsible for protecting the body from invasion by external environmental factors such as Cold, Heat, Damp, and other pathogenic factors that may cause illness.

4. Source of Transformation in the Body

The action of Qi in the body is crucial in transforming food and air into other vital substances, such as Qi itself, Blood, and Body Fluids.

5. Governing Retention and Containment

Healthy and strong Qi is vital in holding the various organs, vessels, and tissues of the body in their correct place, hence facilitating their correct functioning. This would be analogous to the manner in which the correct pressure is needed in a tire to bind it to the wheel and to facilitate the movement of the vehicle.

DISHARMONIES OF QI

THERE ARE generally four characteristic types of Qi disharmony.

1. Deficient Qi (Qi Xu)

In this instance there will be insufficient Qi to carry out adequately the various functions. Thus, for example, in older people a deficiency of Qi resulting from aging can lead to chronic cold because the Qi is not performing its warming function adequately.

2. Sinking Qi (Qi Xian)

If the Qi is very deficient then it may no longer adequately perform its holding function and it may sink. This is most obviously seen in conditions such as organ prolapse.

3. Stagnant Qi (Qi Zhi)

If normal Qi flow is impaired for any reason, this can lead to sluggish flow or blockages. A single bump on the arm will cause localized swelling and pain because of the stagnation of Qi in the meridians. Stagnation can also affect internal organs, leading to more serious disharmonies.

4. Rebellious Qi (Qi Ni)

In this instance, the Qi flows in the wrong direction. For example, Stomach Qi is characteristically considered to flow downward, carrying food to the intestines. If the Stomach Qi "rebels," it will move upward, leading to problems such as hiccups, nausea, and, in extreme cases, vomiting.

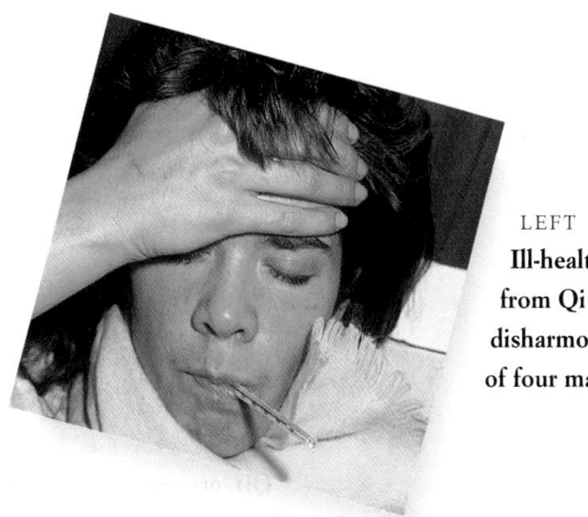

LEFT
Ill-health results from Qi being in disharmony in one of four main ways.

QI AND ENERGY

THE CHINESE tradition is not the only one to have formulated theories of "vital energy." Indian, or Ayurvedic medicine has much in common with Chinese medicine in its historical and philosophical background, and here too health is seen as the result of the harmonious balance of the life energies within us. The life force, comparable to Qi, which flows through individuals as through the universe, is Prana.

HUMAN ENERGY FIELDS

MUCH HAS been written about energy fields. It is suggested that the physical body is merely the densest level of energetic matter that exists within a frequency range that makes it both tangible and visible. There are other levels of energetic matter surrounding the physical with increasingly subtle frequency distributions. The various levels that are believed to exist are: physical, etheric, astral, mental (containing instinctive, intellectual, and spiritual sublevels) and pure spirit or causal.

It has been suggested that the energy levels cannot be considered to have distinct divisions. In this view, each level interacts with its neighbor, and the development and organization of the physical body are preceded by stimulation of the higher-frequency energy bodies. In other words, the organizational field commences at the pure spirit or causal level, which then creates an organizational matrix at the mental level, which in turn causes the same to happen at the astral level, thence at the etheric level; and finally the organizational matrices manifest in physical form – the human body. An energetic view of the body dramatically differs from a mechanistic view, as it suggests that energetic organization precedes the body's physical organization, and not the other way around!

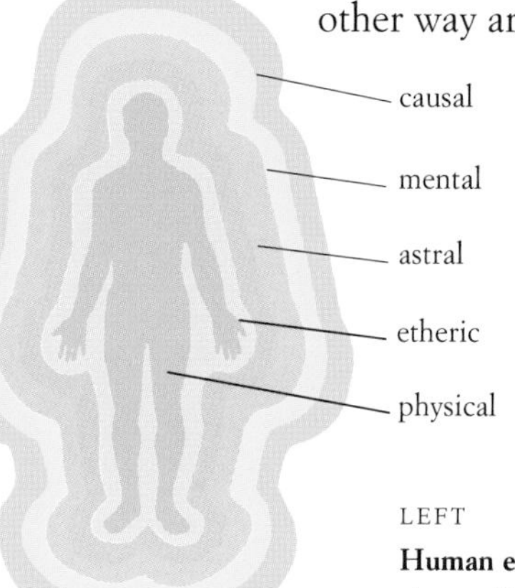

LEFT
Human energy fields, shown diagramatically.

THE QI ENERGY SYSTEM

IT SEEMS that Qi flow in the body and the meridian or channel networks that carry it operate at the cusp between the physical and the nontangible energetic systems. Thus, as the etheric body is seen to be closest to the physical system, the meridians may be seen as forming what Richard Gerber calls the "physical-etheric interface."

The Qi energy of the universe enters through the etheric energy level, accessing the body through the major and minor acupuncture points and flowing to the cellular structures by way of the energy gradients and the concentrations that we term the meridian system. Thus, when a disharmony appears in the body it has firstly manifested itself at the etheric level. Physical illness comes at the end of a chain of energetic processes.

RIGHT
In Western medicine, an electrocardiograph makes visible the electrical variations that occur as the heart contracts.

THE CHAKRA SYSTEM

THE IDEA of the seven major chakra centers of the body and the myriad of minor chakras has long been postulated within the Indian spiritual traditions. Ancient Indian texts suggest that the chakras are like energy vortices or centers that exist within our subtle energy levels and that directly access the cellular structure of the physical body. Chakras may take on the function of "energy transformers," allowing higher-frequency organizational energy fields to function at the relatively lower-frequency levels of the physical body. Each major chakra appears to be associated with a particular gland of the endocrine system giving access to the hormonal flows and changes in the body. It is suggested that the chakras are connected to each other and that they link through the body by subtle energetic channels called "nadis." It is tempting to suggest that chakras and nadis are simply an alternative nomenclature for the meridian system and acupuncture points described in Chinese medicine, but the literature suggests that they function at a more subtle level than the meridian system and may, in effect, complement it.

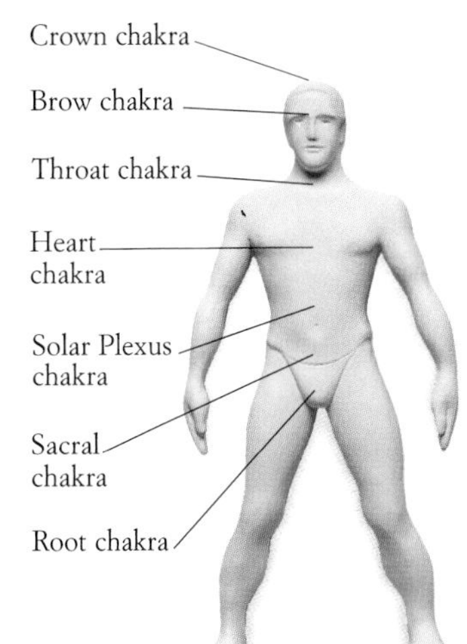

RIGHT
Indian chakras or centers of power in the body are associated with particular glands.

HOW MIGHT CHINESE MEDICINE WORK?

THE PLANT biologist Rupert Sheldrake has introduced the notion of formative "morphogenetic fields" or energy matrices. An illness can be seen as a "blip" in such a matrix, and chronic illness occurs if the "blip" becomes established. This model may help to explain the effects observed in Chinese medicine, which I believe operates firstly at an energetic level. Intervention by acupuncture, herbs and so on, acts firstly on Sheldrake's morphogenetic matrix; this then operates at the cusp between the energetic and the physical, and mollecular and cellular changes result.

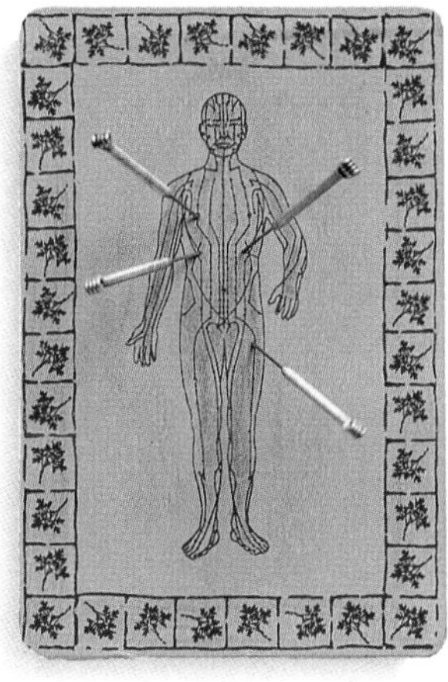

ABOVE
The invisible meridians through which energy flows have minor and major acupuncture points.

A simple analogy would be that of a tuning fork. When the fork is struck, it creates a sympathetic resonance at a certain energetic frequency and when the frequencies are in phase then surprising physical changes may occur, such as the shattering of a glass. The challenge of twenty-first century medicine will be to explore these energetic realms and to give them a status of everyday acceptability. Chinese medicine is pointing our thought processes in the right direction here.

JING

JING, WHICH is usually translated as Essence, is another somewhat difficult concept to understand in Chinese medicine. Jing can be considered as the underpinning of all aspects of organic life. If Jing is plentiful there will be a strong life force and the organism will be healthy and radiant, whereas when Jing is lacking the life force will be weak and the organism will be susceptible to disease and disorders. It is perhaps useful to distinguish Jing from Qi by considering the notion of movement.

As we have seen, Qi is responsible for the on-going, day-to-day movements in the body, whereas Jing can be considered to be associated with the slow, developmental change that characterizes the organism's growth from a fetus, through life, and ultimately to old age and death.

ORIGINS AND TYPES OF JING

BEFORE HEAVEN or Congenital Jing (Xian Tian Zhi Jing) is formed by the coming together of the sexual energies of the man and the woman in the act of conception. Thus, this Congenital Jing forms the basis for prenatal growth in the womb and nourishes the developing embryo and fetus. The quantity and quality of any individual's Congenital Jing is fixed and determines the constitution and characteristics that the person will take through life.

After Heaven or Postnatal Jing (Hou Tian Zhi Jing) is the Jing that is obtained from ingested foods and fluids through the action of the Spleen and the Stomach. This Postnatal Jing serves to supplement Congenital Jing, and together they constitute the overall Jing of the organism.

Chinese medicine closely associates Jing with the function of the Kidneys, and Kidney Jing represents a further distinction arising from both Before Heaven and After Heaven Jing. It will be sufficient for our discussion here to recognize that Kidney Jing promotes the transformation of Kidney Yin into Kidney Qi under the warming influence of Kidney Yang.

LEFT
While Qi is the vital force that governs day-to-day change, long-term change – from prebirth to death – is controlled by Jing. (Drawing by Leonardo da Vinci.)

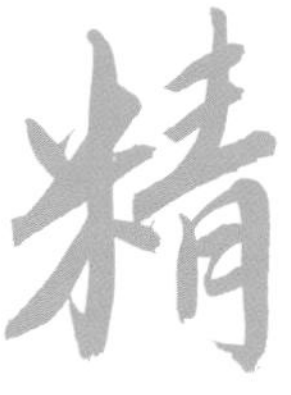

ABOVE
The Chinese character for Jing.

FUNCTIONS OF JING

Governing growth, reproduction, and development

Jing is seen as crucial to the development of the individual through life. In children it is responsible for the growth of bones, teeth, and hair. It also promotes brain development and sexual maturation. In adults, Jing forms the basis of reproduction. Fertility in both the male and the female is dependent upon strong Kidney Jing.

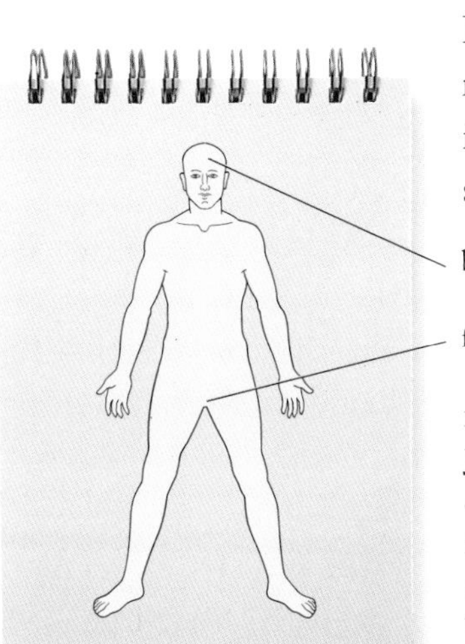

LEFT
Jing, sometimes described as vital force, is with us at birth and corresponds to what the West describes as "Constitution."

Promoting Kidney Qi

The connection between Jing and the Kidneys is very strong. Kidney Qi is the root of all the Qi in the body, and if it is in any way deficient or weak this will lead to deficiency and weakness of the Qi of the whole body.

Producing Marrow

In Chinese medicine the concept of Marrow includes the fundamental make up of the spinal cord and the brain.

Since Jing is responsible for the production of Marrow, there can be serious consequences if this process is weak.

Determining our constitution

The strength of our Jing determines our basic constitutional strength. Thus, the Jing works in concert with the Wei Qi to help protect the body from external factors. If Jing is weak, the individual may be chronically prone to infection and illness.

DYSFUNCTIONS OF JING

JING DISHARMONIES tend to relate directly to development and constitution.

Developmental disorders

Any developmental disorder, such as learning difficulties or physical disabilities in children, is due to a deficiency of Jing. In later life, as Jing diminishes then physical deterioration occurs – commonly with deafness, graying, and balding, as well as general frailty and senility.

Kidney-related disorders

Because of Jing's close association with the Kidneys, any deficiency can lead to Kidney-related problems such as impotence, low-back pain, and tinnitus.

memory loss

allergies

kidney-related problems

Marrow-related disorders

If Jing is weak, then brain dysfunctions such as poor memory, poor concentration, and dizziness can occur.

Constitutional weakness

This can lead to a chronic tendency to external disease patterns and allergies that the individual will find very difficult to shake off.

LEFT
Weakness or deficiency of Jing can be associated with a range of problems and disorders.

BLOOD

THE WESTERN reader who is having difficulty understanding the concepts of Qi and Jing will not find things getting any easier when discussing the nature and significance of Blood in Chinese medicine. Blood in Chinese medicine is not merely the physical substance that is recognized as blood in Western medicine. Closely allied to Qi, it nourishes the body and the Shen.

Chinese medicine sees Blood as a very material and fluid manifestation of Qi. In considering Blood we will slightly alter the focus of our discussion, looking at ✦ ORIGIN OF BLOOD ✦ FUNCTIONS OF BLOOD ✦ INTERRELATIONSHIPS WITH BLOOD ✦ DISHARMONIES OF BLOOD.

ORIGINS OF BLOOD

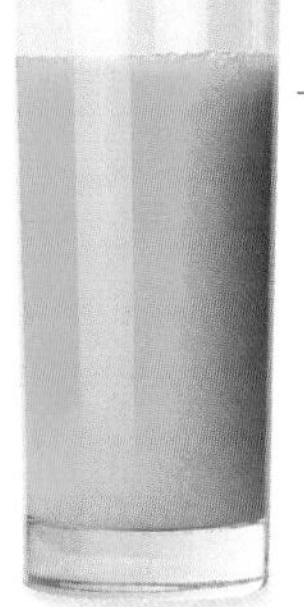

ABOVE
Food and drink are transformed into Blood, starting with the Spleen.

IT IS thought there are two ways in which Blood is produced for use throughout the body.

As will be seen, in Chinese medicine, the Spleen, Stomach, Lungs, Heart, and Kidneys all have important roles to play in the development of Blood.

1. TRANSFORMATION OF FOOD

Food and drink are transformed into Blood, starting with the Spleen.

The Spleen extracts Gu Qi from the food ingested into the Stomach and this is sent upward to the chest area. The Lung Qi begins the process of transformation into Blood, and the Gu Qi is then sent from the Lungs to the Heart where the Yuan Qi and Jing facilitates the further transformation into Blood.

2. THE ACTION OF MARROW

Marrow is also involved in the process of the production of Blood.

In this instance, the Jing that is stored in the Kidneys produces Marrow. This in turn produces Bone Marrow, which further contributes to the manufacture of Blood.

HOW BLOOD IS MANUFACTURED FROM FOOD

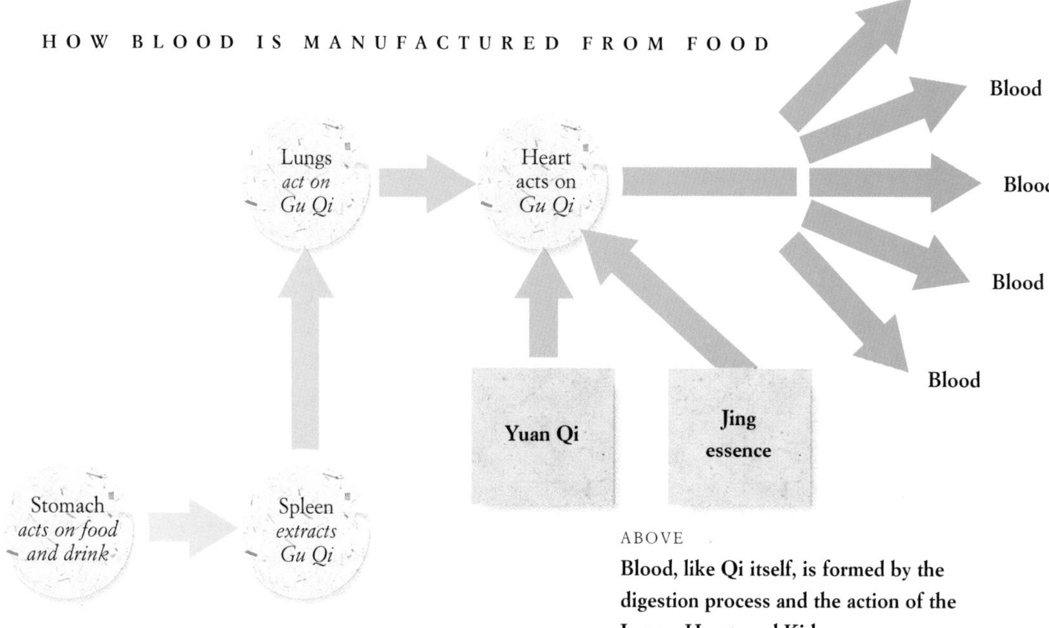

ABOVE
Blood, like Qi itself, is formed by the digestion process and the action of the Lungs, Heart, and Kidneys.

HOW BLOOD IS MANUFACTURED FROM MARROW

RIGHT
Marrow is produced by the action of the Kidneys and leads to the production of Bone Marrow and Blood.

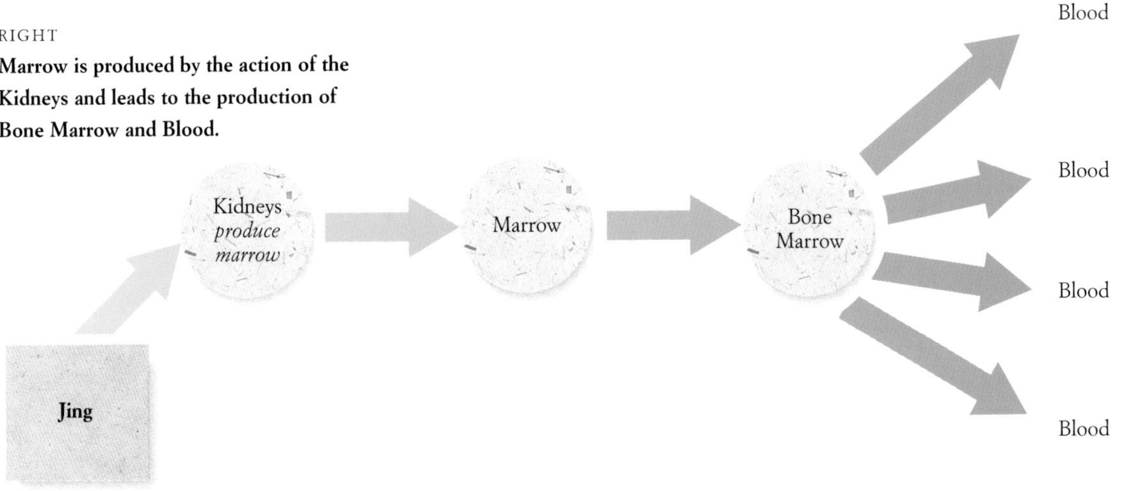

FUNCTIONS OF BLOOD

IT IS thought there are three main functions of Blood in the body.

1. Nourishing the body

Probably the most important function of Blood is that by continuously circulating throughout the body it carries nourishment with it to all the organs, muscles, tendons, and so on. Remember that in Chinese medicine, Blood is seen as an aspect of Qi and as such it helps carry the nutritive aspects of Qi.

2. Moistening the body

Being a fluid, Blood has an important role in moistening and lubricating throughout the body.

3. Aiding the mind (Shen)

Chinese medicine sees the Blood as helping to anchor the mind, allowing for the development of clear and stable thought processes. When an individual is Blood-deficient, there can be a tendency toward irritability and anxiety because the Blood is not adequately anchoring the mind.

RIGHT
Blood nourishes and moistens the body and aids the mind, but it must not be thought of as purely physical.

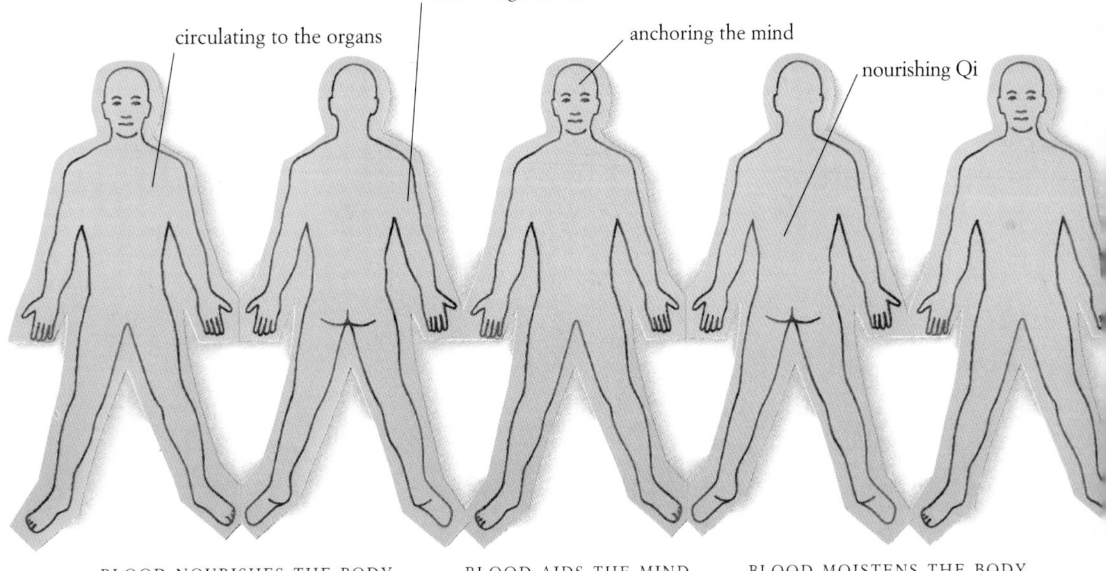

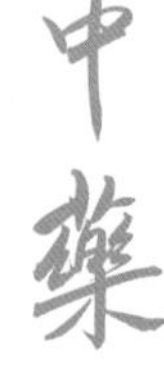

RELATIONSHIP WITH QI

BLOOD HAS important relationships with all the Yin organs (Zang) of the body. This will be discussed in greater detail when we look at the function of the various organs.

It is, however, worth saying a little more about the intimate interdependency between the Blood and Qi. Blood is an aspect of Qi. Qi can be considered Yang with respect to Blood since it is more ethereal; and, by implication, Blood is considered Yin with respect to Qi since it is more tangible. This close relationship can be seen in the following ways.

- Qi produces Blood.
- Qi moves Blood around the body.
- Qi holds the Blood in the blood vessels.
- Blood nourishes Qi.

The Chinese sum up this close relationship between Qi and Blood by stating that "Qi is the commander of Blood, and Blood is the mother of Qi."

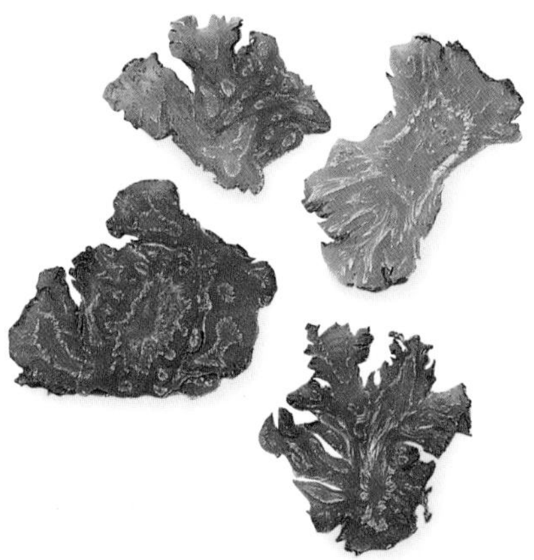

LEFT
A Chinese physician may decide to regulate the Blood with herbal remedies.

CAUTION

DO NOT ATTEMPT SELF-DIAGNOSIS: SEEK THE ADVICE OF A QUALIFIED PHYSICIAN.

DISHARMONIES OF BLOOD

THREE MAIN types of Blood disharmonies are thought to exist.

1. Deficient Blood (Xue Xu)

If Blood is deficient, this is usually connected with the Spleen's ability to move Gu Qi for Blood production. Typically, this can lead to pale complexion, dry skin, and dizziness on occasions.

2. Stagnant Blood (Xue Yu)

If Qi is weak or stagnant, it may fail to move the Blood adequately, thus leading to stagnation of Blood. Typically, this will lead to attacks of sharp and often intense pain. There may also be the development of tumors.

3. Heat in the Blood

This usually results from internal heat generated by the disharmony of another organ – usually the Liver. Heat in the Blood can lead to skin conditions and mental/emotional problems, among many other disharmonies.

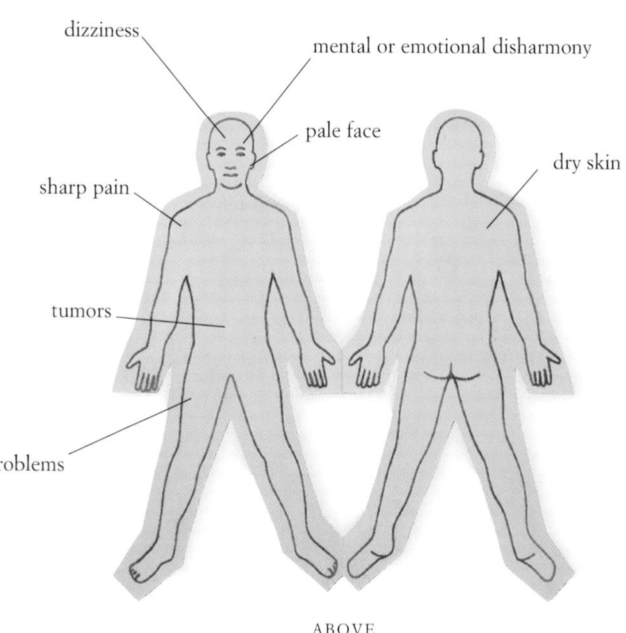

ABOVE
Some problems that can arise from deficient or stagnant Blood.

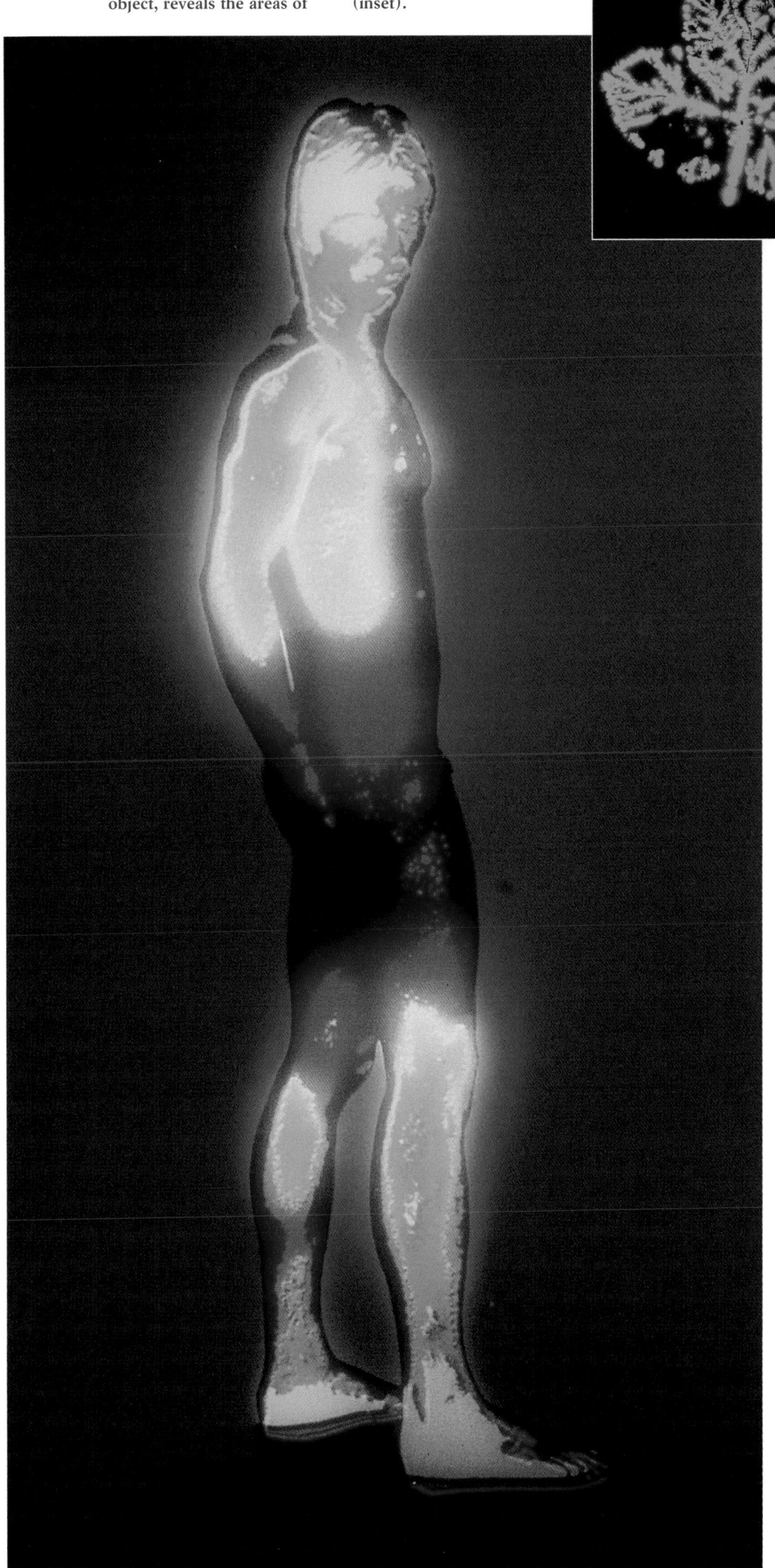

Kirlian photography, which records the electrical discharge emitted by an object, reveals the areas of concentrated energy in a human being (main picture) and in a freshly picked leaf (inset).

BODY FLUIDS

BODY FLUIDS (Jin Ye) are considered to be the other organic liquids that moisten and lubricate the body (in addition to Blood, which, as we have seen, is of great importance in Chinese medicine). Jin Ye originate from the action of the organs on food and drink and act on the body internally and externally. These fluids are of two types – light and watery or dense and heavy – and deficiencies or accumulations of Body Fluids cause their own problems.

ORIGIN AND TYPES OF BODY FLUIDS

THE CYCLE of the origin and transformation of Body Fluids is rather complex but can be simplified as follows.

Body Fluids originate in the process whereby the Spleen and Stomach function on ingested food and drink. In Chinese medicine an important function of the Spleen is to separate "pure" from "impure" fluids that are taken in food. The "pure" fluids are sent upward to the Lungs where they are further separated into "light" fluids and "dense" fluids. These "light" fluids are then dispersed by the Lungs to nourish and moisten the skin and the muscles of the body, while the "dense" fluids are sent downward to the Kidneys. The warming action of Kidney Yang further separates the "dense" fluids, sending the refined fluid back up to moisten the Lungs, while the impure fluids go from the Kidney to the Bladder where they are excreted as urine.

In addition to this process, the "impure" fluids from the Spleen are sent down to the Small Intestine, and this further discriminates between purer fluids, which are sent to the Bladder, and the most impure, which are sent to the Large Intestine for eventual excretion as feces. Even

THE PRODUCTION AND CIRCULATION OF BODY FLUIDS

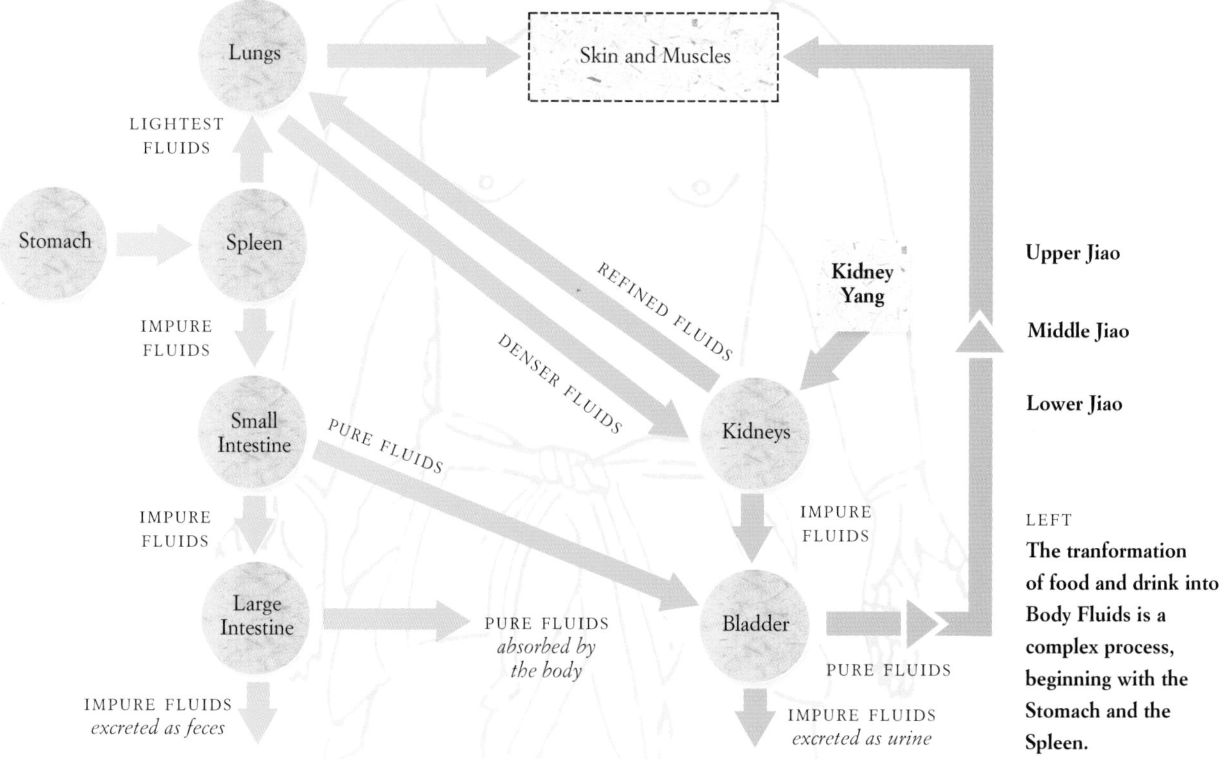

LEFT **The tranformation of food and drink into Body Fluids is a complex process, beginning with the Stomach and the Spleen.**

then, some more pure distillate may be reabsorbed into the body. The final part of the Body Fluid cycle involves yet a further separation in the Bladder where the "pure" is sent back up the body through the action of the San Jiao or Triple Warmer. The "impure" is excreted as urine.

As is obvious, the production and circulation of Body Fluids is a subtle and complex process in Chinese medicine. At all stages there is a continuous process of separation and recycling, in order to ensure that the maximum quantity of beneficial fluid is extracted and used by the body.

Essentially there are two types of Body Fluids.

1. **Light fluids (Jin)**
Light and watery fluids that circulate with the Wei Qi around the skin and muscles on the exterior of the body, under the control of the Lungs.

2. **Dense fluids (Ye)**
These are much heavier and thicker. They are seen as circulating throughout the interior of the body with the Ying Qi under the influence of the Spleen and the Kidneys.

FUNCTION OF BODY FLUIDS

The function of all Body Fluids is basically to moisten and nourish the body.

The Jin fluids perform this function for the skin, the muscles, and the hair. They can appear as fluids that flow directly from the body such as sweat, tears, and saliva.

The Ye fluids perform this function for the joints and the brain.

BODY FLUIDS, QI, AND BLOOD

As should be becoming increasingly evident, in Chinese medicine we cannot think of any one of the vital substances as existing functionally on its own. Their mutual functions continually interact and interrelate, and this is well illustrated in thinking about Qi, Blood, and the Body Fluids.

Qi is crucial in both the production and the transportation of Body Fluids, and it is responsible for holding the fluids in place. Conversely, if Body Fluids become deficient, then this can damage Qi; thus Body Fluids are themselves essential for maintaining healthy Qi.

Body Fluids and Blood are seen as nourishing each other, and Body Fluids are essential to maintaining Blood at the right consistency so that it will not stagnate, causing illness.

DISORDERS OF BODY FLUIDS

Essentially, there are two types of disorder that can arise with Body Fluids.

1. **Deficient Body Fluids**
This can lead to a whole range of problems arising from a lack of a nourishing and moistening function. For example, a deficiency of fluids in the Intestines can lead to constipation.

2. **Accumulation of Fluids**
If Body Fluids accumulate this can lead to problems described in Chinese medicine as Dampness and Phlegm. This can have a variety of causes and outcomes. For example, if the Spleen is damaged by poor diet, this can lead to Dampness that may manifest itself as lethargy with a feeling of heaviness in the lower abdomen.

SHEN

THE LAST basic substance that we will briefly discuss is the Shen, which can be translated as the Mind or the Spirit of the individual. Mind is perhaps the most appropriate term to use since Chinese philosophy distinguishes between several aspects of spirit, a discussion of which goes beyond the scope of this book. However, we should not think of the Shen as simply the mind that thinks, memorizes, and carries out logical processing. Hence, Shen is not human consciousness as such, but we can say that the existence of human consciousness is evidence of the action and presence of the Shen.

It is perhaps best to consider Shen in terms of its relationship with Qi and Jing. Jing, Qi, and Shen are referred to collectively in Chinese medicine as the "Three Treasures" and are believed to be the essential components of the life of the individual.

- Jing is the densest component and is responsible for the developmental processes of the body.
- Qi is the next stage and is responsible for the more immediate animate life of the body.
- Shen is the most refined level responsible for human consciousness.

When the Three Treasures are in harmony the individual will be radiant with life: physically fit, mentally sharp, and alert. The driving force of the Shen suggests the personality of the individual.

Disharmonies of Shen

A minor Shen disturbance may present as slow and muddled thinking, anxiety, or insomnia. In extreme instances, a Shen disharmony can produce a serious personality disorder, psychiatric disturbances, and even unconsciousness.

SHEN
This is the mental or spiritual aspect.
QI
Qi is the animating force, from within and without.
JING
This is the aspect that accounts for constitution and development.

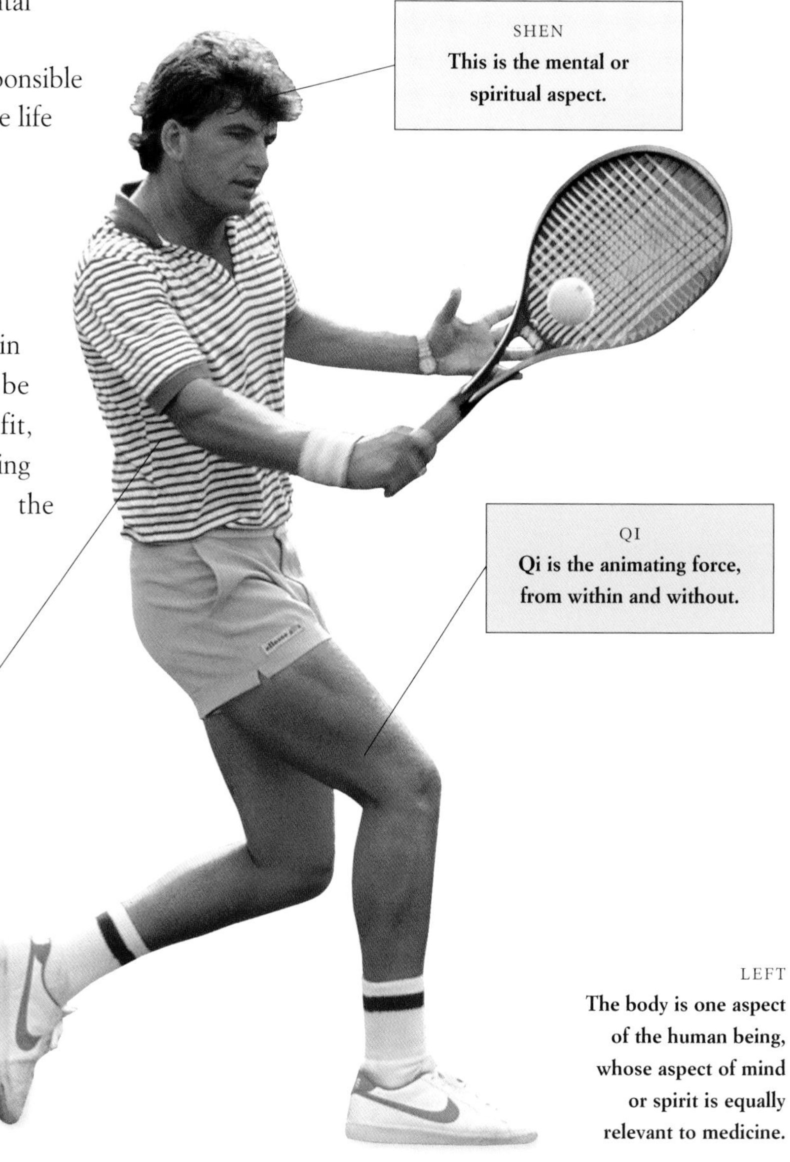

神

ABOVE
The Chinese character for Shen.

LEFT
The body is one aspect of the human being, whose aspect of mind or spirit is equally relevant to medicine.

SUMMARY

THIS CHAPTER has introduced to you at some length the basic substances of Chinese medicine. As will be apparent, it presents a very different picture to that of the Western tradition, but one that is certainly no less subtle or comprehensive.

It may be useful to summarize the various origins and functions of the fundamental substances in tabular form. A good rule of thumb to help ease you into these ideas is not to get caught up in trying to see Qi, Jing, Blood, Body Fluids, and Shen as "things" that make up the human being, but rather, to recognize that, above all, process is being described by these ideas and that these basic substances exist in a constant dynamic equilibrium – they are the "dance of life" in Chinese medicine.

THE BASIC SUBSTANCES

SUBSTANCE	ORIGINS	FUNCTIONS
Qi	Before Heaven – parents After Heaven – food/air	*movement and activity* *warming, transformation, protection, containment*
Jing	Before Heaven – parents After Heaven – ingested foods	*growth, reproduction development, promotes Kidney Qi, produces Marrow, forms constitution.*
Blood	Transformation of food Action of Marrow	*nourishes, moistens* *aids Shen*
Body Fluids	Distilled from ingested foods	*moistens, nourishes via:* *Jin – light fluids* *Ye – dense fluids*
Shen	Manifestation of consciousness	*keeps mind sharp and alert*

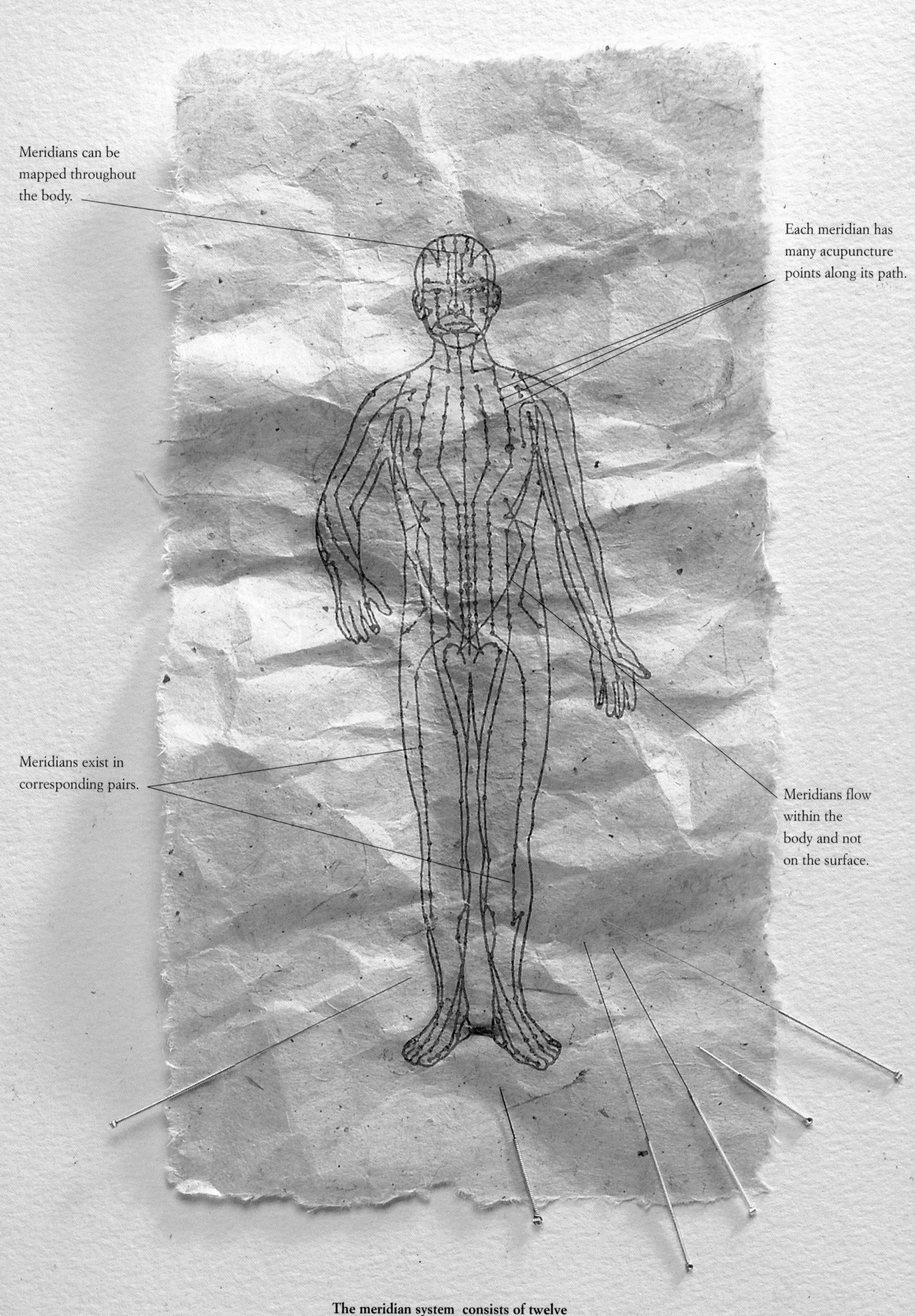

The meridian system consists of twelve main channels. Each has many specific, recognized acupuncture points.

THE MERIDIAN SYSTEM

THE AIM of this chapter is to bring some clarity and logic to the understanding of the energy-distribution system of Chinese medicine and to relate it to the overall discussion of Chinese medicine so far. The term "meridian" has been chosen to describe the overall system, but often the meridians themselves will be described as "channels," or even "vessels," referring to specific pathways in the body. The choice is often simply one of personal preference, but using the terms "channels" and "vessels" tends to suggest the idea of carrying, holding, and transporting, whereas "meridian" is functionally a more neutral term.

WHAT ARE THE CHANNELS?

IT WILL have been clear from the discussion on the basic substances that there must be a way in which these substances permeate the whole body. Chinese medicine describes a complex system of channels and their connecting vessels as the distribution system that carries Qi, Blood, and the Body Fluids around the body.

It is tempting to think of the channels in the same way as we think of the system of blood vessels – arteries, veins, capillaries – that carry blood around the body. This is both a useful and a misleading analogy. It is useful to the extent that the channel system is indeed responsible for the distribution of the basic substances through the body, but it can be misleading in as much as conventional anatomy and physiology would not be able to identify these pathways in a physical sense in the way that blood vessels can be identified.

It is necessary to remember that Chinese medicine operates very much at a subtle energy level. Qi, Blood, Jing, and Shen are all four essentially energetic properties that continually oscillate around the cusp of the physical and the energetic. The effects of the processes that they drive will manifest themselves in the physical body, with all its strengths, weaknesses, idiosyncrasies, and disharmonies, but they themselves remain essentially energetic in nature. Thus, it is perhaps more useful to consider the meridian system as an energetic distribution network that in itself tends toward an energetic manifestation. In much the same way that we try to understand Qi by its effects, similarly, the meridian system can best be understood as process rather than structure.

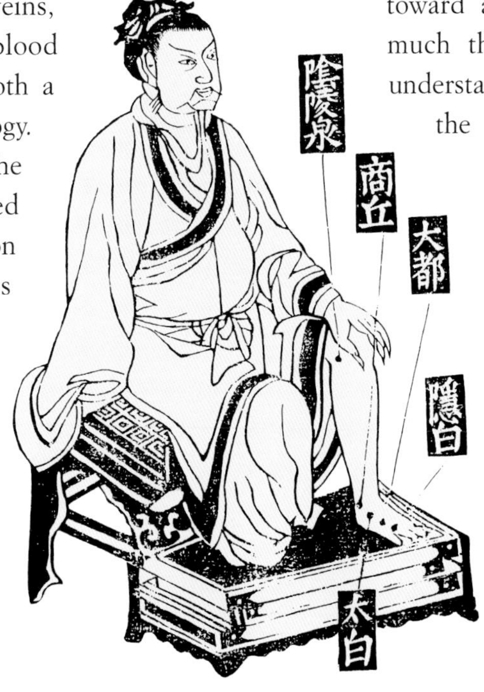

ABOVE
Acupuncture points relating to specific organs are located along the meridians.

A useful analogy that is often used to describe Qi flow in Chinese medicine is that of a river. A river has a source and it follows its course ultimately toward the ocean. As it flows it will vary from shallow to deep, quick-flowing to slow-flowing, while always following the most "natural" path.

Chinese philosophy believes that Qi permeates everything in the universe – there is nothing that is not a manifestation of Qi.

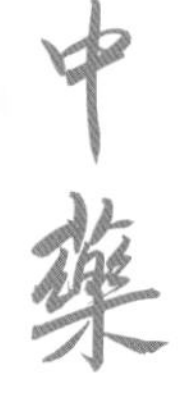

There will, however, be varying concentrations of Qi, and it is perhaps useful to consider the meridian system as representing areas or pathways of high Qi concentration. Thus, as you move away from any given channel, you do not suddenly reach an "edge" – it is more a matter of moving from areas of high Qi concentration to ones of lower Qi concentration. This is similar to the way in which, as you move away from the center of a river, the water becomes progressively more shallow, and even when you move beyond the obvious physical boundary of the river there is still moisture which is contained within the soil. The water is, therefore, present beyond the limits of the river boundaries.

Thus, we have the picture of the body being permeated by an energy system that concentrates around areas of high-density energy, which are termed channels. This energy is in constant dynamic movement in quite specific ways, as will be described later, driving the myriad of processes that manifest themselves as that physical organism. If anything occurs to weaken or block this energy flow in any way, then the result will be an energetic imbalance that in turn will manifest itself in the physical organism as disease or illness.

WHAT ARE ACUPUNCTURE POINTS?

THE OTHER feature that is always present on a meridian chart of the human body is the specific points that are marked upon the individual channels. Some channels appear to have many, some have fewer; some points appear grouped close together and others appear more discrete. These represent what are commonly described as acupuncture points, but how do they relate to the dynamic energy system that we have been describing above?

It would appear that along many of the channels there are what could be best described as "access points." Going back again to the analogy of the river, consider how a whirlpool effect draws everything down into the heart of the river – it gives access to the depth of the river in effect. Following the analogy, we can consider acupuncture points as "energy vortices" that draw Qi into or out of the body's energy flow and that provide access points whereby the Qi flow of the body can be directly influenced by these vortices.

ABOVE
An acupuncture point can be compared to a miniature whirlpool or vortex, through which energy can be drawn.

Even simple pressure on a specific "energy vortex" will produce changes in the energy system, with consequent physical effects. This, of course, provides the basis for simple acupressure treatment. It is likely that we instinctively use a form of acupressure techniques when suffering from a minor disharmony in everyday life. For example, rubbing the temple area on the side of our head when we are suffering a headache would stimulate the "energy vortex" or acupuncture point known as Taiyang. Acupuncture simply takes this a stage further.

In acupuncture, fine needles are inserted into the patient's energy system at a series of appropriately selected vortices, or acupuncture points.

BELOW
A patient is given acupuncture in a modern Kowloon clinic.

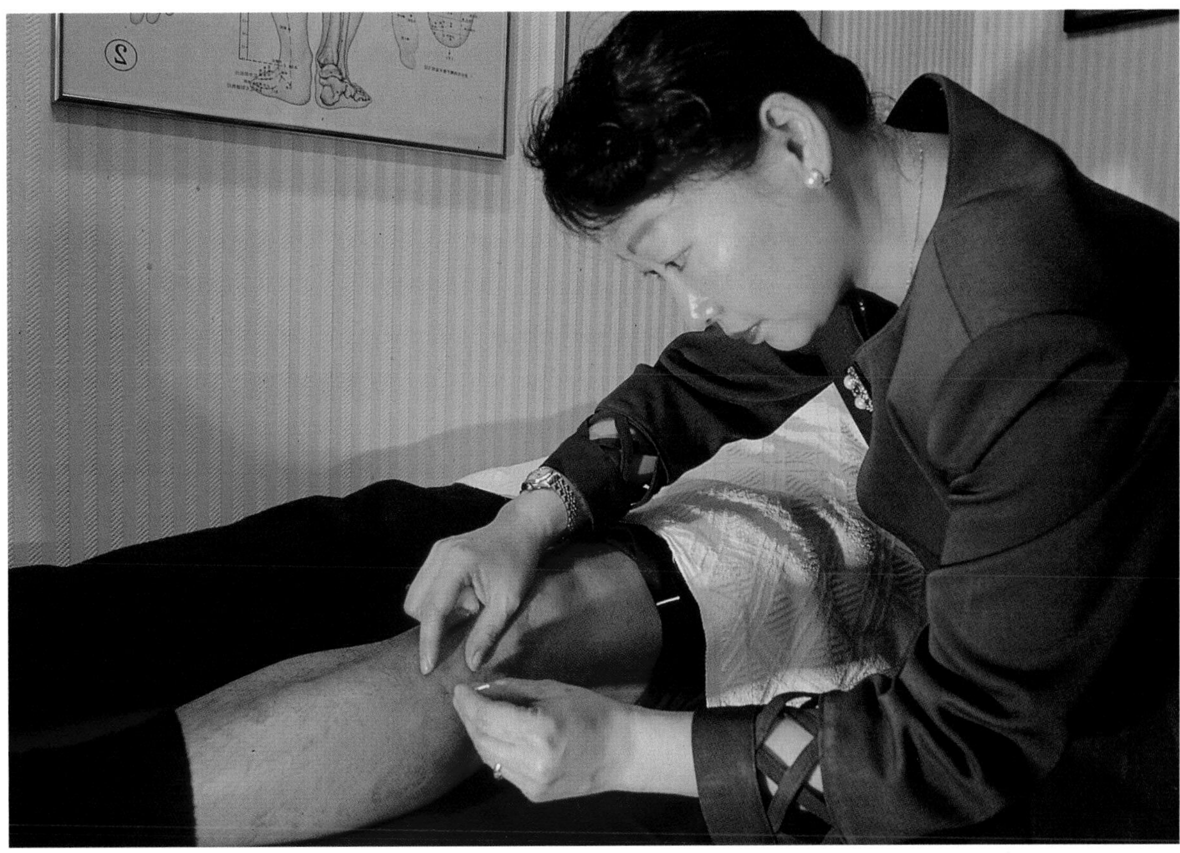

The effect of the needling is expected to cause changes in the pattern of the patient's energy system with the result, it is to be hoped, that beneficial changes will take place at the physical level. It is thought likely that the practitioner's own energy system is also a factor in the process, the needle in effect becoming an extension of that energy system.

Ideally, by now the reader will have a more dynamic view of the body's energy system that will help in understanding the concept of the meridian system as a form of "energy anatomy."

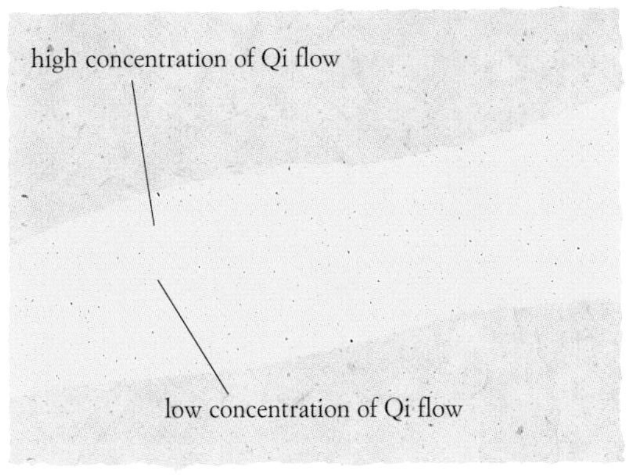

CHANNEL TOP VIEW

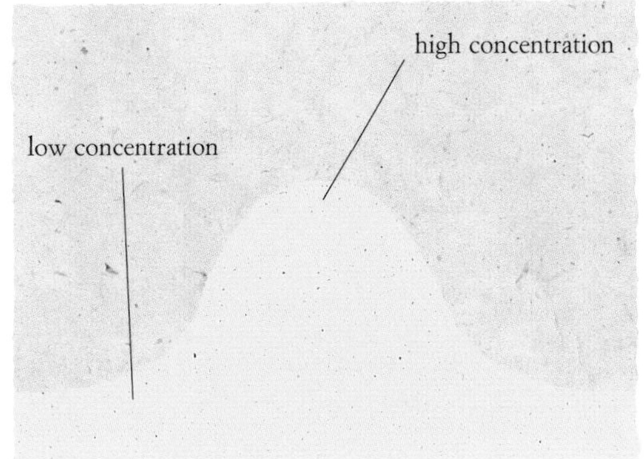

CHANNEL CROSS-SECTION

ABOVE RIGHT
Within a channel or meridian, higher and lower concentrations of energy can be detected.

RIGHT
A cross-sectional representation of the Qi energy flow shows how a high concentration of Qi in one area disrupts the flow.

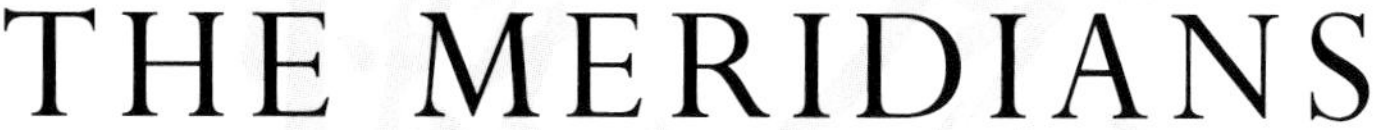

THE MERIDIANS

IN THIS section the channels or meridians will be described in terms of their relationships and their functions. It is worth noting that the practitioner of Chinese medicine must be as knowledgeable about these networks as the Western doctor is about the anatomy and physiology of the physical body. Without that understanding, successful intervention would be very difficult. An anatomical diagram of the meridian system appears to show that the system is made up of a series of independent channels that run on the surface of the body – nothing could be further from the truth.

THE TWELVE REGULAR CHANNELS

THE TWELVE regular channels correspond to the five Yin organs, the six Yang organs, and the Pericardium. (The Pericardium is functionally considered to be a Yin organ in Chinese medicine.) The San Jiao is an organ that has no anatomical counterpart in Western medicine, and the other organs should not be thought of as being identical with the physical organs.

There are three Yin organs and three Yang organs relating to both the arm and the leg. Each Yin organ is paired with its corresponding Yang organ: the Yin Lung organ, for example, corresponds with the Yang Large Intestine.

Taking the limbs as an example, there are six paired Yin channels and six paired Yang channels (three of each on the arm and the leg respectively). The main channels are listed below.

Arm Tai Yin Channel:	*Lung (Lu)*
Leg Tai Yin Channel:	*Spleen (Sp)*
Arm Shao Yin Channel:	*Heart (He)*
Leg Shao Yin Channel:	*Kidney (Kid)*
Arm Jue Yin Channel:	*Pericardium (Per)*
Leg Jue Yin Channel:	*Liver (Liv)*
Arm Yang Ming Channel:	*Large Intestine (LI)*
Leg Yang Ming Channel:	*Stomach (St)*
Arm Tai Yang Channel:	*Small Intestine (SI)*
Leg Tai Yang Channel:	*Bladder (Bl)*
Arm Shao Yang Channel:	*San Jiao (SJ)*
Leg Shao Yang Channel:	*Gall Bladder (GB)*

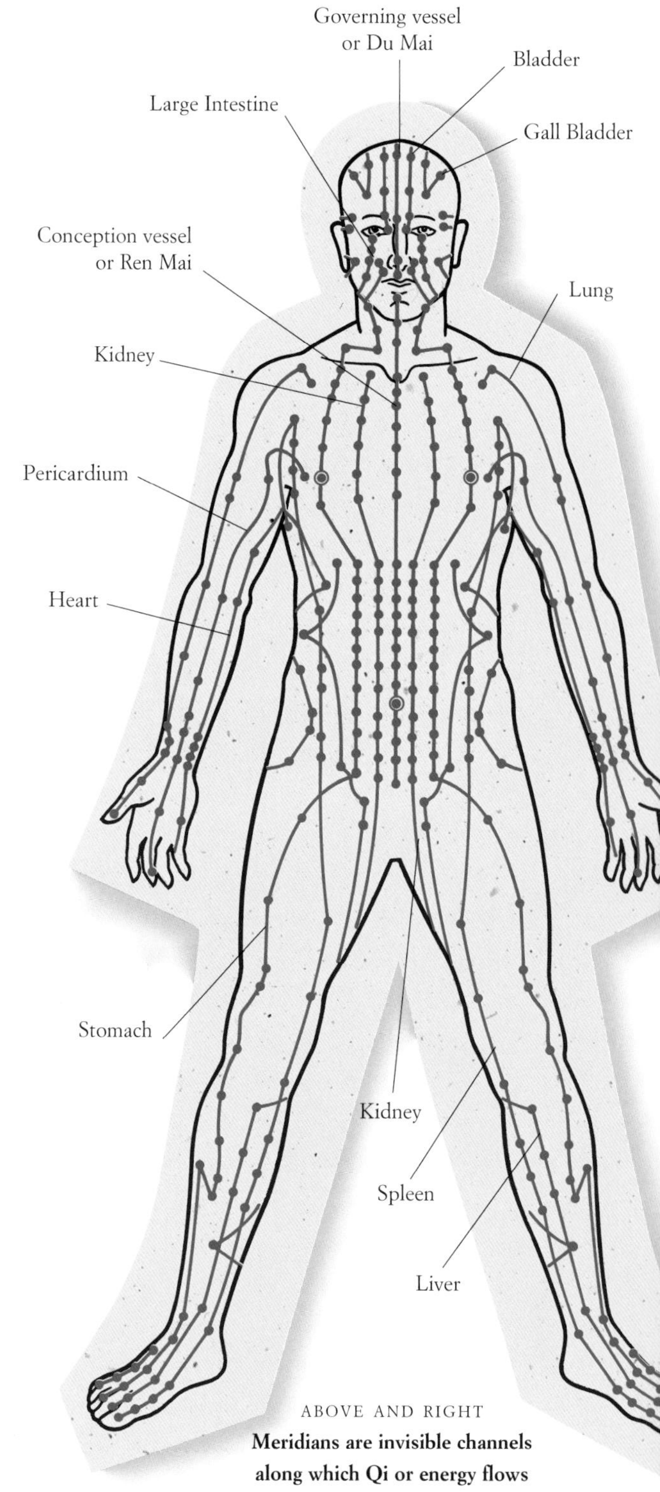

ABOVE AND RIGHT
Meridians are invisible channels along which Qi or energy flows around the body. There are twelve main meridians.

Yin Organ	Yang Organ
Lung	Large Intestine
Heart	Small Intestine
Pericardium	San Jiao
Liver	Gall Bladder
Kidney	Bladder
Spleen	Stomach

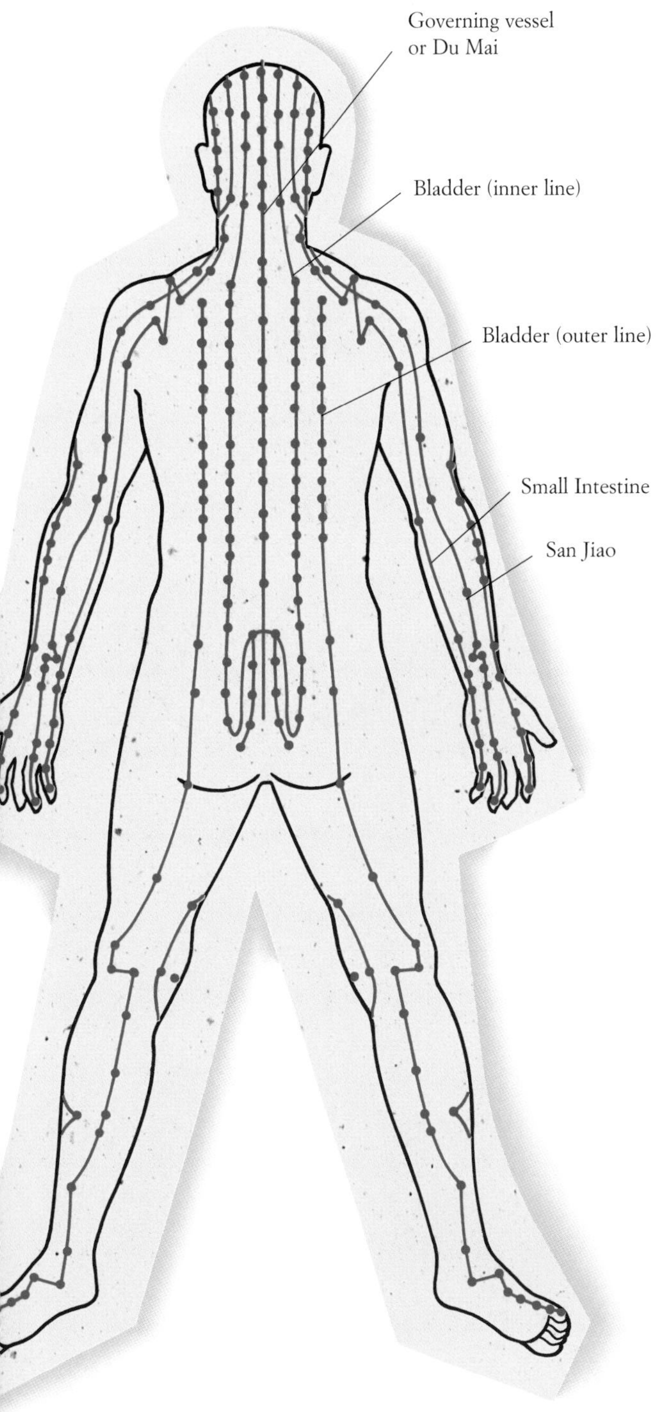

Qi flow circulation in the twelve regular channels

Qi flows from the chest area along the three arm Yin channels (Lu; Per; He) to the hands. There they connect with the three paired arm Yang channels (LI; SJ; SI) and flow upward to the head. In the head they connect with their three corresponding leg Yang channels (St; GB; Bl) and flow down the body to the feet. In the feet they connect with their corresponding leg Yin channels (Sp; Liv; Kid) and flow up again to the chest to complete the cycle of Qi circulation.

Although Qi is continuously circulating through the twelve regular channels at all times, there are recognized times when the Qi and Blood flow is at its maximum in each given channel. Thus, the maximum flow in each channel in relation to the daily cycle is as follows:

LUNG (3 a.m.–5 a.m.), LARGE INTESTINE (5 a.m.–7 a.m.), STOMACH (7 a.m.–9 a.m.), SPLEEN (9 a.m.–11 a.m.), HEART (11 a.m.–1 p.m.), SMALL INTESTINE (1 p.m.–3 p.m.), BLADDER (3 p.m.–5 p.m.), KIDNEY (5 p.m.–7 p.m.), PERICARDIUM (7 p.m.–9 p.m.), SAN JIAO (9 p.m.–11 p.m.), GALL BLADDER (11 p.m.–1 a.m.), LIVER (1 a.m.–3 a.m.).

This information can be of great assistance to the practitioner in considering diagnosis and treatment strategies.

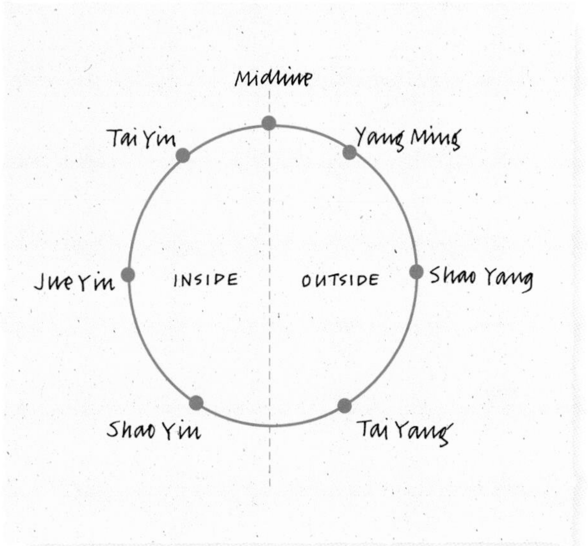

ABOVE
Each limb is traversed by six channels, three Yin on the inside and three Yang on the outside, along which Qi flows.

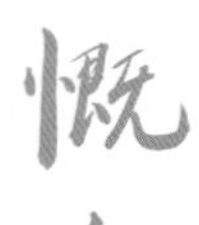
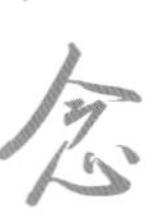

Channel functions

The channels have the function of being the energetic unification structures of the whole body. They connect the interior with the exterior and are the pathways and concentrations of Qi and Blood flow throughout the body. They carry the protective Wei Qi throughout the body, but at the same time they also provide the route through which external pathogenic factors can invade the body and cause harm, initially to the exterior but also, ultimately, to the interior. Importantly, the channels also provide the practitioner with the "entry points" to access the Qi flow with acupuncture.

Channel communication

The arm and leg channels of the same name are considered to "communicate" with each other in Chinese medicine. Thus, problems in a given channel or organ can be treated by using various points on the communication partner. As an example, a disharmony in the Lungs can be treated by using points on the Spleen channel – they are both Tai Yin channels.

Each channel also relates to its corresponding organ. This is an example of an interior/interior communication. Finally each channel will relate to its paired Yin or Yang organ. This can be illustrated with a couple of examples.

1. If there is a problem on the Large Intestine channel this can be treated by points on the Large Intestine channel and also by points on the Lung Channel (paired Yin of Large Intestine).

2. If the Kidneys have a problem, this can be treated by points on the Kidney channel and it can also be treated by points on the Bladder channel (paired Yang of the Kidneys).

Regular channel disharmonies

It should be borne in mind that when a disharmony occurs in a given organ, the problem can spill over into related organs through the channel system.

For example, someone who follows an excessively "cold" diet of, say, salads, cold and raw foods, fruit and iced drinks, can cause the Stomach to become Qi deficient. This can affect the Yang energy of the Spleen (the paired organ) resulting in the Spleen Qi being unable to rise. In consequence, the Spleen energy will fall, leading to problems such as diarrhea.

The connection of the Stomach with the Large Intestine (Yang Ming channels) will also exacerbate the disharmony.

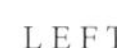

LEFT
Parallels can be drawn between Reflexology, a method of treatment involving pressure on specific points on the foot, related to specific areas of the body, and the treatment of specific areas of the body through the meridian system.

THE EIGHT EXTRAORDINARY CHANNELS

THESE EIGHT channels are not directly linked to the major organ systems and only two of them have acupuncture points on them. The eight extraordinary channels are ✦ Ren Mai, *Conception vessel,* ✦ Du Mai, *Governing vessel,* ✦ Chong Mai, *Penetrating vessel,* ✦ Dai Mai, *Girdle vessel,* ✦ Yin Wei Mai, *Yin linking vessel,* ✦ Yang Wei Mai, *Yang linking vessel,* ✦ Yin Qiao Mai, *Yin heel vessel,* and ✦ Yang Qiao Mai, *Yang heel vessel.*

The most important of these channels are the Du Mai and Ren Mai. These both have acupuncture points that are independent of the twelve regular channels. The other six are considered less important and they share points with points on the twelve regular channels.

FUNCTIONS OF THE EXTRAORDINARY CHANNELS

These channels have various specific functions that can be highlighted.

1. *They act as reservoirs of Qi and Blood for the twelve regular channels, filling and emptying as required.*
2. *They circulate Jing around the body because they have a strong connection with the Kidneys.*
3. *They help circulate the defensive Wei Qi over the trunk of the body and, as such, play an important role in maintaining health.*
4. *They provide further connections between the twelve regular channels.*

DIVERGENT CHANNELS

Each of the twelve regular channels has a divergent channel, thus providing connections from the Yin channels to their associated Zang organs and from the Yang channels to their associated Fu organs *(see page 58).*

FINER NETWORK CHANNELS (LUO)

Blood flow has major distribution vessels – arteries and veins – but there is also a myriad of tiny connecting capillaries that ensure that blood flows to every corner of the body. In the same way, the meridian system is made up of a network of small connecting channels.

FIFTEEN CONNECTING CHANNELS

These channels provide the connection between the Yin and Yang channel pairs, for example between the Heart and the Small Intestine channels. Each of the twelve regular channels has a connecting channel; the Spleen channel has two, and the Ren Mai and Du Mai have one each, making fifteen channels in total.

MINUTE CHANNELS

These are a myriad of tiny connecting channels. All together they make up the full matrix of the meridian system.

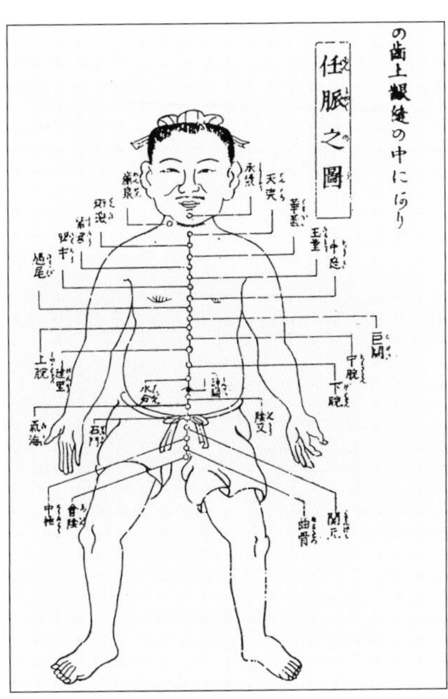

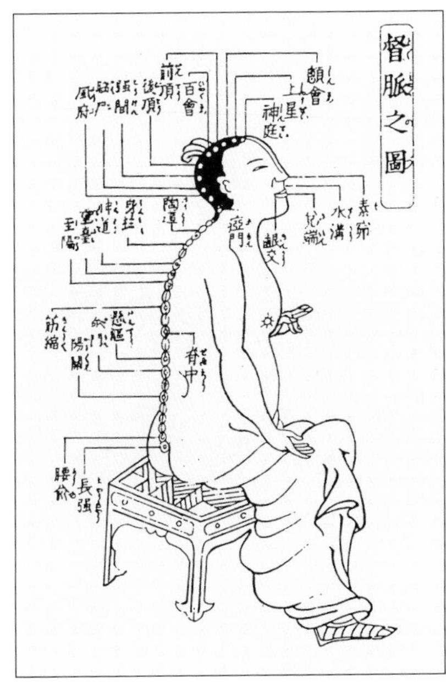

The Ren Mai or Conception vessel (right) acts mainly on Yin energy, while the Du Mai or Governing vessel (far right) acts mainly on Yang energy.

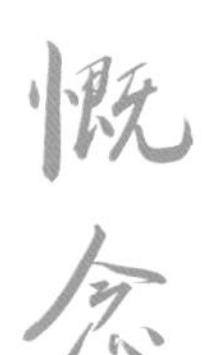

EXPERIENCE YOUR OWN QI FLOW

CHINESE MEDICINE

ONE OF the main problems that people have with Chinese medicine is in coming to terms with the idea of a system and a process that cannot be directly observed. We can easily experience our blood flow by pricking our finger, but experiencing our Qi flow is not so easy.

This is a simple Qigong exercise that may allow you to begin to experience the effects of Qi flow.

1 *Sit comfortably with your feet resting flat on the floor and your back upright. Place your hands face up in your lap.*

2 *Take two or three minutes just to relax, keeping still and breathing gently.*

3 *Bring your arms to about chest height with the palms facing each other about 6 to 8 inches apart. The arms should be relaxed. Avoid having them straight out with the muscles tense. Imagine you are holding a soft, flexible beach ball between your hands.*

4 *Breathe naturally, expanding your lower abdomen – the area known in Chinese medicine as the lower Dan tien – on the inhalation. Imagine your Qi moving from this area, about two finger-widths below your umbilicus. This point on the Ren channel is called Qihai, or "sea of Qi."*

5 *Imagine the Qi rising up the Ren channel and out along the Yin channels on the inside of your arm. In particular, pay attention to the Pericardium channel that runs right down the center of the inside arm to end at the tip of the middle finger.*

6 *With each exhalation imagine the Qi flowing down the Pericardium channel to the palm of the hand. Focus on the Laogong point in the center of the palm. This is Pericardium 8.*

7 *Begin to become aware of your experience at the Laogong points on the two opposite palms as you continue to relax and breathe easily. You may have a variety of experiences – warmth, coolness, tingling, heaviness, a sense of attraction between the palms, and so on. Just be aware of the feeling.*

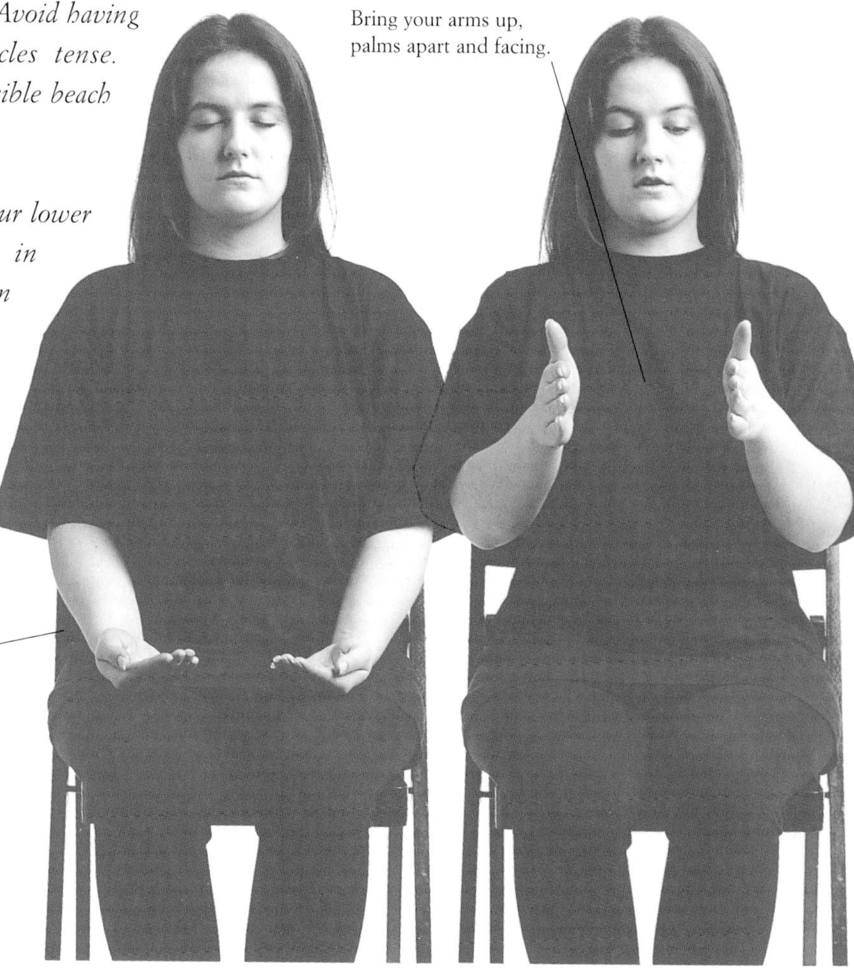

LEFT TO RIGHT
Qigong exercises enable you to become aware of the flow of Qi in your body.

8 Play with the experience by bringing the two palms closer together and then pulling them apart. You may like to run the palm of one hand up the outside of the opposite arm from the thumb to the elbow. Keep it about an inch above the arm. Be aware if you experience any "hot spots" as you go, where Laogong seems to be making a connection with a point on the opposite arm. This may well be noticed at the point Hegu (on the fleshy mound between the thumb and the forefinger) or at the point Quchi, which is at the elbow.

As you do this simple exercise you will begin to experience the effect of Qi flow, whether as heat, cold, or whatever. Remember, the sensation is not the Qi, it is the effect of Qi.

Think of this analogy. If electricity passes through a wire it will meet resistance. If the resistance rises, the current flow will cause the wire to heat up. The heat in the wire is not the electricity, it is the effect of the electricity flow.

Think of your experience in this exercise in the same way. What you are experiencing is the effect of Qi flow. The point to emphasize is that there is no one sensation to be looking for. The sensations experienced can vary, but some form of warmth tends to be the most common. If you practice Qigong exercises on a regular basis then your ability to become aware of your own Qi flow, and indeed of that of other people, will develop markedly. More about Qigong can be found on pages 189–205.

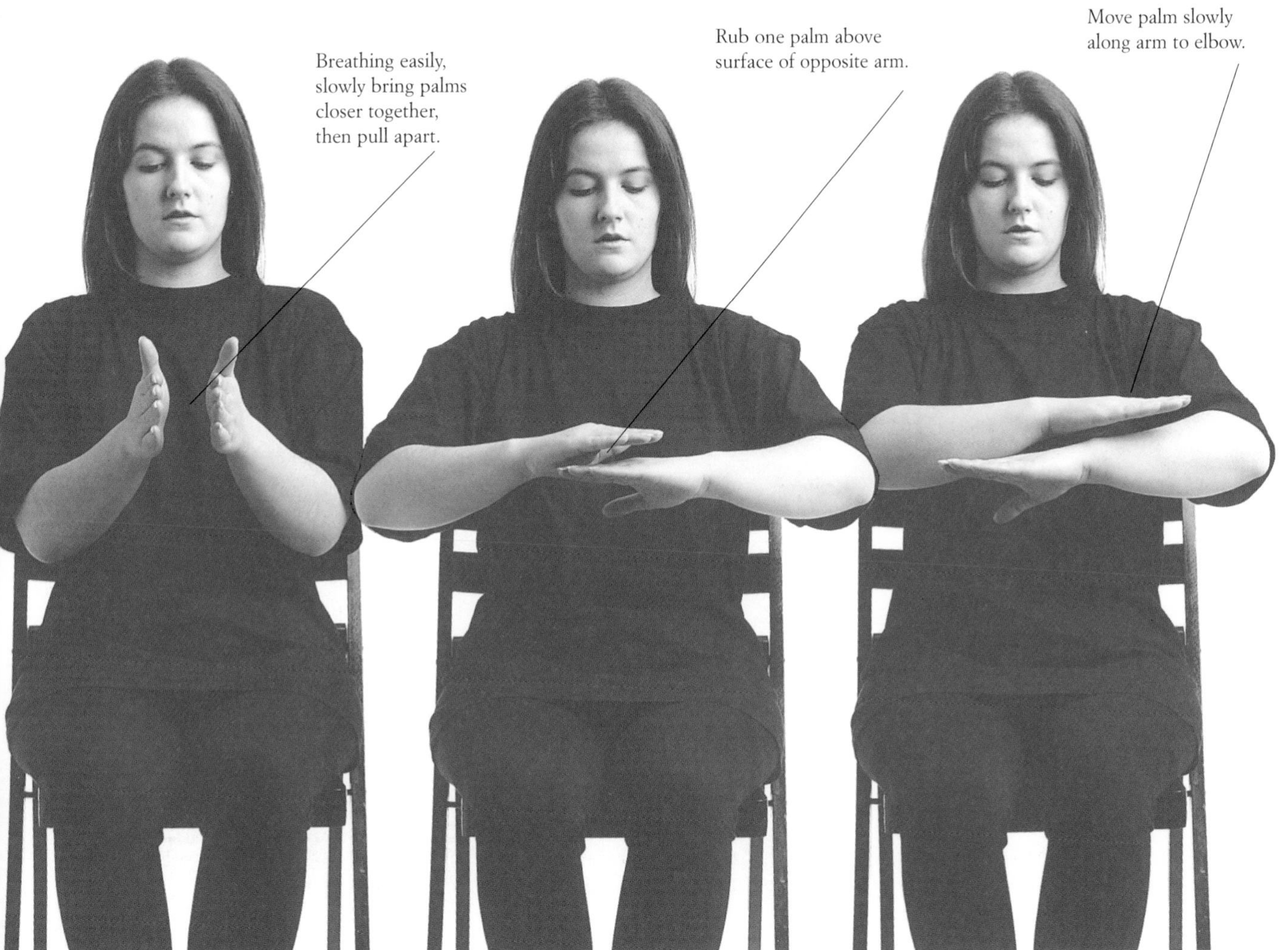

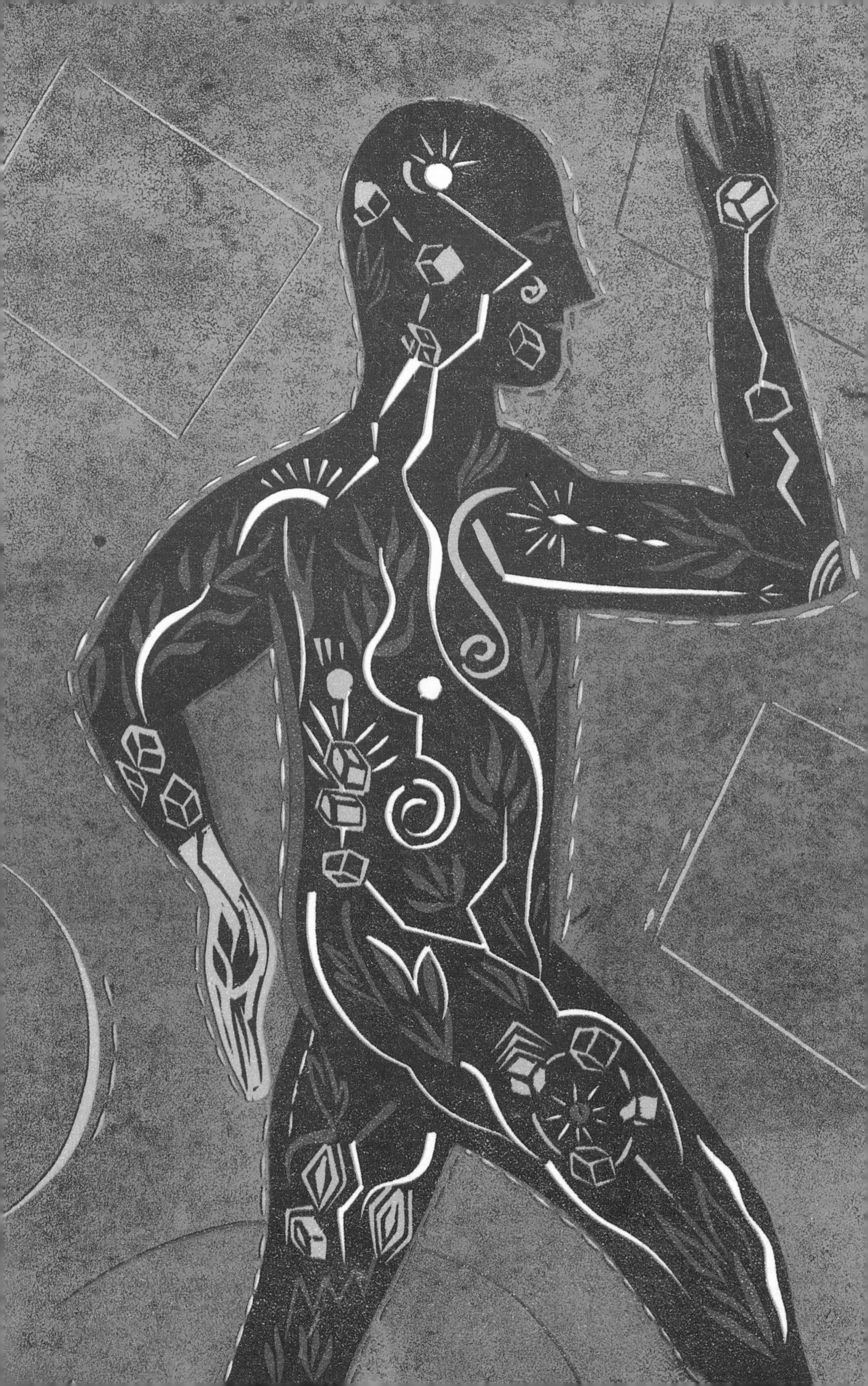

THE ZANGFU SYSTEM

IN THIS chapter we will look at a system that is of fundamental importance in understanding the way in which Chinese medicine sees the functioning of the human body. The Zang or Yin organs and the Fu or Yang organs work in combination, to assure the health of mind and body. Together, these organ systems are known as Zangfu. We will explore the basic ideas of the Zangfu first, and then look in more detail at the features of the system with respect to each organ of the Zangfu in turn.

PROCESS AND STRUCTURE

THE FIRST point that needs addressing is that of the difference between process and structure.

THE BODY ORGANS AS PHYSICAL STRUCTURES

The idea that the organs are physical entities seems so self-evident to the Western mind that we have to wonder, why state it at all? It is important to state the obvious in order to emphasize just what a difference the nonobvious implies.

The gift that Western anatomy and physiology has given to the world is an immensely sophisticated view of the structures of the physical body. Among these structures the individual organs are emphasized in terms of their biology and function. Thus, for example, the Heart is seen as a very complex and reliable pump that ensures a constant flow of blood around the whole body.

The Western approach to medicine has concerned itself, almost exclusively, with trying to understand how these structures function when normal and the ways in which this normal functioning can break down. Therapy, then, has the goal of trying to restore the malfunctioning structure to good working order.

It is important to understand that there is absolutely nothing wrong with this way of seeing the body. It has undeniably brought us some remarkable medical breakthroughs that would have been inconceivable a few decades ago.

We will, however, find this "commonsense" understanding stretched to the limit when we begin to consider the Chinese model. Indeed, a good rule of thumb to adopt when looking at the Chinese approach to medicine is to leave our conventional wisdom to one side. Experience dictates that if you try to combine the two systems then the conceptual problems that follow only hinder understanding.

THE BODY ORGANS AS PROCESSES

In Chinese medicine the first thing that will become obvious is that very little is said about organs as structures, but an awful lot is said about how an organ system is part of the overall dynamic energy process of the human body. In every instance the emphasis will be on how the organs ensure the constant ebb and flow of the fundamental substances of the body. Illness is seen as a process disharmony that needs alleviating, not as a "machinery breakdown" that requires fixing. Now this distinction may seem like semantic juggling, but the full significance will emerge as we explore the process function of each of the organ systems in turn.

WHAT ARE THE ZANGFU?

The term Zangfu can be considered as the collective name for the series of Yin and Yang organ systems that are identified in Chinese medicine. These systems are those of the solid Yin organs, the hollow Yang organs, and the extra Fu organs, as they are described in the following paragraphs.

LEFT
The body is seen as an interplay of energy forces – a network of processes rather than a simple physical structure.

The Yin organs – the Zang

In the theory of Chinese medicine, the Zang consist of the five solid (Yin) organs. These are ✦ *Lungs* ✦ *Heart* ✦ *Spleen* ✦ *Liver* ✦ *Kidneys*. There is also considered to be a sixth Yin organ, namely the Pericardium. This has its own Qi meridian, but to all intents and purposes its function is closely associated with the Heart.

In general, Chinese medicine considers the Zang to be deeper in the body and to be concerned with the manufacture, storage, and regulation of the fundamental substances.

The Yang organs – the Fu

In the theory of Chinese medicine, the Fu consist of the six hollow (Yang) organs. These are ✦ *Small Intestine* ✦ *Large Intestine* ✦ *Gall Bladder* ✦ *Bladder* ✦ *Stomach* ✦ *San Jiao* (sometimes called Triple Warmer or Triple Heater).

The San Jiao is considered an organ in Chinese medicine because its processes can be identified, but at the same time there is obviously no anatomical structure that can be identified with it. Once you are able to appreciate the concept of the San Jiao, then you can be confident that you are well on your way to gaining a complete understanding of the whole system that comprises Chinese medicine.

In general, Chinese medicine considers the Fu to be closer to the surface of the body and to have the functions of receiving, separating, distributing, and excreting body substances. The Fu are not considered as storage organs but as organs involved in an on-going process of movement and change. The Fu demonstrate the first interesting distinction between the Western and Chinese view regarding structure and process.

The Extra Fu (or Extraordinary Fu)

In addition to the main breakdown into the Zangfu, the traditional Chinese medicine system also identifies a series of less important organs in terms of process. They are ✦ *Brain* ✦ *Uterus* ✦ *Marrow* ✦ *Bone* ✦ *Blood Vessels* ✦ *Gall Bladder*. (Note: The Gall Bladder is considered both a Fu and an Extra Fu – just to complicate the picture!)

It will be useful at this stage in our discussion of the Zangfu to consider the functions and processes of each of the Zang and Fu organs in turn. With each description of the Zangfu, simple examples will be given of the most commonly found types of disharmony of that particular organ. This will be for illustrative purposes and will be elaborated upon when Zangfu disharmonies are considered in more detail later in the book.

FUNCTIONS OF THE ZANG

Ancient texts speak of the body as a kingdom governed by twelve state officials or ministers, which correspond to the six solid Yin organs (the Zang) and the six hollow Yang organs (the Fu). The Heart (sometimes translated as Heart-Mind) is the chief official and is concerned with the Shen or spirits. The other officials act as messengers, take responsibility for transportation and storage, deal with excess and waste, control internal connections, make decisions and verdicts, and activate the body. In Chinese medicine today, the functions of the Zang organs are seen as similar to those of the physical organs known to Western medicine, but they have important additional functions, including those relating to Qi. Additionally, each Zang is linked to an emotion. All Zang act as storage places or reservoirs, and Fu are paired with Zang.

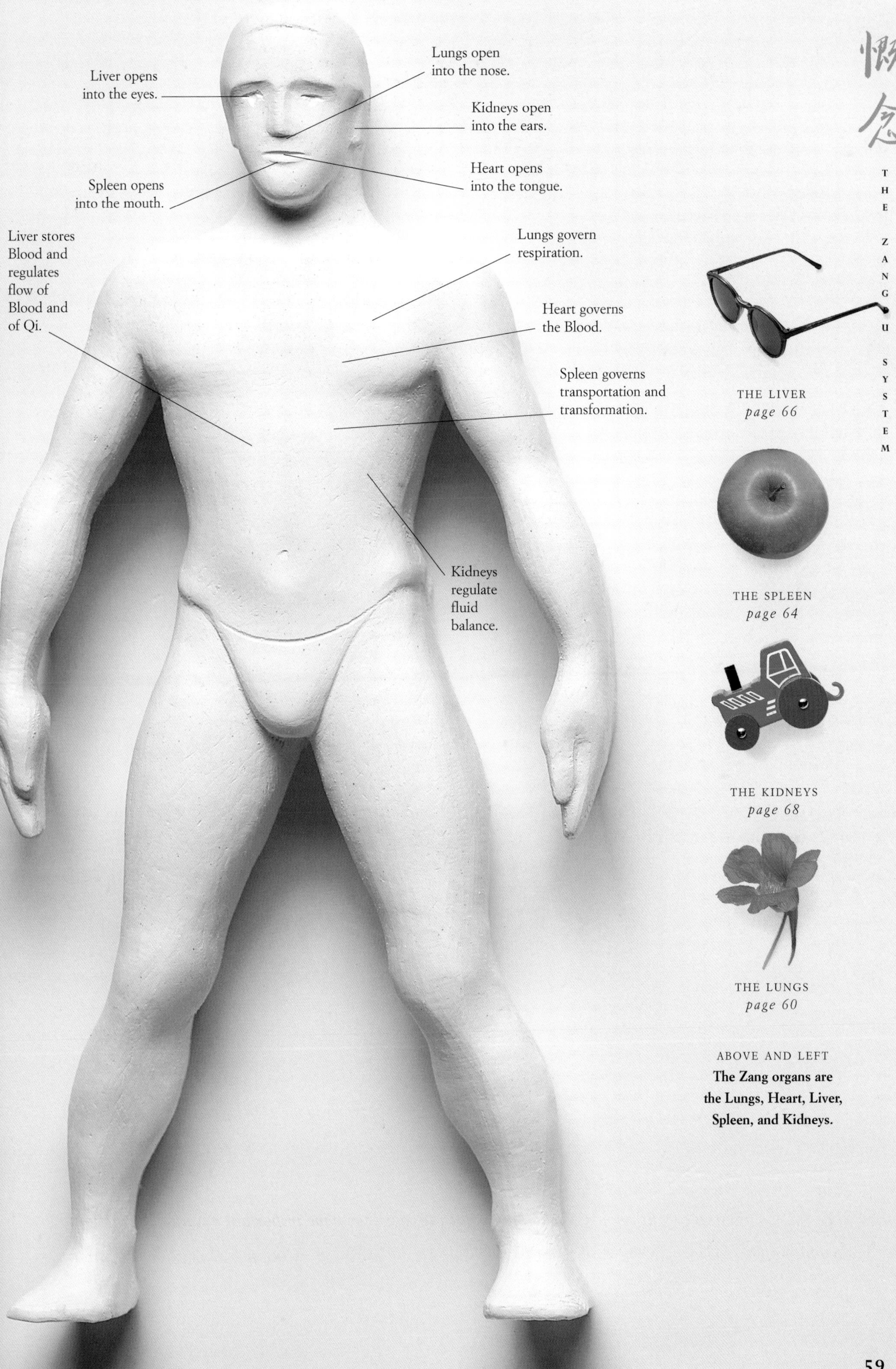

THE LIVER
page 66

THE SPLEEN
page 64

THE KIDNEYS
page 68

THE LUNGS
page 60

ABOVE AND LEFT
The Zang organs are the Lungs, Heart, Liver, Spleen, and Kidneys.

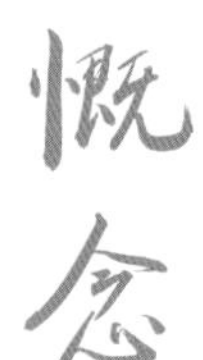

THE LUNGS

THE LUNGS GOVERN QI AND RESPIRATION

The most important function of the Lungs is both similar to, and different from, that of the conventional Western view. The Lungs govern the inhalation of pure Qi from the air and the exhalation of impure Qi. The crucial difference lies in the Chinese-medicine view that it is the Qi we get from the air that is important, and not just the oxygen.

The second aspect lies in the role that the Lungs take in the formation of the Qi we use in our bodies. The Spleen sends up the Qi extracted from food to the Lungs, where it combines with the pure Qi inhaled in the air to form what is called Zong Qi. This is the aspect that ensures that the Lungs help to spread Qi to all parts of the body. If there is any imbalance in the Lungs, then this can lead to general symptoms of Qi deficiency affecting the whole body and causing general weakness and tiredness.

When the Lungs are functioning well, then the respiration pattern is smooth and regular.

THE LUNGS CONTROL DISPERSION AND DESCENDING

The Lungs disperse defensive Qi (Wei Qi) and the Body Fluids throughout the outermost layers of

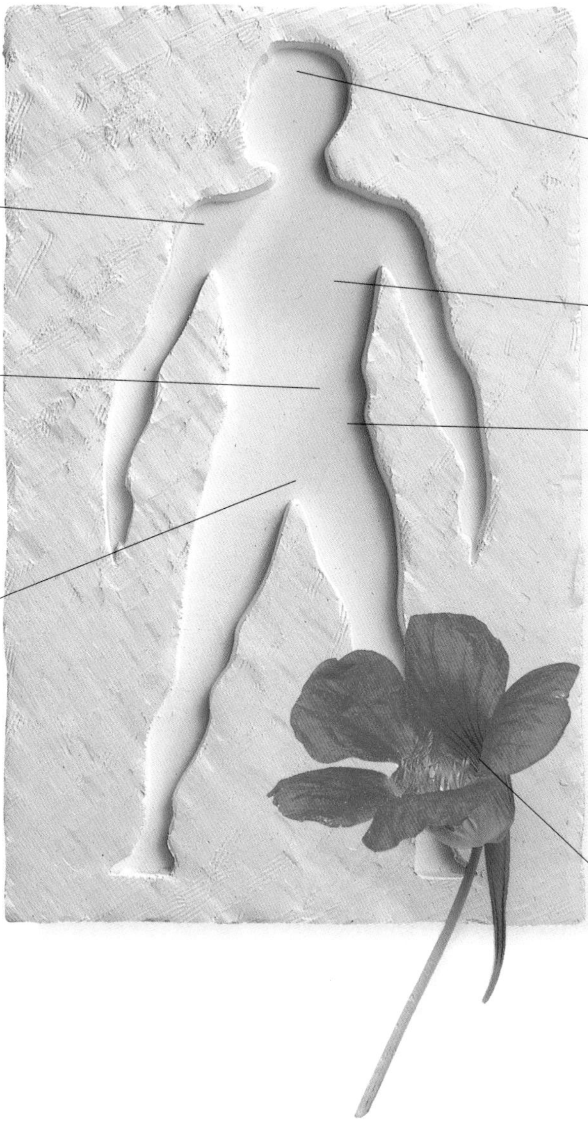

Skin and sweat glands are affected by Lung function.

Weakness and tiredness result from Qi deficiency.

Lungs distribute Qi to all parts of body.

Spleen sends Qi from food to Lungs.

Qi descends from Lungs to Kidneys.

Lungs help healthy dispersal of Body Fluids.

Every living thing extracts Qi from the air.

RIGHT
Respiration draws Qi from the air into our bodies.

the body. If the Lungs are healthy then this keeps the body at an even temperature and also protects the body from invasion by external pathogenic factors such as Cold, Wind, and Damp. If the Lung Qi is weak then the body is liable to be very susceptible to disease. Thus, for example, when we "catch a cold" our Lung Qi is likely to be depleted, thus allowing the cold to invade the body. The organ that is then most immediately affected is, of course, the Lungs. In terms of the Body Fluids, the Lungs control the healthy functioning of sweating, and if abnormal sweating occurs, the Lungs are likely to be affected.

Chinese medicine describes the Lungs as the uppermost Zang in the body, and because of this the natural function of the Lungs is a descending one. The Lungs send the Qi down to the Kidneys (the lowest Zang) where it is "held down." This dynamic between the Lungs and the Kidneys is vital to healthy respiration. If the descending function is impaired, then this may lead to chest problems including coughing, congestion, and even asthma.

The Lungs also send down Body Fluids to the Kidneys, where they are separated into pure and impure. Healthy Lungs will ensure healthy fluid metabolism, whereas an impaired Lung function will lead to swelling and edema in the upper part of the body, mainly the face.

The Lungs regulate the passage of water through the body

As discussed above, the Lungs have a role to play in ensuring that Body Fluids are dispersed healthily throughout the body. Impaired Lung function can lead to retention of urine.

The Lungs control the skin and the hair

As has been pointed out, the Lungs have a vital role to play in ensuring that Qi and fluids flow smoothly and effectively in the outermost parts of the body. Thus, it is seen in Chinese medicine that the Lungs have a powerful influence over the skin and the sweat glands. If Lung function is impaired then this may lead to rough and dry skin. In Chinese medicine, skin conditions are always seen as being evidence of a Lung disharmony. It is interesting to note that Chinese medicine provides a strong basis for the observed connection between skin allergies and Lung allergies, for example asthma and eczema.

In terms of hair, the Lungs control the condition of general body hair, while the hair on our head is seen as being related to Kidney function. The health of general body hair is closely related to the condition of the skin.

The Lungs open into the nose

The nose is seen as the opening of the Lungs, and the condition of the Lungs will therefore determine factors such as how clear the nose is and how acute our sense of smell is. Clearly, when Lung function is impaired then so are these factors.

The Lungs bring us a sense of connection to the world

The theory of Chinese medicine sees the Lungs as being responsible for the extent to which we make healthy and constructive connections with the world we live in. With healthy Lung function we are able to maintain structures in our dealing with others. Impaired Lung function can lead to a sense of alienation. In particular, the emotion associated with the Lungs is Grief. When we deal with loss and change in a healthy way, our sense and experience of Grief can be controlled and helpful. If the Lungs are impaired we may find it very difficult to cope with Grief and change.

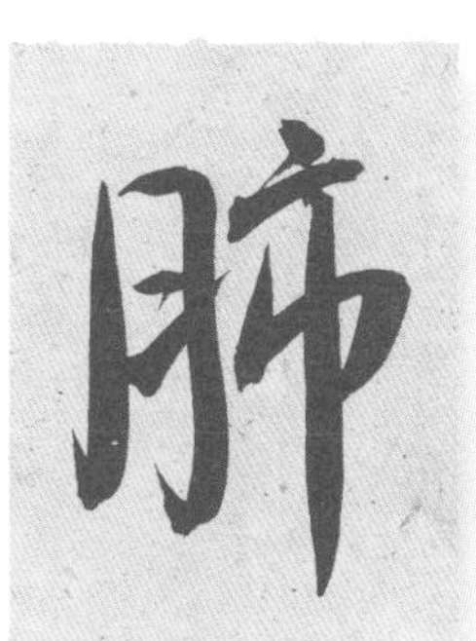

LEFT
The Chinese character for Lungs.

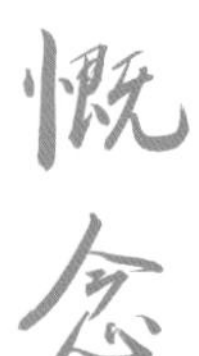

THE HEART

The Heart governs the Blood

This function of the Heart is the closest to the conventional Western view. The Heart controls and regulates the flow of Blood through the vessels of the body. This is essential to ensure a healthy supply of Blood to all the tissues of the body. A healthy functioning of the heart will result in an even warmth in the extremities of the body and a regular and even pulse. Impaired functioning may lead to cold extremities and abnormal pulse patterns, and, in serious cases, classic heart-related chest pains.

The Heart also has the function of transforming the Qi from food (Gu Qi) into Blood, and a poor diet can be seen as having a role in impairing Heart function.

Heartbeat, which moves the blood, is aided by the Zong Qi of the chest, which also has a role in respiration of the Lungs.

The Heart controls the blood vessels

The function of the Heart is reflected in the healthy functioning of the blood vessels, which in Chinese medicine are seen as an extension of the Heart. Good functioning will lead to healthy circulation, while impaired functioning may lead to conditions such as hardening of the arteries.

The Heart houses the Shen

As we have already seen, the concept of the Shen is a complex one in Chinese medicine and can have a variety of meanings. For our purposes here it is important to consider that the Shen represents the myriad of mental, psychological, and also spiritual faculties that constitute a central feature of the human condition. It is probably best described as the force that shapes our personalities. When the Heart has the Shen under control then we can use the attributes of our personality in a constructive and healthy fashion. If the Heart fails to house the Shen, then this can lead to a whole range of mental and psychological disorders. It is often said in Chinese medicine that the health of the Shen can be viewed in the eyes.

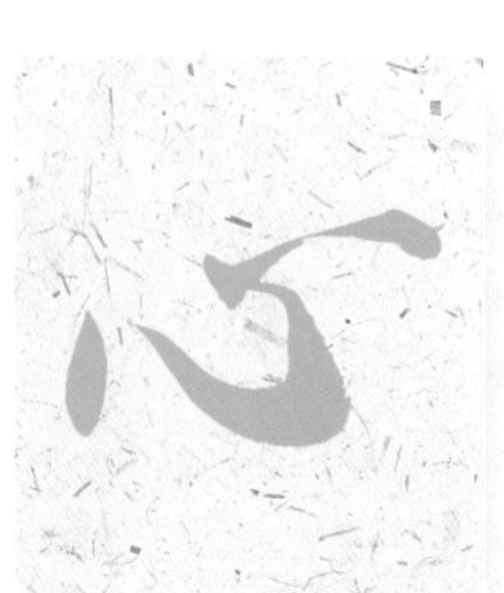

LEFT
The Chinese character for Heart.

The Heart is manifested in the complexion

Since it is the function of the Heart to ensure the smooth flow of Blood around the body and through the vessels, it is considered important to gauge the functioning of the Heart by looking at the complexion. When the Heart is healthy there will be a strong, rosy, and lustrous complexion, whereas if there is deficient Heart function then the complexion will be dull. If the function is impaired to the point of Blood stagnation then the complexion may be blue or purple in tinge.

The Heart opens into the tongue

It is often said in Chinese medicine that "the tongue is the mirror of the Heart." Although the condition of other organs can be gauged from the tongue, it is the Heart function that most readily shows in the tongue – especially in the tip. If Heart Blood is deficient then the tongue will be pale, and if there is stagnation of Heart Blood, then the tongue will appear purple in color.

The Heart controls sweat

In Chinese medicine, Blood and Body Fluids are seen as having a common origin and there is a continuous interchange between the two.

Thus, if a patient is sweating in an abnormal way then consideration has to be given to the role that the Heart Blood has in this.

The Heart maintains Joy

The emotion that is associated with the Heart in the Chinese system is Joy. The extent to which people manifest appropriate Joy in their lives will often reflect the health of their Heart function. As with everything in Chinese medicine, emotions are seen in balance and not as extremes. Thus, a tendency to overexpress joyful emotions in an inappropriate manner can be seen as a disharmony just as much as an overly negative and pessimistic disposition.

Joy is an emotion of the Heart.

A rosy complexion is a sign of a well-functioning Heart.

Warm extremities indicate a healthy functioning of the Heart.

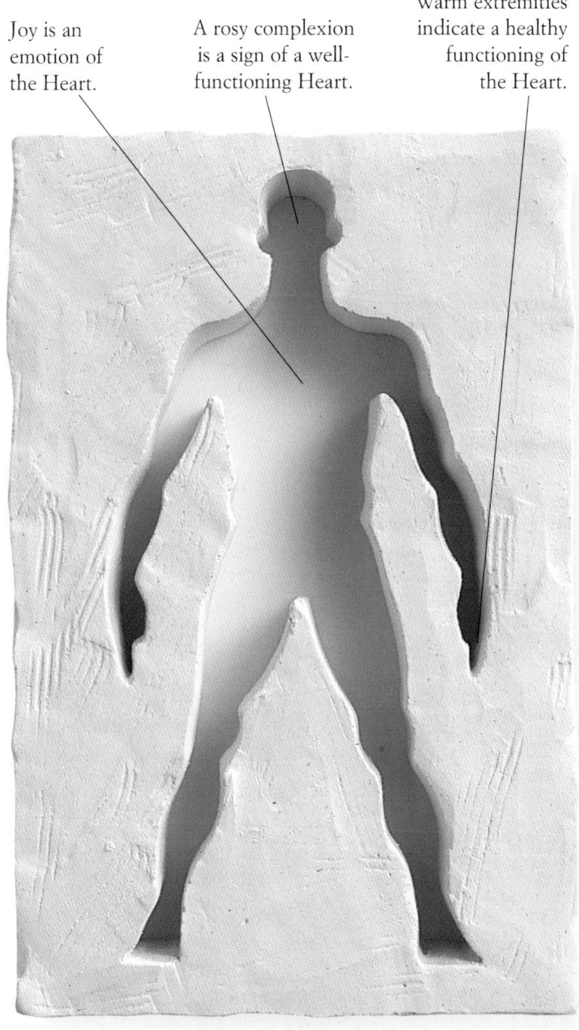

ABOVE
As well as regulating the flow of Blood, the Heart controls the Shen, which can be said to form our personality.

THE PERICARDIUM

It is important to mention the first anomaly at this point. In traditional Chinese medicine the Pericardium is considered to be a Yin organ, but it is not considered to be one of the five major Zang organs. In practical terms, the Pericardium is closely allied to the Heart.

The Pericardium protects the Heart

In Western medicine the Pericardium is seen as the protective outer covering of the Heart. This is mirrored in Chinese medicine, which sees the Pericardium as protecting the Heart from invasion by external pathogenic factors, such as high fever. The Heat in such an instance would be contained by the Pericardium, thus protecting the major Yin organ, the Heart.

The Pericardium guides Joy and pleasures

This somewhat vague function of the Pericardium seems to relate to the Heart's association with the emotion of Joy. It is important to realize that Chinese medicine would consider either too little or too much Joy in one's life as an example of a disharmony. Thus, in its role as protecting the Heart, the Pericardium seeks to guide us through life to experience Joy and pleasures in a manner that is balanced.

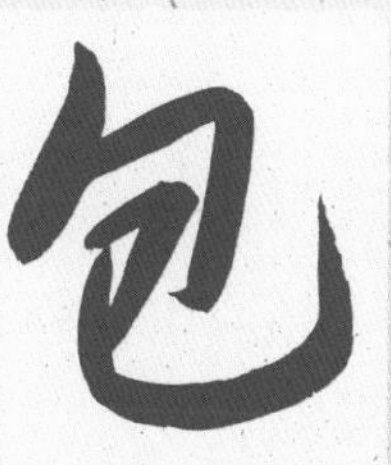

ABOVE
The Chinese character for Pericardium.

THE SPLEEN

THE SPLEEN GOVERNS TRANSPORTATION AND TRANSFORMATION

In Chinese medicine, the Spleen is seen as the primary organ of digestion. The Spleen extracts the nutrients from food in the Stomach (Gu Qi), which forms the basis of Qi and Blood, and transports it to the Lungs and the Heart for transformation into Qi and Blood. A healthy Spleen will mean good appetite, digestion, energy, and muscle tone. When the Spleen's function is impaired this will lead to fatigue, abdominal distension, poor digestion, and diarrhea. The Spleen also transforms and transports fluids throughout the body. When the Spleen is impaired this will lead to an accumulation of body fluids, ultimately leading to internal Damp. This may manifest itself as edema, obesity, and also phlegm-related disorders.

THE SPLEEN CONTAINS THE BLOOD

The Spleen has the function of ensuring that the Blood flow is controlled within the blood vessels. This is distinct from the Heart function, which ensures that the Blood flows, that is, that it is "pumped." If Spleen function is impaired then this can result in Blood leakages that can manifest themselves as blood in the stools and urine or a tendency to bruise easily. Varicose veins may also be seen as a Spleen-related disorder.

THE SPLEEN DOMINATES THE MUSCLES AND THE LIMBS

The Spleen has the function of transporting refined Qi throughout the body, and this ensures that the muscles and the limbs have good tone and shape. If the Spleen Qi is deficient in any way, then the refined Qi will not adequately tonify the flesh – resulting in fatigue and then weak and flabby muscles. In any condition where tiredness or weakness is present, then it will be important to work with the Spleen.

THE SPLEEN OPENS INTO THE MOUTH AND MANIFESTS ITSELF IN THE LIPS

The mouth has a crucial role in preparing food for digestion, and as such it is closely related to the Spleen in Chinese medicine. When the Spleen is healthy then the sense of taste will be sharp and the lips moist and rosy.

If there is a Spleen disharmony then the sense of taste will be dulled and the lips will become pale and dry.

THE SPLEEN CONTROLS THE RAISING OF THE QI

A general feature of Spleen function is that it has a lifting effect on the energy of the body from the midline. Thus, the well-functioning Spleen will hold internal organs in place.

When there is a Spleen disharmony then this is likely to lead to such conditions as internal prolapse and an imbalance of normal function producing problems such as diarrhea.

THE SPLEEN HOUSES THOUGHT

As a result of its raising function, the Spleen has the role of sending clear energy to the head and brain. This results in a clarity of thought that can give the sense of lightness and well-being. Thus the ability to think clearly and concentrate well is dependent on a healthy Spleen function.

When the Spleen is impaired there will be a deficiency of clear energy reaching the head,

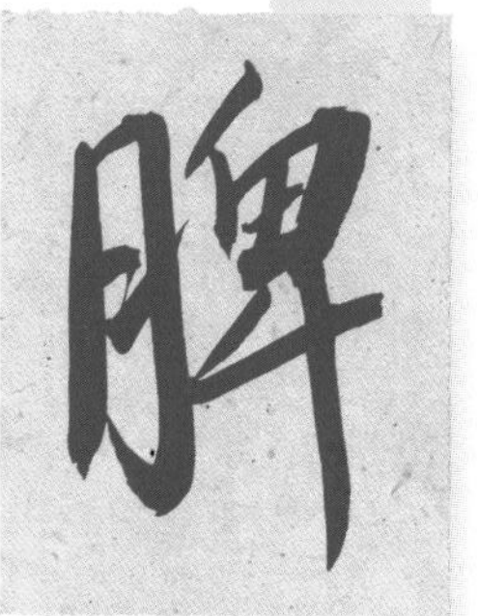

ABOVE
The Chinese character for Spleen.

which can result in muzzy and, at times, disordered thinking. This can lead to a form of psychological block, where it becomes difficult to make decisions and move on in any facet of life. In the same way, excess of concentration and thinking (for example when a student is cramming for an exam) causes damage to the Spleen, leading to fatigue and lethargy.

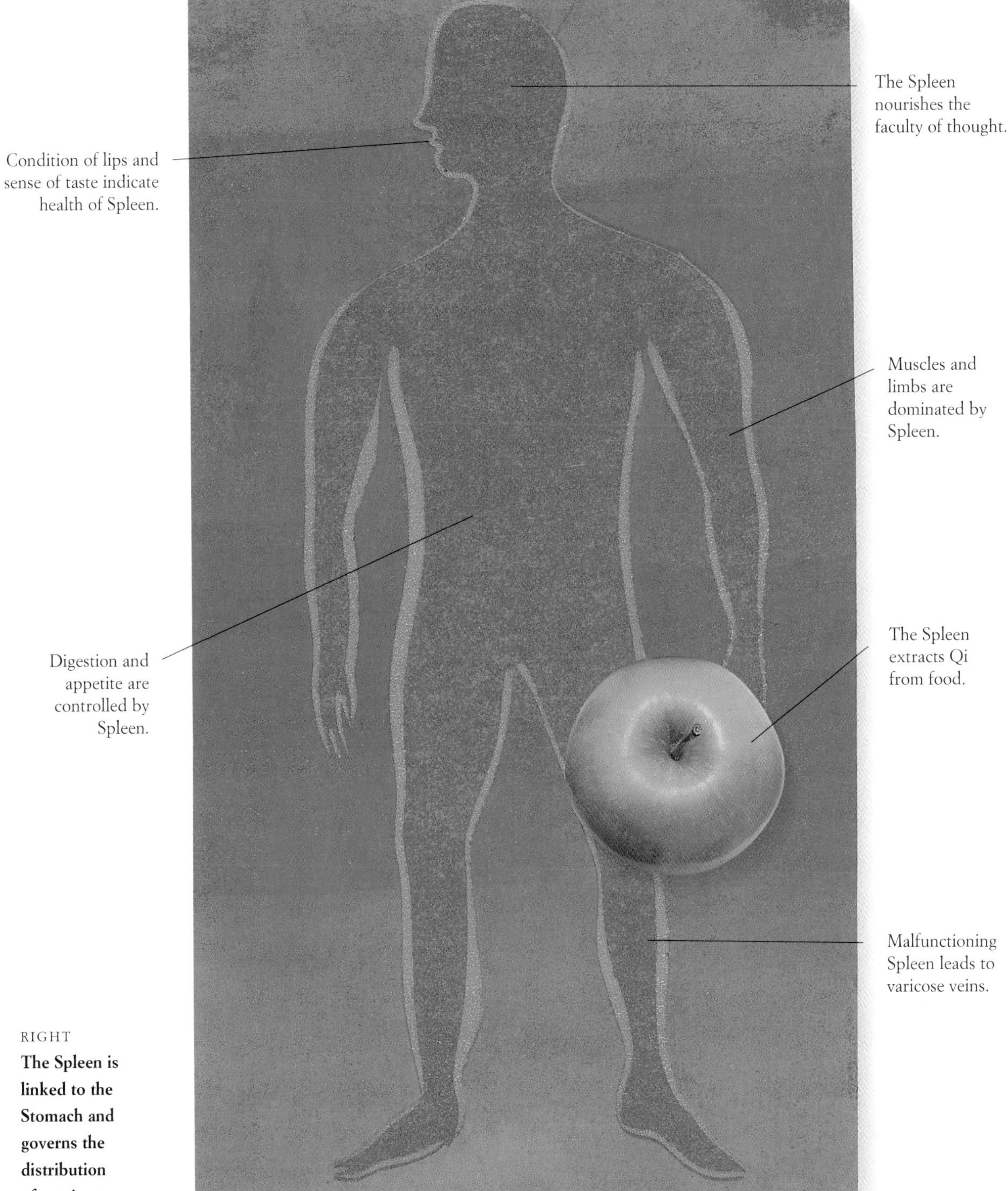

RIGHT
The Spleen is linked to the Stomach and governs the distribution of nutrients.

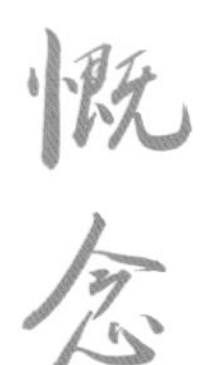

THE LIVER

The Liver stores Blood

A major function of the Liver is to regulate the amount of Blood in circulation. This will naturally vary, depending upon the demands of physical activity. Thus, when the body needs increased Blood flow, the Liver will release Blood, and when the body requires less Blood flow it is the role of the Liver to store the excess until it is needed again. In healthy Liver function the body will receive a good Blood supply and will be healthy, strong, and flexible. If there is impaired Liver function then weakness and stiffness may ensue.

In women, because of this role in storing and releasing Blood, the Liver is closely associated with menstruation and due to this many gynecological problems are likely to be related to the Liver function.

The Liver controls the smooth flow of Qi

This is by far one of the most important functions of the Liver. The free flow of Qi throughout the body is crucial to the health of all functions in the body, and it is because of this that stagnant Liver Qi is often associated with many other disharmonies that may be observed. Clinically, it is probably the most common disharmony that a practitioner of Chinese medicine will see. Problems arising from stagnant Liver Qi will be discussed in greater detail later in this book.

This smoothing and flowing function of the Liver is also seen as relating closely to the harmonization of the emotions and to preventing emotional stagnation. At the same time, Anger and feelings of frustration can harm the liver.

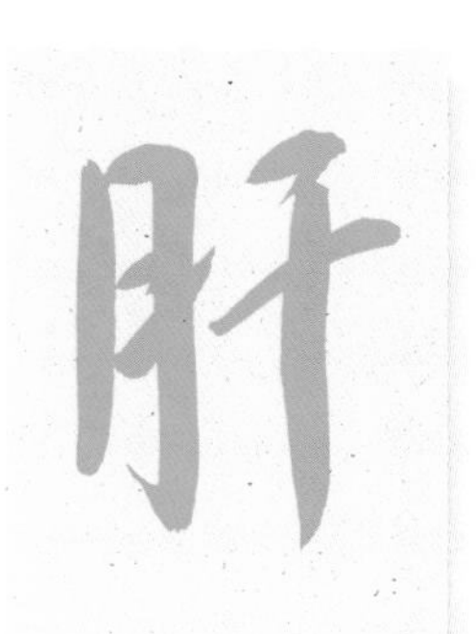

LEFT
The Chinese character for Liver.

The Liver controls the tendons

In Chinese medicine, the concept of "tendons" covers ligaments and tendons and the manner in which they interact with the muscles. Thus, the Liver is seen as being very important in terms of our capacity for movement and flexibility. The capacity of the tendons to expand and contract effectively depends on the nourishment from Liver Blood, which in turn requires the smooth flow of Liver Qi.

The Liver manifests itself in the nails

Chinese medicine sees the nails as belonging to the tendons, hence the connection with the Liver. If Liver Blood is healthy, then the nails will be strong and moist. If there is a problem with Liver Blood, then this is likely to lead to thin, brittle, and pale nails.

The Liver opens into the eyes

The eyes require the nourishment of Liver Blood in order to see clearly. Thus, the condition and health of the eyes is seen as being dependent on the health of the Liver function. When Liver Blood is deficient, then it is possible that this may lead to a variety of eye disorders.

The Liver exercises control

In Chinese medicine, the Liver is seen as the Zang that helps us keep control of our life in all its facets. When the Liver is balanced and functioning well, then we can exercise effective control over the events in our life and we respond to sudden changes in a considered and flexible manner. On the other hand, if the Liver function is in any way impaired, there can be a tendency to become overcontrolling, rigid, and inflexible, or to become undercontrolling, which may lead to outbursts of Anger and irrational emotional reactions. Liver disharmonies are always present in any stress-related disorder.

BELOW
The Liver regulates the Blood, and its functioning is associated with emotions and stress.

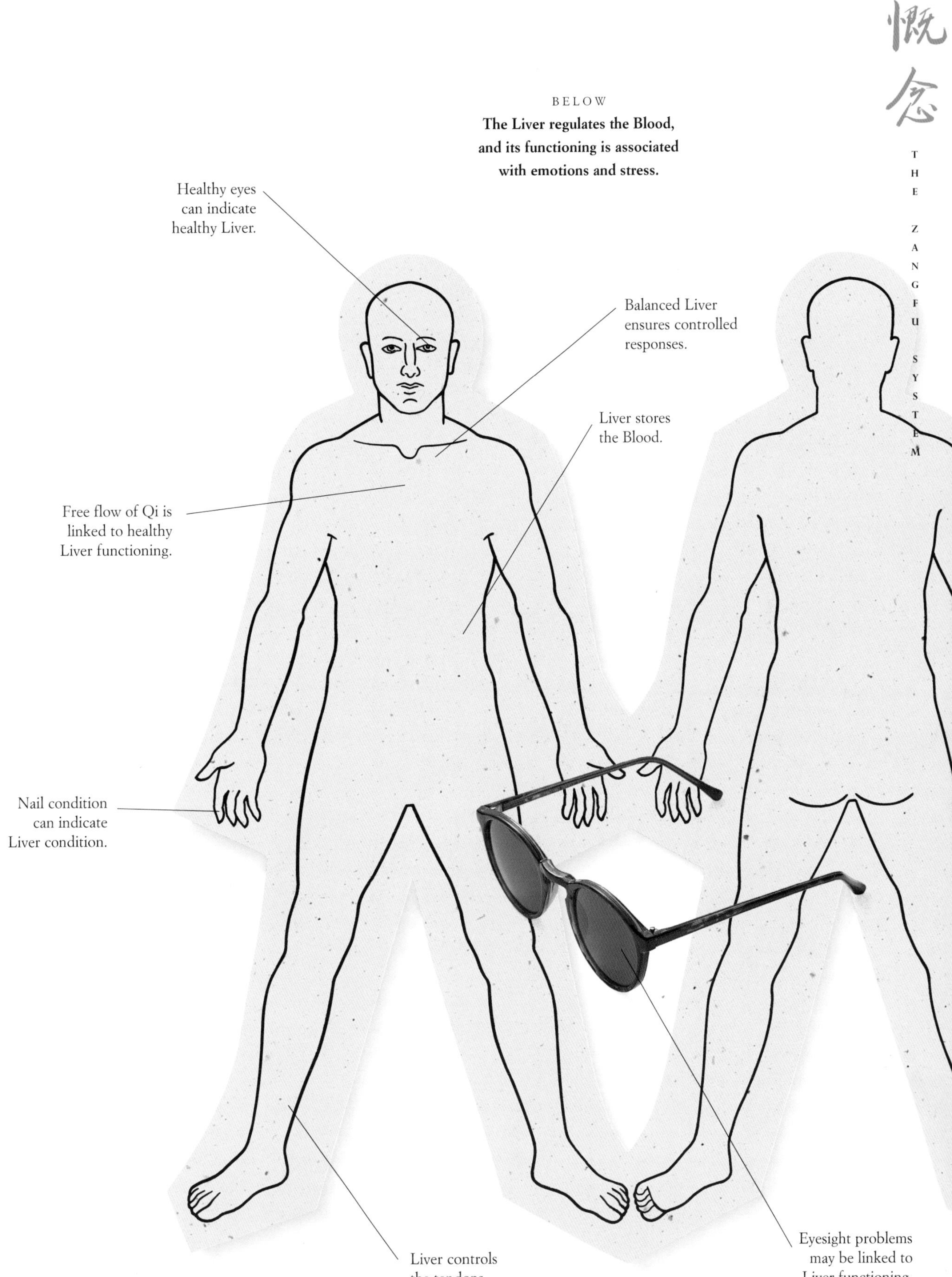

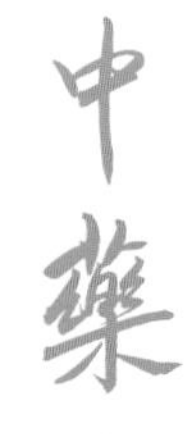

THE KIDNEYS

THE KIDNEYS STORE JING AND DOMINATE REPRODUCTION, GROWTH, AND DEVELOPMENT

As was pointed out before, Jing is the essence of life and is stored in the Kidneys. It is in part inherited from our parents and in part refined essence extracted from food.

Jing determines our constitutional strength and is an essential component of every aspect of the body. It is particularly the basis of growth and development through childhood and also fundamental to normal sexual and reproductive functioning throughout life.

When Kidney Jing is impaired in any way – often for constitutional reasons – then this can lead to retarded growth, learning difficulties, infertility, sexual disorders, or premature senility.

THE KIDNEYS PRODUCE MARROW, FILL UP THE BRAIN, DOMINATE THE BONES, AND MANUFACTURE BLOOD

There is a set of connections between these apparently disparate functions that connects them all to the Kidneys. Kidney Jing is responsible for the production of Marrow. In Chinese medicine, Marrow is the essential element of bone, Bone Marrow, the spinal cord, and brain structure. Thus, healthy Kidney Jing will result in strong bones and teeth and efficient brain function.

If Marrow production is impaired in any way then this may result in a whole variety of problems, including tinnitus, blurred vision, impaired thinking, and aching low back. Marrow also has a role in manufacturing Blood, so very often impaired Kidney function can also lead to Blood deficiency.

THE KIDNEYS MAINTAIN THE GATE OF VITALITY (MINGMEN FIRE)

In Chinese medicine, the Mingmen Fire is the source of all heat in the body. The maintenance of this essential Fire represents the Yang aspect of Kidney function. If the Kidney Yang energy is deficient then this will affect the Mingmen Fire, possibly resulting in general coldness, lethargy, and/or impaired sexual function; and, by damaging the Spleen, in some cases it can also lead to poor digestion.

THE KIDNEYS GOVERN WATER

A central function of the Kidneys is that of regulating the fluid balance in the body. The Kidneys dominate the Lower Jiao, often called "the drainage ditch," and they can therefore be seen as having the function of eliminating any waste water from the body.

When the Kidneys are functioning well they are able to send the clear fluids back to the Lungs and excrete the impure fluids through the Bladder. If the Kidney function is at all impaired then this can lead to a whole range of urinary problems.

THE KIDNEYS CONTROL THE RECEPTION OF QI

This function represents the harmonious relationship between the Kidneys and the Lungs. The Lungs send Qi downward and the Kidneys have the function of holding the Qi down, thus facilitating the healthy breathing process.

If the Kidney function is impaired, then this can lead to the Qi rebelling upward, causing breathing difficulties and leading, in extreme cases, to chronic asthma. Thus, in Chinese medicine, the Kidneys play a very important part in the facilitation of healthy breathing.

LEFT
The Chinese character for Kidneys.

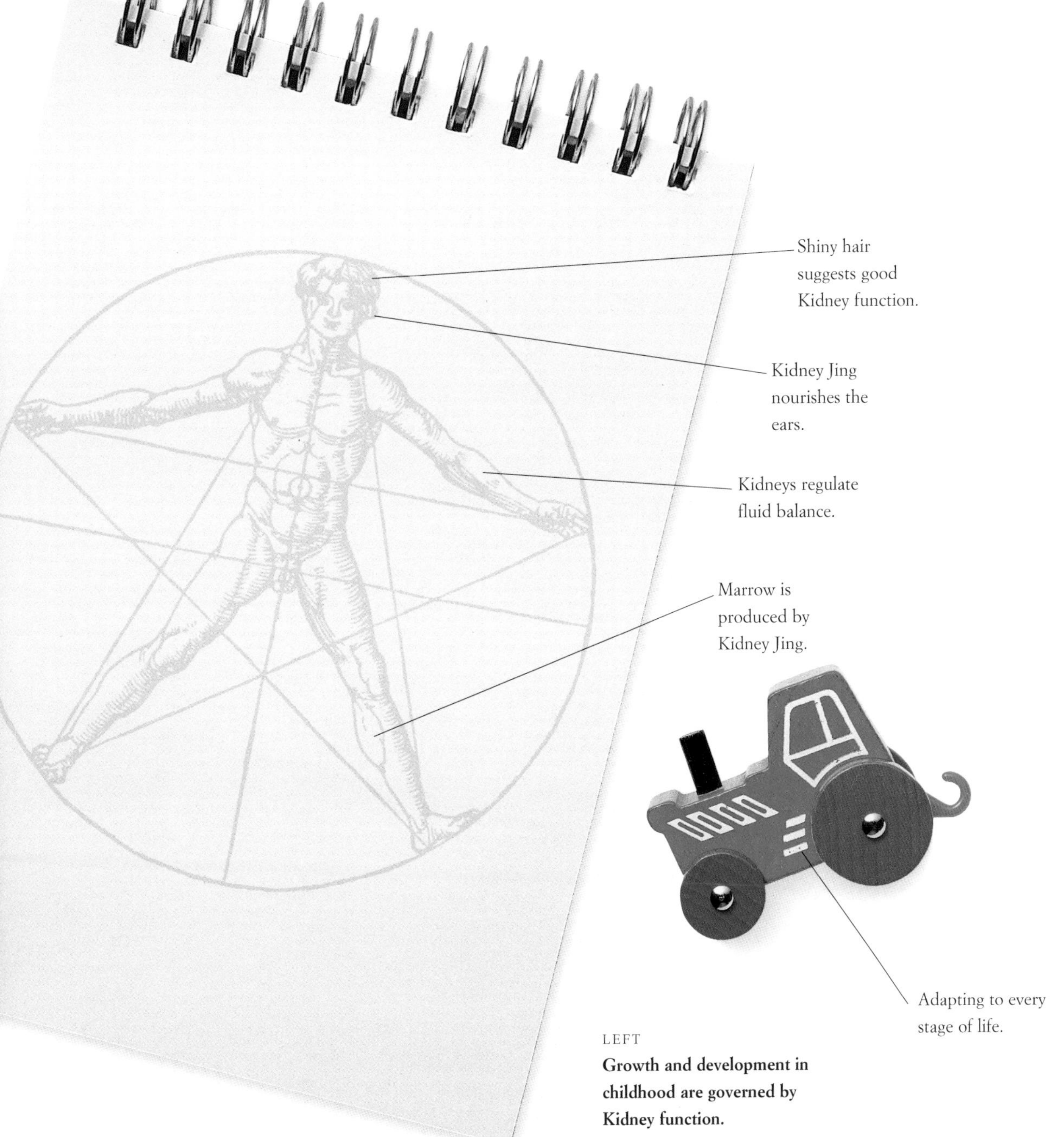

LEFT
Growth and development in childhood are governed by Kidney function.

The Kidneys open into the ear

The ears rely on Kidney Jing for nourishment, and if this is in any way lacking, then it can lead to tinnitus and deafness. As Jing diminishes with age, it is seen that older people often start to have problems with their hearing.

The Kidneys are made manifest in the hair

The hair also relies on Kidney Jing for nourishment. In normal functioning, the hair will be healthy and glossy. If, on the other hand, there is a deficiency, then this is liable to lead to dull, lifeless, and brittle hair. It can also lead to premature graying and thinning.

The Kidneys house the will and control Fear

The connection between will power and the emotion of Fear is seen in the Kidneys. The Kidneys are seen as the root of life, and thus our sense of personal power and will to succeed in life are rooted in healthy Kidney functioning. Consequently, poor Kidney functioning will lead to feelings of weakness and timidity – of being unable to face the demands made by life itself.

FUNCTIONS OF THE FU

*B*EFORE GOING *on to consider the factors that cause disharmony in the intricate Zangfu system, we should take a brief look at the functions of the Yang organs of the body – the Fu. For the purposes of this book the main focus will be upon the Zang organs, but an awareness of the Fu is important.*

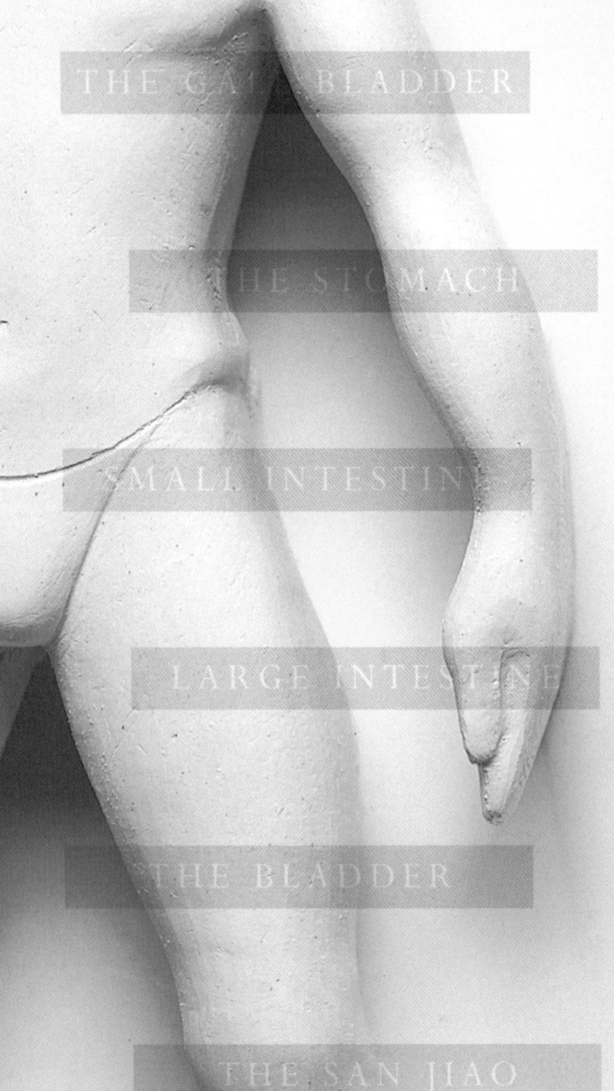

ABOVE
The body's Yang organs, the Fu, are generally considered less vital than the Zang (the Yin organs), but the Fu and Zang are coupled.

THE GALL BLADDER

The Gall Bladder stores Bile
This is stored and excreted into the digestive tract to aid digestion.

The Gall Bladder dominates decision-making
The theory of Chinese medicine sees the Gall Bladder as bestowing the capacity to make judgments. Gall Bladder impairment can lead to either an inability to make decisions or to the making of ill-thought-out decisions. The Gall Bladder is paired with the Liver.

THE STOMACH

The Stomach receives and stores food
The Stomach has the function of receiving food, separating out the pure essence that it passes on to the Spleen, where it is refined into Gu Qi, and passing on the impure to the Small Intestine for eventual excretion.

The Stomach Qi descends
The natural function of the Stomach is to send Qi downward for further processing. If this function is in any way impaired, then the Stomach Qi is said to be "rebelling upward." This leads to belching, hiccups, regurgitation, nausea, and vomiting. The Stomach is paired with the Spleen.

THE SMALL INTESTINE

The Small Intestine separates the pure from the impure
The Small Intestine receives partially digested food from the Stomach. The pure is extracted under the control of the Spleen, and the impure is then passed either to the Large Intestine or to the Bladder for excretion. The Small Intestine also

performs this function with the Body Fluids. The Small Intestine is paired with the Heart.

The Large Intestine

The Large Intestine absorbs the pure and excretes the impure
The Large Intestine receives the impure from the Small Intestine and further refines it to extract any further pure fluids or essence; it excretes the impure as feces. The Large Intestine is paired with the Lungs.

The Bladder

The Bladder stores urine and controls excretion
The Bladder receives waste Body Fluids from the Lungs, and the Small and Large Intestines, and, under the influence of the Kidneys, it stores and excretes this as urine. The Bladder is paired with the Kidneys.

The San Jiao

The San Jiao coordinates transformation and transportation of fluids in the body
The San Jiao coordinates water functions in the upper, middle, and lower Jiao areas of the body. The San Jiao can perhaps be likened to the manager who oversees the day-to-day workings of his or her "team."

The San Jiao regulates the warming function of the body
By ensuring that the Yang energy of the Kidneys is coordinated appropriately, the San Jiao helps move Qi and maintain the ambient temperature in the body. This function is recognized in its alternative name the Triple Heater, Triple Burner, or Triple Warmer. The San Jiao is related to the Pericardium in Chinese medicine.

FUNCTIONS OF THE EXTRA FU

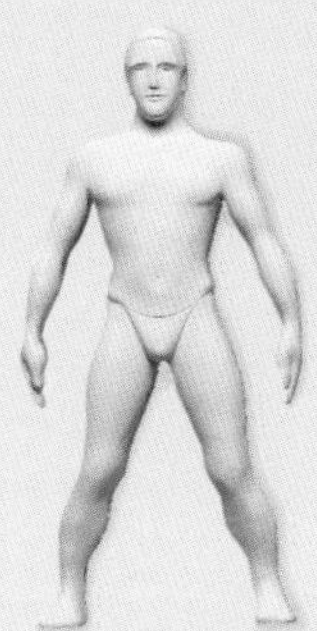

ABOVE
Some of the minor storage places are considered as Extra Fu.

As if the Zangfu were not enough to have to contend with, Chinese medicine also talks about the Extra or Extraordinary Fu (sometimes referred to as the Curious Fu). These resemble the Fu in as much as they are considered hollow, yet they have functions of storage that relate them more to the Zang. They tend to store the Yin essences of the body, namely, Jing, Marrow, and Blood.

We can very briefly mention their functions as follows:

- The Uterus regulates menstruation and promotes conception. (There is considered to be a male equivalent in the Dan Tien area called the Jing or Semen Palace.)
- The Brain stores Marrow – it is known as the "Sea of Marrow."
- The Bones store Bone Marrow.
- The Blood vessels contain the Blood.
- The Gall Bladder is also considered an Extra Fu since it has a storage function in respect of Bile.

This brief mention of the Extra Fu is included here merely for completeness – they will not be discussed in any further detail in this book.

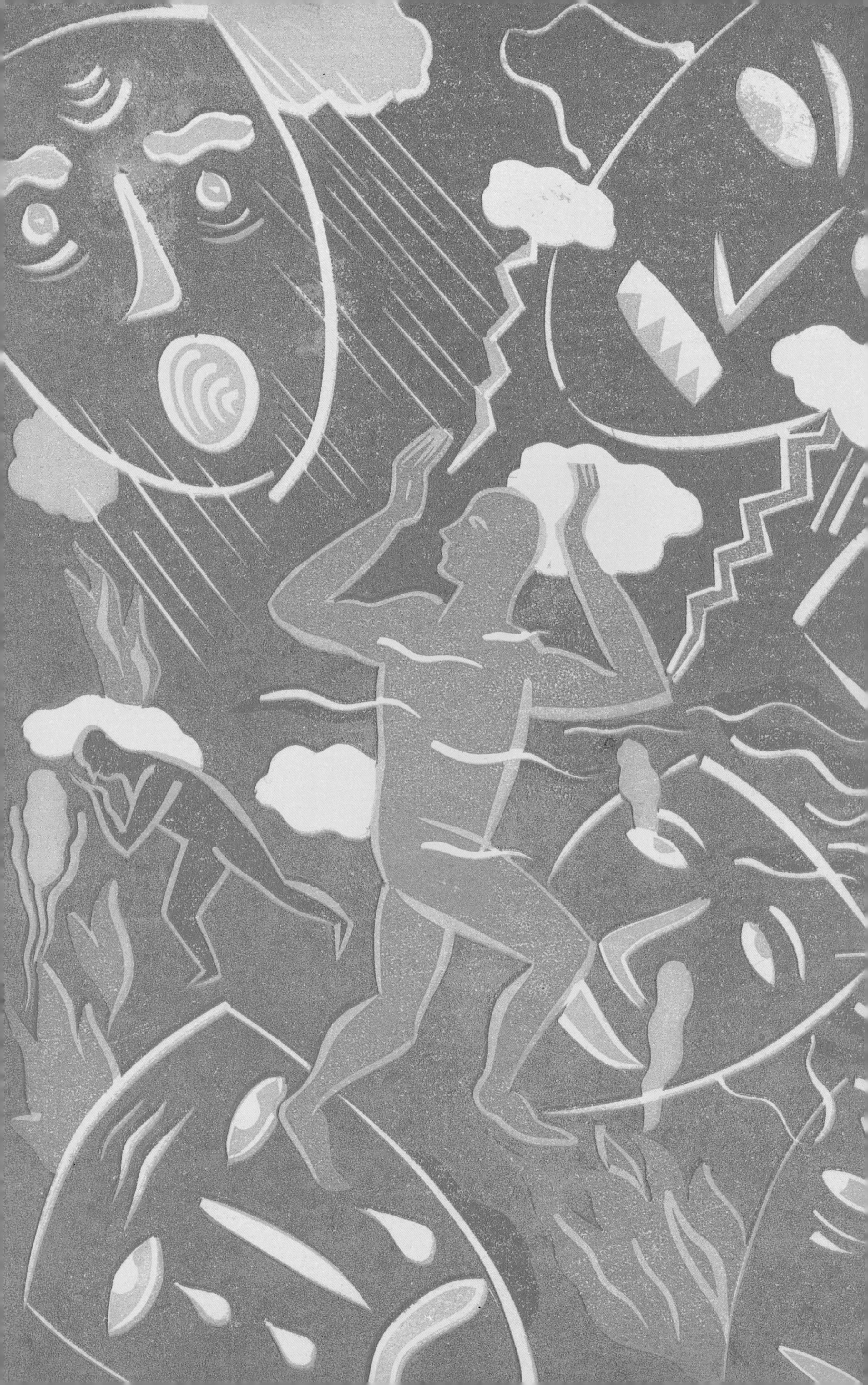

CAUSES OF DISHARMONY

概念

HAVING LOOKED at the elaborate system that Chinese medicine uses to understand the body and its processes, it will now be clear that the central concept is that this system exists in a dynamic equilibrium. The more mechanistic view of Western medicine leads us into a way of thinking that equates illness with something that has caused some part of our biological mechanism to "break down," so treatment focuses primarily on the "damaged bit." There are occasions when this view is appropriate and it can lead to valuable and effective treatments, but it does create a psychological set that can at times be counterproductive.

Chinese medicine, on the other hand, begins by thinking of disease as arising from influences that have disturbed the harmony and the balance of the whole energy system, and although they may appear as symptom-specific, we are encouraged never to lose sight of the "balanced whole." In this part of the book we will look at the influences that Chinese medicine considers important when disharmonies occur.

For the purposes of our discussion, the causes of disharmony will be divided into three broad areas: ✦ INTERNAL CAUSES ✦ EXTERNAL CAUSES ✦ MISCELLANEOUS CAUSES; and these in turn will be divided into their component parts.

INTERNAL CAUSES

AS WILL have been clear from our discussion of the Zangfu system, Chinese medicine considers the internal organs as influencing not only the physical functions of the body but also the psychological and spiritual aspects. The major internal causes of disharmony are considered psychological in nature and are termed the "seven emotions." These seven emotions are ✦ *Anger* ✦ *Joy* ✦ *Sadness* ✦ *Grief* ✦ *Pensiveness* ✦ *Fear* ✦ *Fright.*

In some instances there are clear overlaps between some of these emotions, and with certain pairs the distinction is more a matter of degree, for example, Sadness and Grief, Fear and Fright. As always, Chinese medicine does not neatly compartmentalize emotions, and such overlaps are not considered problematical.

Relating back to the systems of Five Element correspondences, the emotions can be associated with the organ system as shown.

The seven emotions are considered neither "good" nor "bad"; it is how they balance that is important. So too much Joy is as imbalanced as too much Grief, but the disharmony will appear in a different way. We now consider the seven emotions in turn. Most people experience a wide range of emotions that vary in intensity. Some are appropriate and adaptive, others less so. It is important to be aware of how emotions may influence the balance of Qi in the body and how this may exacerbate disharmonies.

EMOTION	ZANG	FU
Anger	*Liver*	*Gall Bladder*
Joy	*Heart*	*Small Intestine*
Sadness *Grief*	*Lungs*	*Large Intestine*
Pensiveness	*Spleen*	*Stomach*
Fear *Fright*	*Kidney*	*Bladder*

LEFT
The key to good health lies in maintaining balance or equilibrium, within and without.

欢樂

JOY

Joy leads to Heart Fire.

LEFT
Joy, in Chinese medicine, refers to an active state of excitement. Too much Joy can lead to palpitations of the Heart.

JOY

IN CHINESE medicine the concept of Joy more readily refers to a state of agitation or overexcitement, rather than to the more passive notion of deep contentment. The organ most directly affected here is the Heart. Such overstimulation can lead to problems of Heart Fire connected with such symptoms as feelings of agitation, insomnia, and palpitations.

ANGER

ANGER AS described by Chinese medicine covers the full range of associated emotions including resentment, irritability, and frustration. Anger will affect the Liver, resulting in the stagnation of Liver Qi. This can lead to the Liver energy rising to the head, resulting in headaches, dizziness, and other symptoms. In the long run it can result in high blood pressure and can cause problems with the Stomach and the Spleen.

SADNESS AND GRIEF

THE LUNGS are more directly involved with these emotions. A normal and healthy expression of Sadness or Grief can be expressed as a sobbing that originates in the depths of the Lungs – deep breaths and the expulsion of air with the sob. However, Sadness that remains unresolved and becomes chronic can create a disharmony in the Lungs, making the Lung Qi weak. This in turn can interfere with the Lungs' function of circulating the Qi around the body.

Grief and Sadness must be resolved.

LEFT
Long-term, unresolved Grief causes disharmony affecting the function of the Lung Qi.

悲傷

GRIEF

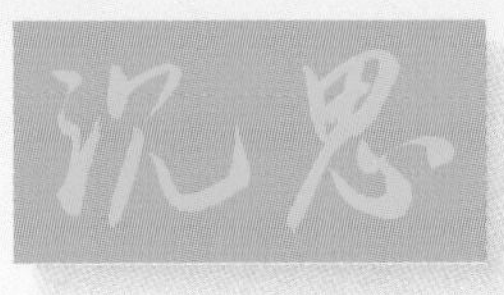

PENSIVENESS

Pensiveness affects the Spleen.

Anger affects the Liver and causes headaches.

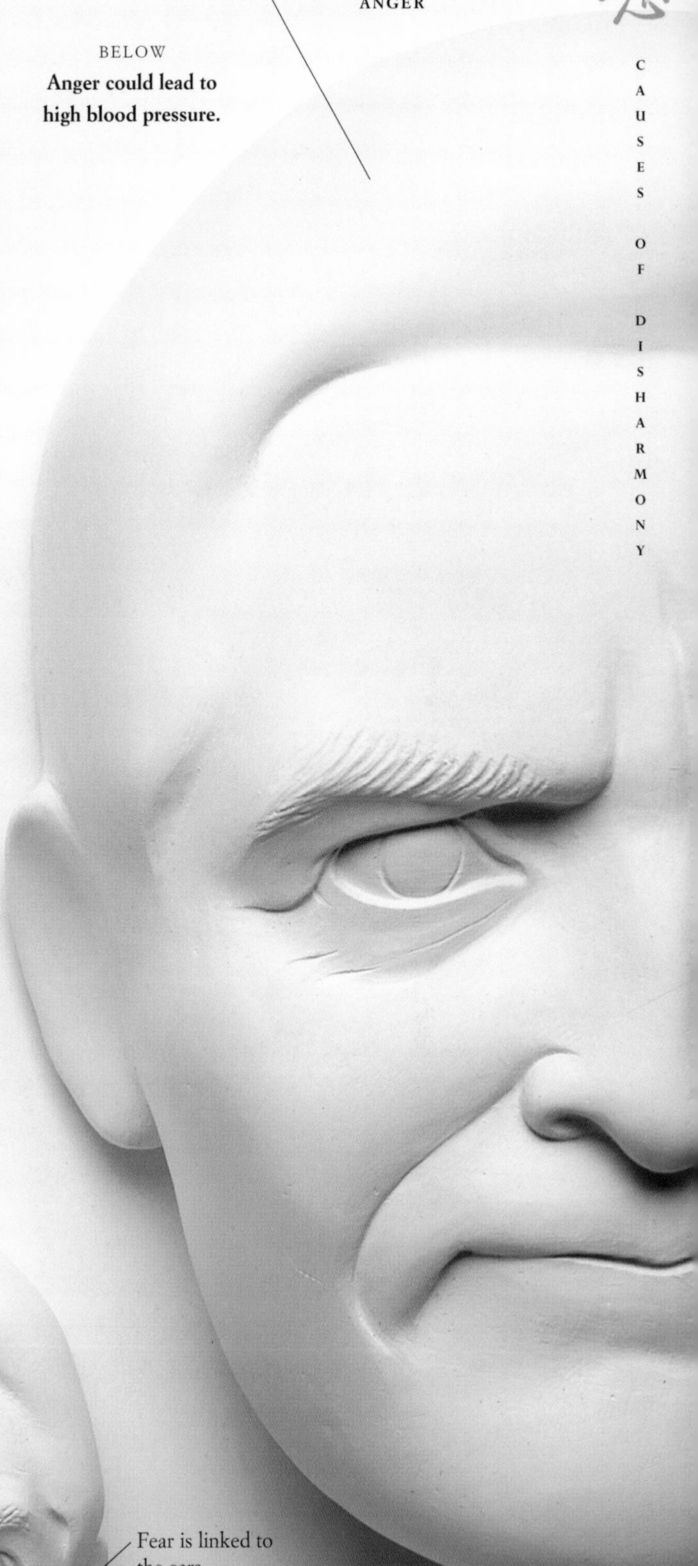

怒氣

ANGER

PENSIVENESS

IN CHINESE medicine, Pensiveness is considered to be the result of overthinking or too much mental and intellectual stimulation. Any activity that involves a lot of mental effort will run the risk of causing a disharmony. The organ most directly at risk here is the Spleen. This can lead to a deficiency of Spleen Qi, in turn causing worry and resulting in fatigue, lethargy, and inability to concentrate. This can be exacerbated by poor eating habits that can damage the Spleen.

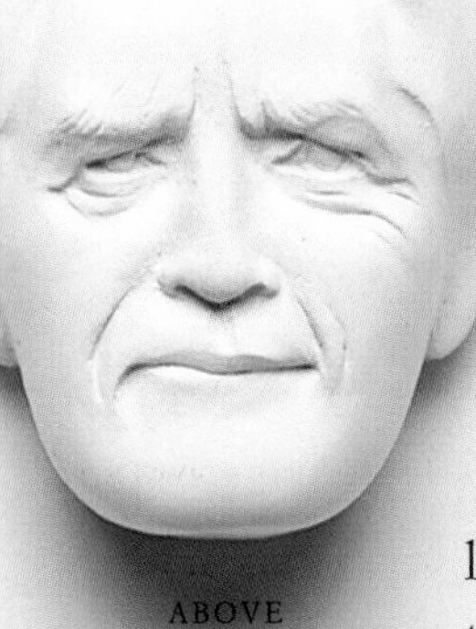

ABOVE
Too much intellectual stimulation can cause Pensiveness.

BELOW
Anger could lead to high blood pressure.

FEAR AND FRIGHT

FEAR IS a normal and adaptive human emotion, but when Fear becomes chronic and when the perceived cause of the Fear cannot be directly addressed, then this is likely to lead to disharmony. The organs most at risk here are the Kidneys. In cases of extreme fright the Kidneys' ability to hold Qi may be impaired leading to enuresis. This can be a particular problem with children. Kidney Qi becomes less, leading to less Kidney Yin.

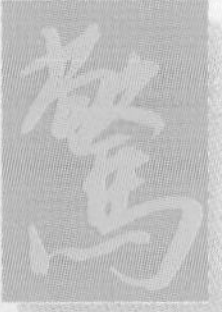

FEAR

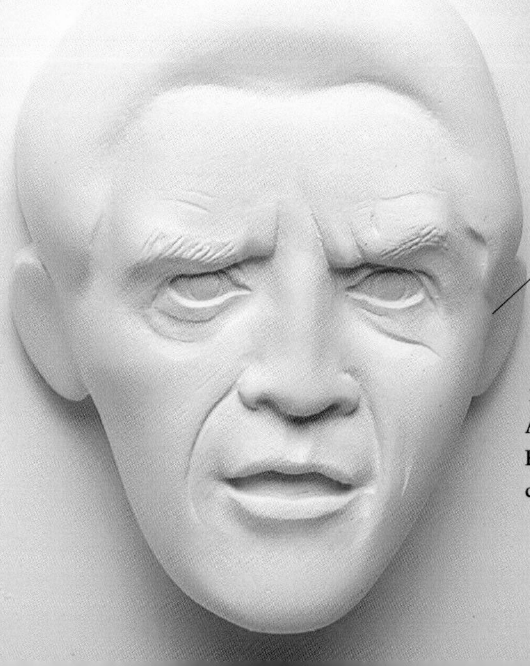

Fear is linked to the ears.

LEFT
A deficiency of the Kidney Yin could be caused by chronic Fear.

EXTERNAL CAUSES

IN CHINESE medicine there are considered to be six external causes of disharmony that relate to climatic conditions. They are variously known as the "six pernicious influences," the "six pathogenic factors," or the "six outside evils." They are ✦ WIND ✦ FIRE AND HEAT ✦ COLD ✦ DRYNESS ✦ DAMP ✦ SUMMER HEAT. In temperate climate, the most commonly observed factors are Cold, Damp, Wind, and to some extent Heat.

WIND

WIND IS considered a Yang pathogenic influence, with similar characteristics in the body to those in nature. Most especially:

> *Wind causes movement.*
> *Wind causes sudden change.*
> *Wind causes shaking and swaying.*

Wind is a very influential external factor and has the effect of penetrating the exterior of the body. It can often combine with other external factors – especially Cold – to invade the body.

Wind disharmonies are often characterized by their sudden onset. A very common condition related to Wind is the common cold. If the Wei Qi is weak then Wind and Cold can readily penetrate the surface of the body and rapidly penetrate to the most "external" of the internal Zang, namely the Lungs. This leads to the classic symptoms of sneezing, shivering, and free-flowing clear mucus. It is interesting to note that if the Wind-Cold disharmony takes hold, then the Cold symptoms will turn to Heat symptoms – as Yin transforms into Yang.

Thus, the disharmony will then change to show as fever, sore throat, dry mouth, and thick yellow phlegm.

In Chinese medicine, Wind can also be related to an internal disharmony, usually to do with the Liver. Internal Liver Wind tends to be a considerably more serious disharmony that can result in conditions such as epilepsy, stroke, or Parkinson's disease. The internal Liver Wind rises and causes the body to shake and tremble or shiver.

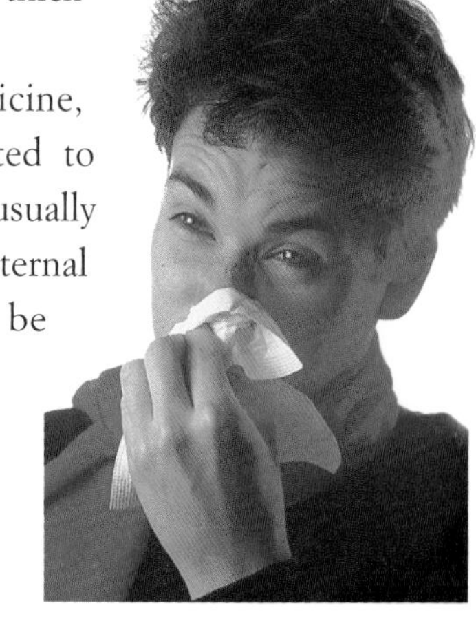

ABOVE
Windy weather – external Wind – can cause a cold, but inner Wind – a disharmony within the body – can give rise to more serious symptoms.

Wind is related to the Spring according to Five Element correspondences, and this suggests that in Chinese medicine an individual is more likely to be susceptible to external Wind disharmonies in the Spring.

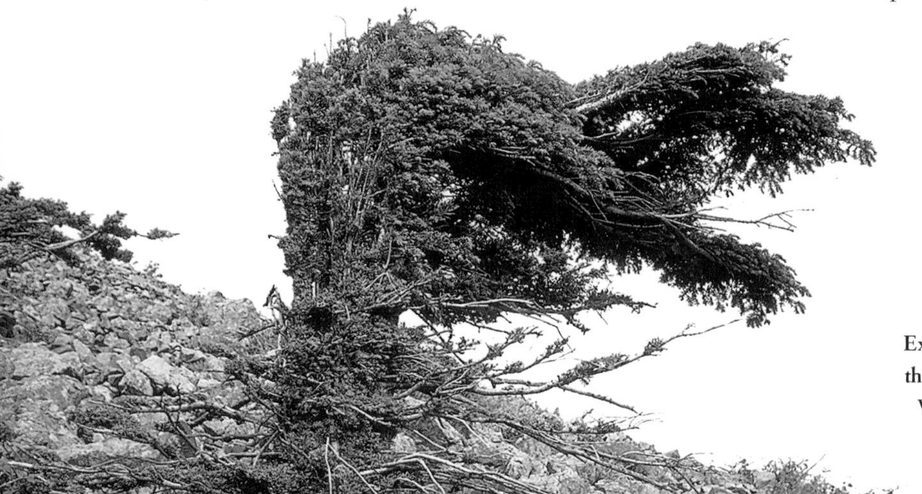

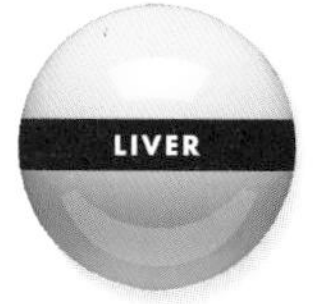

LEFT AND ABOVE
External Wind can affect the Lungs while Internal Wind can cause Liver disharmonies.

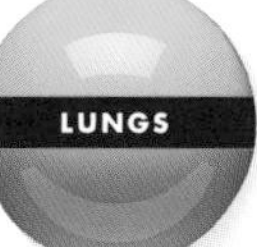

COLD

COLD IS considered a Yin pathogenic influence. The main effects are that

> *Cold constrains movement.*
> *Cold constrains warmth in the body.*
> *Cold causes contraction of the body.*
> *Cold can lead to stagnation.*

An invasion by Cold will be of sudden onset and will leave the individual feeling chilly, headachy, and with an aversion to cold. The body may ache generally, and there is likely to be no evidence of sweating.

If it is not dealt with, invading Cold can affect the Lungs, and also the Stomach and the Spleen, possibly leading to abdominal pain, vomiting, or diarrhea. It can also affect the Liver channel, especially in the genital area, causing pain and discomfort in this area.

Internal Cold usually results from a chronic Yang deficiency that may have a variety of causes, one of which would be long-term exposure to external Cold. As might be expected, the element Cold is associated with the season of Winter.

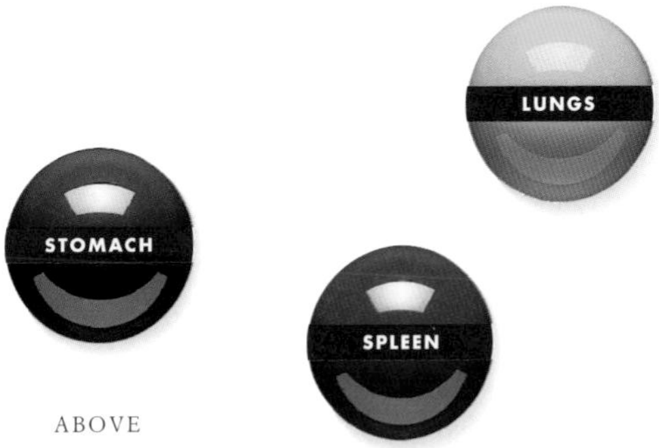

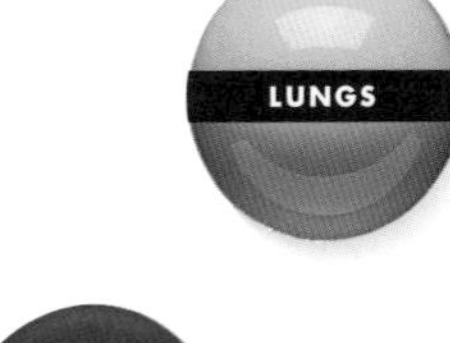

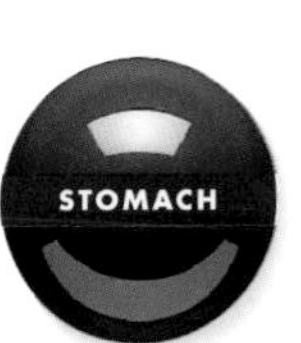

ABOVE
Headaches and abdominal pains can be caused by external Cold, which damages the Yang energy. Inner Cold can be related to eating too much cold food or to Stomach and Spleen disharmonies.

BELOW
Exposure to external Cold causes a chilling of the body. At the emotional level, Cold is associated with Fear, in Chinese and in Western thought.

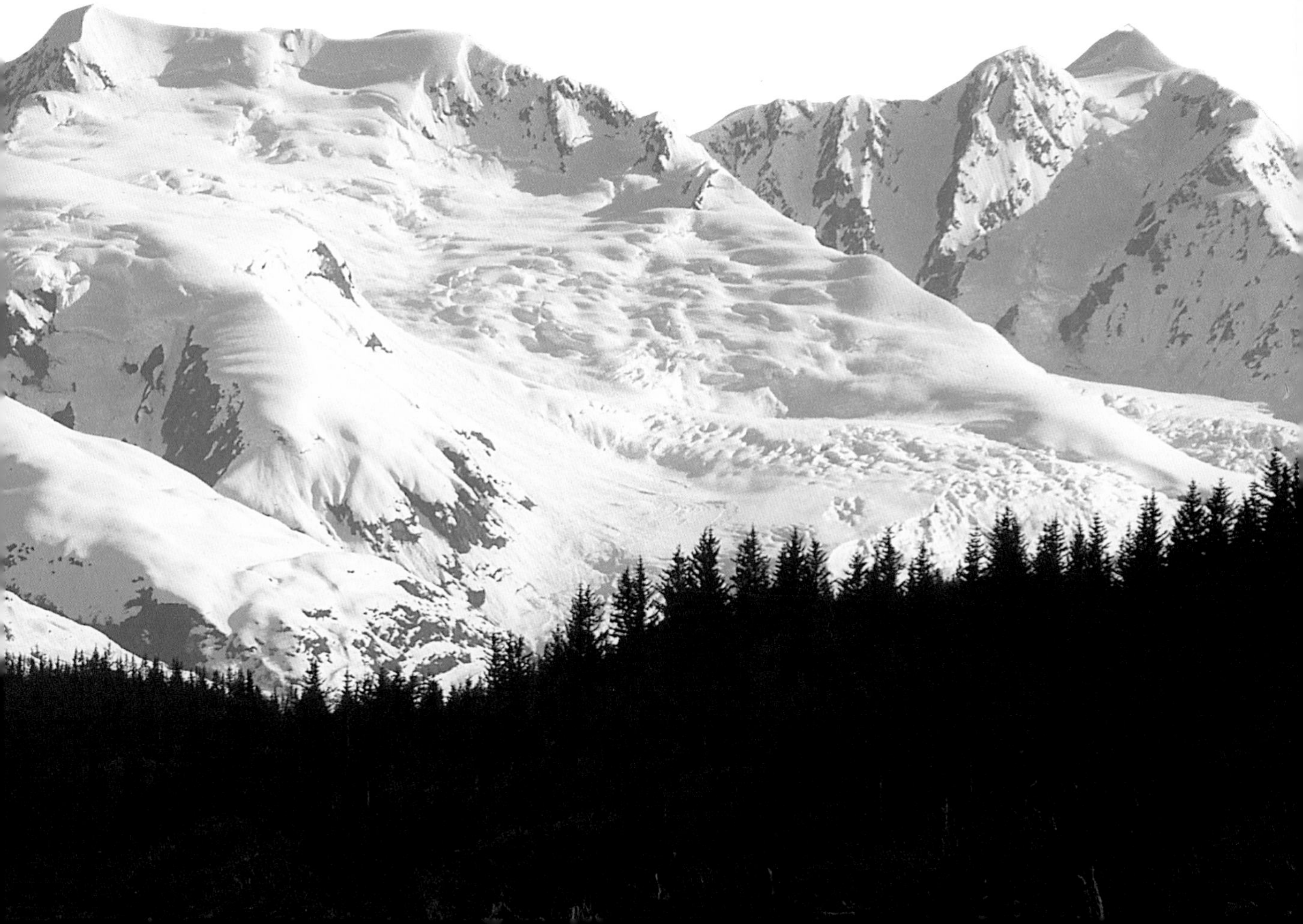

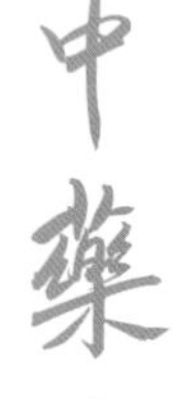

DAMP

DAMP IS considered a Yin pathogenic influence. The idea of Damp in Chinese medicine shares many of the qualities that would be associated with damp in the environment, notably:

Damp is wet.
Damp is heavy and lingering.
Damp is slow to clear.

When Damp invades the body it leads to sluggishness, tired and heavy limbs, muzzy-headedness, and general lethargy. Any bodily discharges will tend to be sticky and turbid, and the tongue will tend to have a sticky coat. The Spleen is especially susceptible to Damp, which will inhibit the transporting and transformational functions of the Spleen. This can lead to abdominal distension and possibly diarrhea.

Damp can affect the joints, leading to stiffness – especially in the morning on rising – and the joints can become aching and swollen, as is found in some arthritic conditions. Damp also tends to combine readily with both Cold and Heat.

If the Spleen becomes damaged because of invasion by external Damp or possibly through poor diet, this can lead to a more chronic internal Damp condition that in turn can lead to the accumulation of Phlegm. Internal "invisible" Phlegm can be particularly problematical in Chinese medicine, and this can contribute to such problems as chronic dizziness and hypertension (high blood pressure).

In the Chinese calendar, Damp is associated with the late Summer, which can be wet.

However, it is reasonable to say that Damp can occur at any season of the year, depending upon the local climatic conditions.

BELOW
A damp climate is popularly believed to cause rheumatism. The associated mental state is over-Pensiveness.

BELOW RIGHT
Damp as an external force causes symptoms from lethargy to stiff and aching joints. Inner Damp is related to the Spleen.

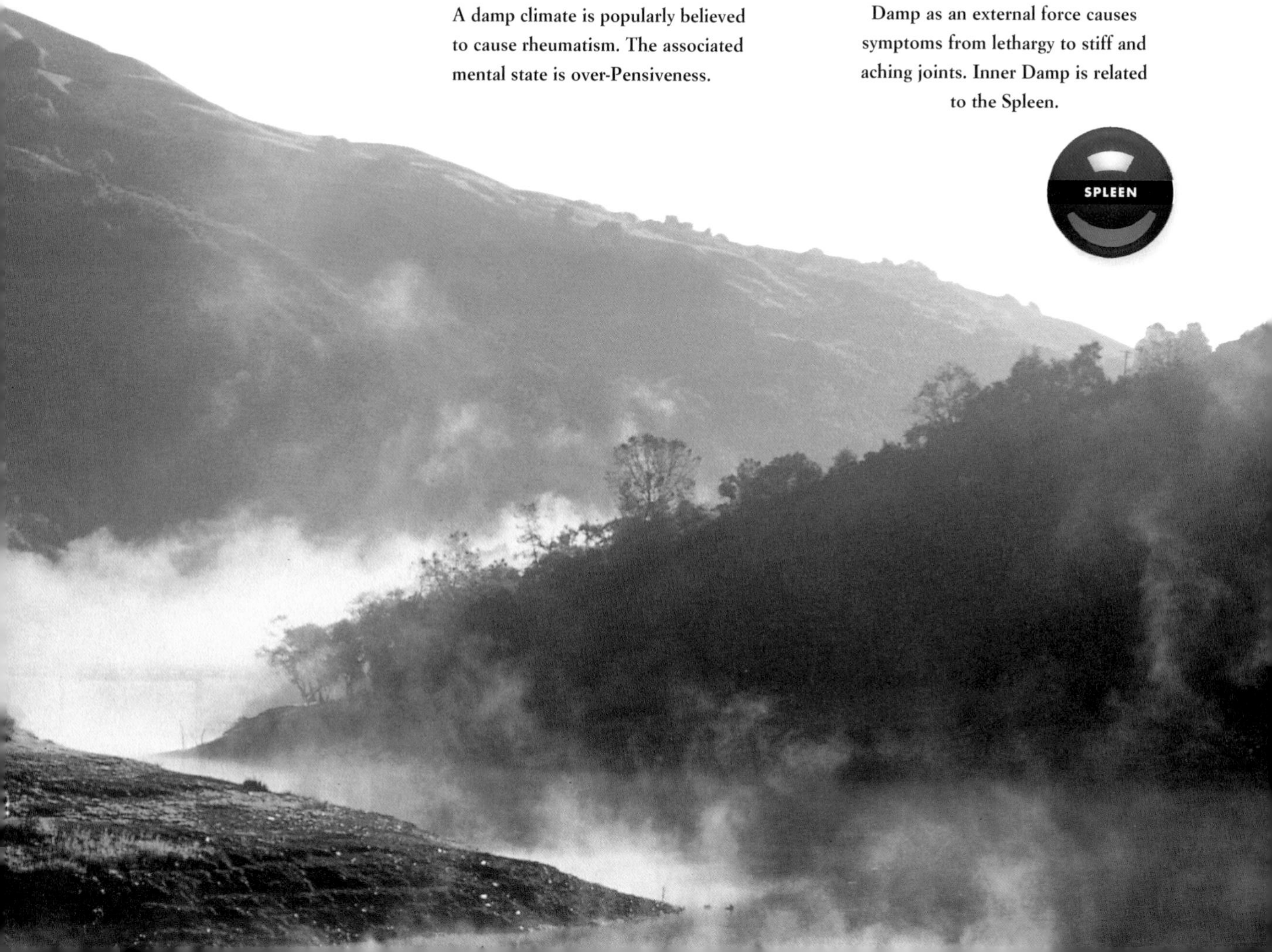

SPLEEN

FIRE AND HEAT

IN CHINESE medicine it is not unusual to use the terms Fire and Heat interchangeably. They are considered Yang pathogenic influences. The main characteristics of both these influences are fairly obvious:

> *Fire and Heat are hot.*
> *Fire and Heat induce movement.*
> *Fire and Heat are drying.*

Fire and Heat lead to a whole plethora of heat-type symptoms, including fevers, inflammation, red eyes, aversion to heat, hot skin eruptions, and so on. They have a very drying effect on the Body Fluids, with dry skin, constipation, and scanty yellow urine as common examples. Fire and Heat can also lead to disturbing psychological patterns, including hyperactivity, mental agitation and, in severe cases, delirium and mania, caused by the Heat disturbing the Shen.

There can also be internal Fire and Heat conditions. A Yin deficiency, usually termed "Empty Heat," will affect a number of Zangfu organs, although in all instances there is usually an underlying Kidney Yin deficiency.

Fire conditions tend to be associated with the Liver, the Stomach, and the Lungs and lead to conditions where Fire blazes upward, often affecting the head. For example, Stomach Fire can result in acute toothache as the Fire rises up the Stomach channel to the face.

Fire and Heat are associated with the Summer, heat stroke being a good example. Obviously, there will be climatic variations that will influence this. However, individuals who live in cool, and also damp, climates are potentially often quite susceptible to invasion by Fire and Heat if they go to a hot country – on vacation, for example – and if they do not take appropriate and sensible precautions.

ABOVE
Externally, Fire and Heat are drying and cause fevers and inflamed skin. Inner Fire or Heat is linked to Liver, Stomach, and Lungs and can rise to the head.

LEFT
Emotionally, Heat is linked to Joy. Too much Joy is an imbalance as damaging as too much physical Heat.

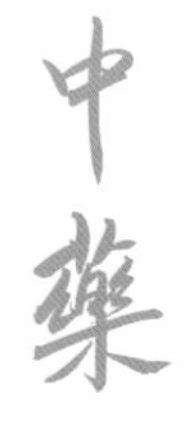

DRYNESS AND SUMMER HEAT

WE WILL consider these last two external influences together. They are much less common and less important than the others discussed above. Both of these are are considered to be Yang pathogenic influences.

Dryness is really on a continuum with Heat, and the symptoms are similar, but with a greater emphasis on the drying up of Body Fluids. It can lead to cracked skin, dry lips and nose, and a dry cough with little or no phlegm. The Lungs can be particularly susceptible, especially if the Heat is accompanied by a drying wind.

Dryness is associated with the Fall, but again this is geographically specific.

Summer Heat is associated with the height of Summer and again is on a continuum with Fire and Heat. It is often associated with very hot and humid climates, thus adding an element of Damp. It readily depletes the Qi and Body Fluids, leading to exhaustion and dehydration.

As can be seen, the external cause of disharmony represents the environmental experiences that go along with living. Which factors individuals will be exposed to will naturally depend on the climate where they live, but nevertheless the extent to which the factors lead to disharmonies will be a function of the general robustness of an individual's Qi and that person's behavioral patterns. None of us can avoid exposure to these influences, but how we look after ourselves will to a large extent determine how they affect us.

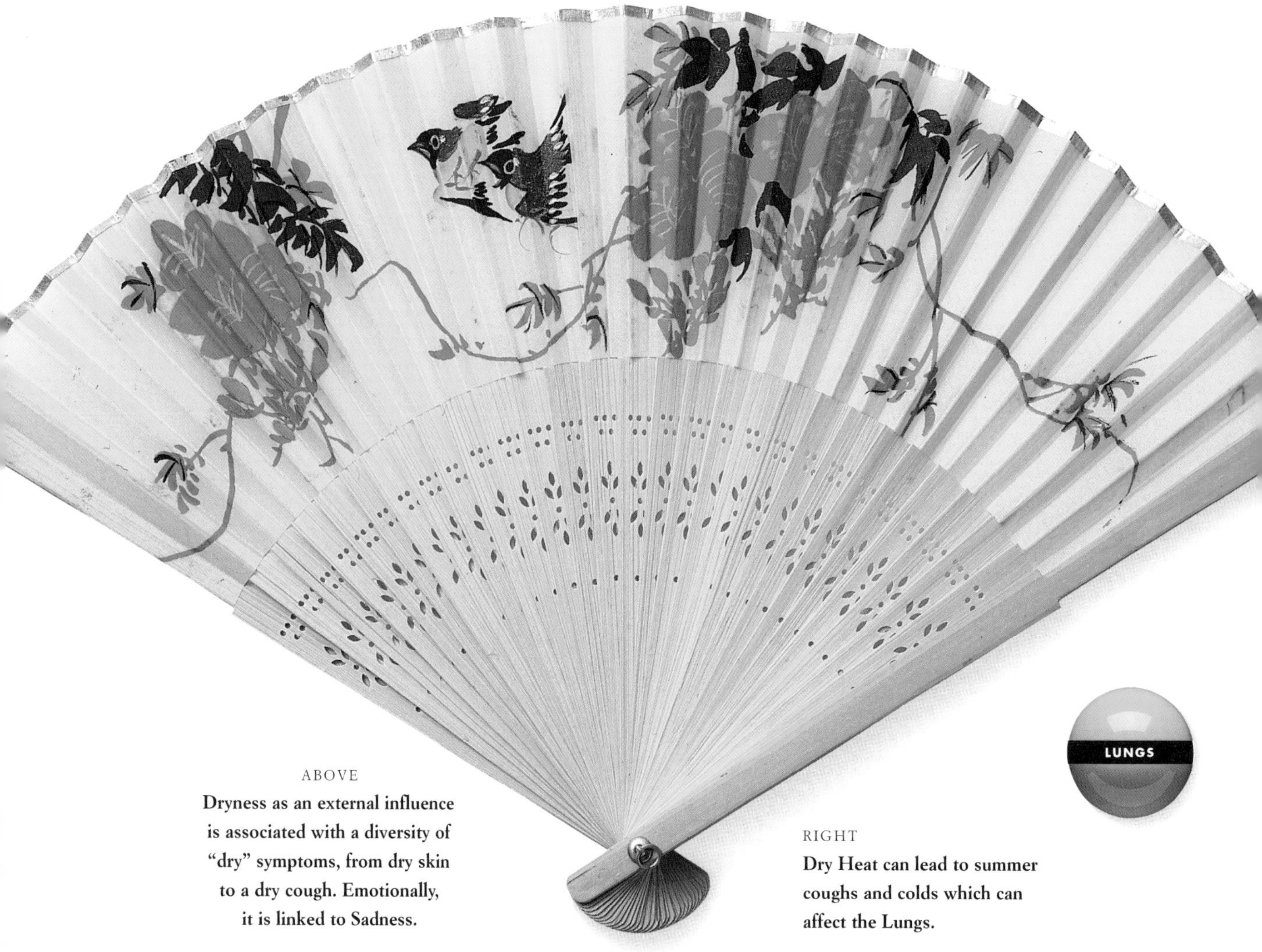

ABOVE

Dryness as an external influence is associated with a diversity of "dry" symptoms, from dry skin to a dry cough. Emotionally, it is linked to Sadness.

LUNGS

RIGHT

Dry Heat can lead to summer coughs and colds which can affect the Lungs.

MISCELLANEOUS CAUSES

WE HAVE now seen that the main causes of disharmony are the internal ones of the emotions, or of degrees of emotions, causing an imbalance, and the external ones of hostile climatic conditions influencing the body. However, in addition to the main internal and external factors that have been described, there are a number of other factors that need to be taken into consideration. These will be briefly outlined below.

CONSTITUTIONAL FACTORS

AS WAS discussed under a consideration of Basic Substances earlier on, Chinese medicine recognizes that an individual's energy system comprises pre-Heaven Qi and Jing as well as that produced through life. Our pre-Heaven inheritance represents our constitution, which depends on our parents. If the pre-Heaven inheritance is deficient, this will leave the individual more susceptible to the whole range of external and internal factors, which can possibly cause a disharmony.

Therefore, if we believe that we have any constitutional weakness, we need to take particular care to ensure that any other potential causes of disharmony in our lives are avoided if at all possible – or at least minimized.

LIFESTYLE FACTORS

WE ARE all aware of the general stresses that accompany normal daily life, and Western medicine readily recognizes that these "lifestyle factors" can be very influential in terms of health and well-being. In the same way Chinese medicine likewise recognizes the importance of lifestyle, although this will be interpreted in a completely different manner.

WORK

THE KIND of work we do – or the lack of work in the case of someone who is unemployed – can have a profound influence on our energy system. Too much physical work can impair the Qi, and with excessive lifting the Lungs become deficient. Too much mental activity can damage the Spleen and make the Yin deficient. Someone who works outdoors is more liable to be at risk from Cold, Damp, Wind, Heat, and so on.

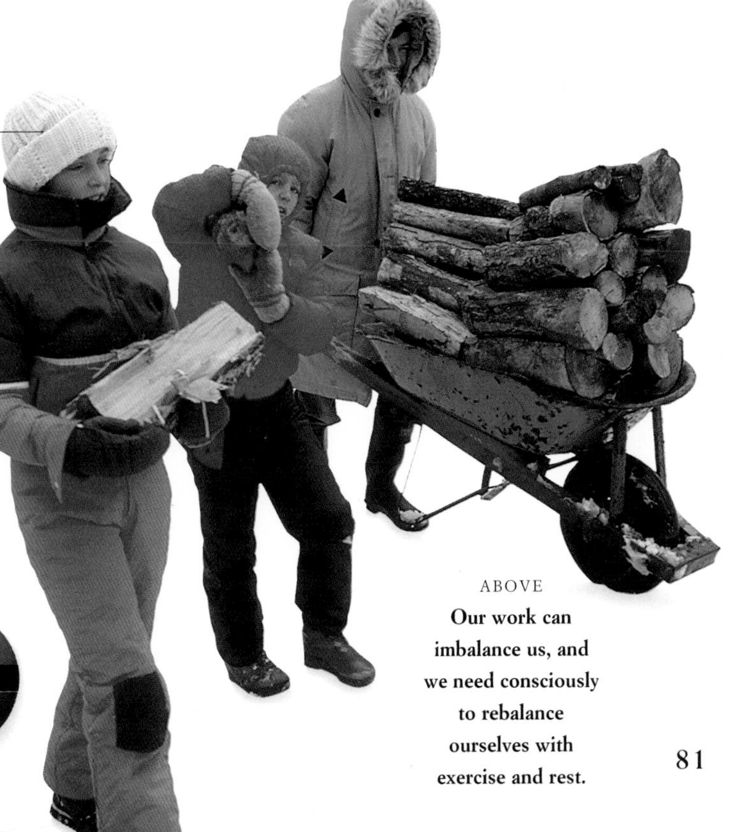

RIGHT
Unrelieved mental work can harm the Spleen.

ABOVE
Our work can imbalance us, and we need consciously to rebalance ourselves with exercise and rest.

EXERCISE

THE AMOUNT and kind of exercise – not to mention the lack of exercise – we take can have an influence that can cause Qi stagnation over time. As with everything in Chinese philosophy, it is a matter of balance. It is not a matter of any particular exercise being good or bad, but if the exercise is undertaken to an extreme this can cause a clear disharmony.

For example, many athletes who train to an excessive degree, and on the face of it appear very fit, are often very susceptible to infections and injuries. In the long run they may become chronically Qi deficient because of overstressing the Kidneys. It will be noted that many of the Chinese exercise regimes such as Qigong and Taiji are not obviously aerobic in nature like many Western forms of exercise. These Chinese exercise regimes do, however, offer a more balanced approach to exercise consistent with the principles of Chinese medicine. It is evident that good health and longevity are notable in the practitioners of such activities, which cannot always be said for practitioners of Western forms of exercise.

LEFT
Although exercise is considered to be "good for us," too much exercise or overstressful exercise can cause exhaustion and be detrimental to the Qi.

DIET

DIET IS afforded a very important place in Chinese medicine and a discussion of diet would be a whole book in itself.

The Stomach and the Spleen have the responsibility for processing the ingested food and extracting the Gu Qi, which is then passed to the Lungs as a central part of the production of Qi in the body. If the Spleen has to work against poor and damaging foods, then it will suffer – especially from Damp – and the follow-on effect will deplete the Qi of the body as a whole.

Again, balance rather than specific do's and don'ts represents the Chinese approach to diet. If an individual follows a healthy, balanced diet, then the Spleen will remain healthy and the Qi of the body will be sufficient. The overemphasis on sweet and processed foods in many Western diets does not lend itself to such a balance.

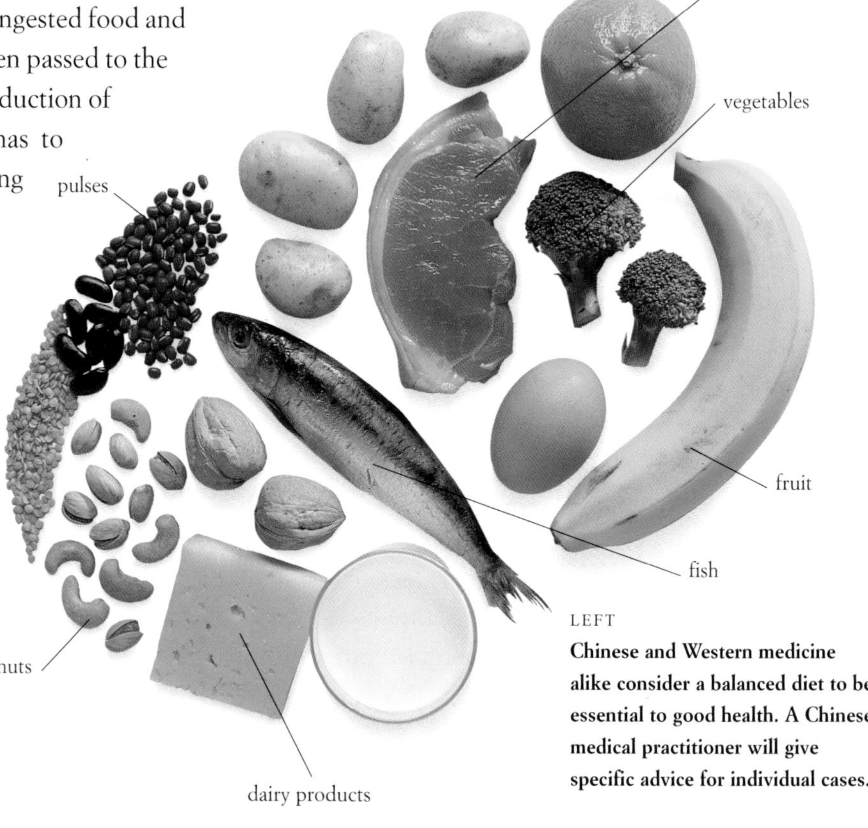

LEFT
Chinese and Western medicine alike consider a balanced diet to be essential to good health. A Chinese medical practitioner will give specific advice for individual cases.

SEXUAL ACTIVITY

IN CHINESE medicine, excessive sexual activity is considered to be damaging to the Kidney Jing and to lead to long-term deficiency problems. An excessive number of pregnancies can seriously deplete a woman's Blood and Jing. There are various prescriptions as to what is excessive sexual activity, and many Westerners would have different ideas on this subject, but generally the Chinese system emphasizes a natural decline in this activity as part of the aging process.

BELOW
The need for regulation in all things also applies to sexual activity.

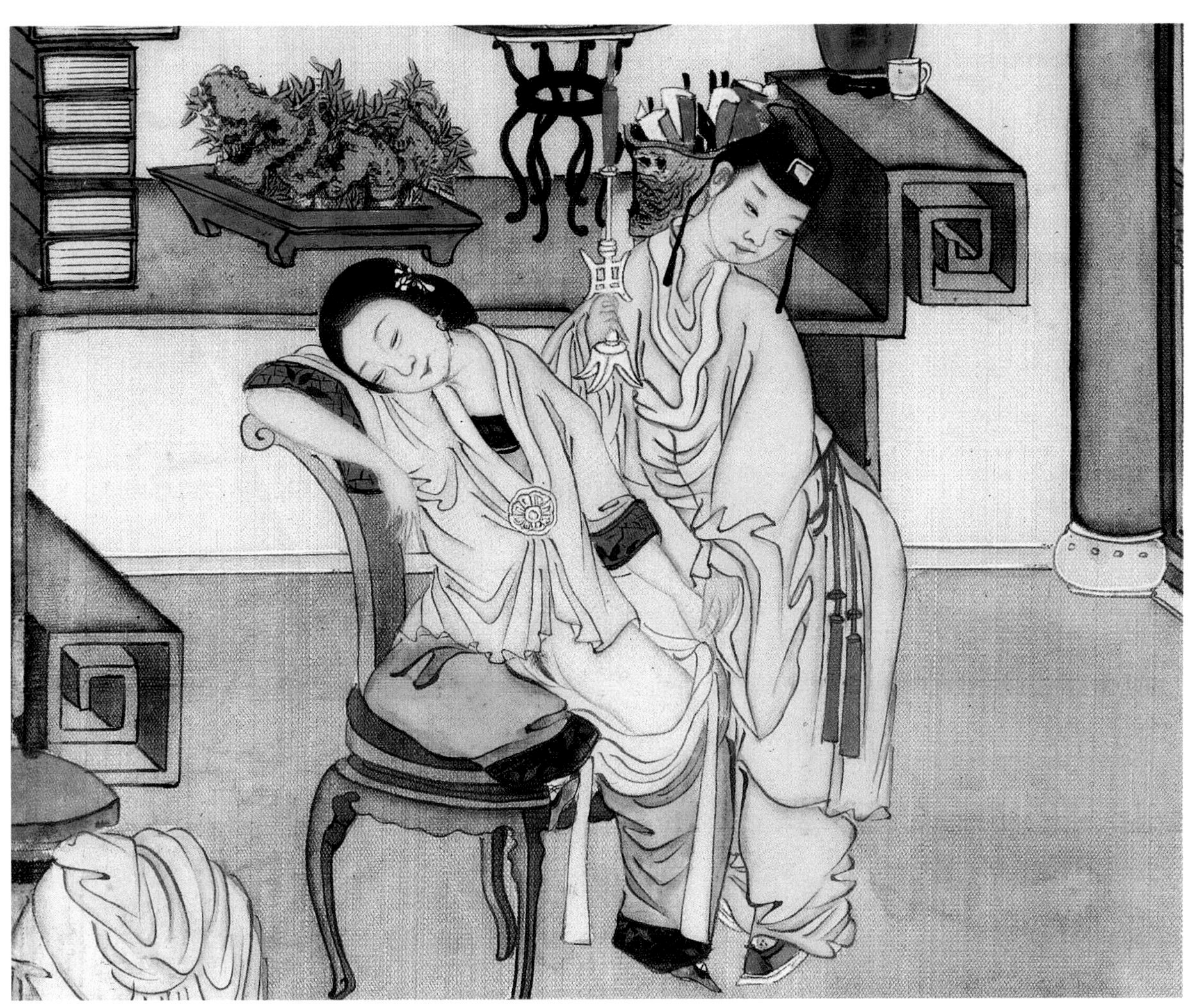

UNFORESEEN EVENTS

THE LAST general category that should be mentioned includes accidents and injuries, which obviously can affect the Qi of the body depending on their type and severity. The Chinese would also consider events such as plagues and epidemics as belonging here and, although they may be a problem in certain parts of the world, they are generally not an issue for the West. Of course accidents and injuries also occur in the West, and we have plenty of other problems such as pollution and contamination of food that can readily be placed in this category.

SELF-REFLECTIVE EXERCISE

THIS PART of the book has highlighted the ways in which Chinese medicine sees disharmonies occurring in the body; some involving internal causes, some external causes, some miscellaneous causes; some causes being avoidable, some less so.

In this exercise you are invited to consider yourself, your lifestyle, and your environment and to make a judgment about the areas of "risk" in your life from the perspective of Chinese medicine. Take time to reflect on your responses to this very simple questionnaire but do not take it too seriously! All it can do is offer some very general pointers that you may wish to be aware of.

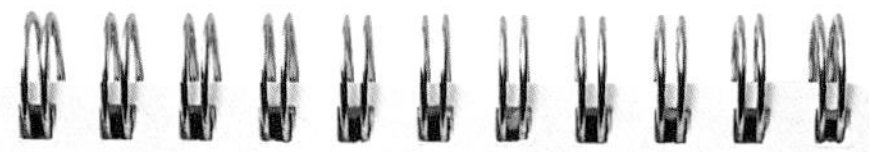

EMOTION	SCORE
Joy	
Anger	
Grief	
Sadness	
Pensiveness	
Fear	
Fright	

INTERNAL FACTORS

For each of the seven emotions listed, give yourself a score on a five-point scale as follows:

1. *I handle this emotion very well.*
2. *I handle this emotion quite well most of the time.*
3. *Sometimes I handle this emotion well; sometimes I don't handle it well at all.*
4. *I tend not to handle this emotion too well.*
5. *I handle this emotion very badly.*

You will find it interesting to have a friend or relative – someone who knows you well – complete this about you as well. The comparison of opinions can reveal a lot!

Look at the final pattern that emerges. It will serve to give you a very rough guide to where disharmonies may occur and what Zangfu may be affected as a result of your internal factors.

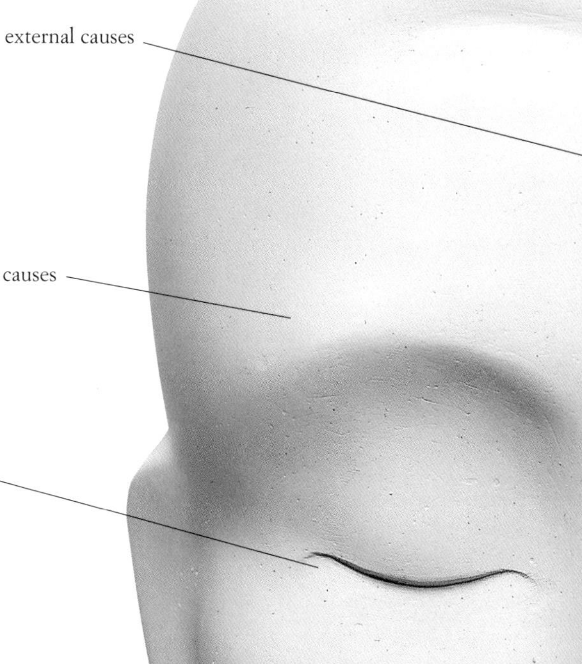

RIGHT
How do you handle your emotions? All the emotions – even Joy – can be a challenge and can be treated in a balanced or an inharmonious way.

概念

Disharmonies in the body are neither necessary nor inevitable. We can control external factors by protecting ourselves from them, even if we cannot always avoid being exposed to them. And by taking preventive steps – watching our diet, taking the kind of exercise that balances us mentally as well as physically – to guard against disharmony, we can keep our internal forces in harmony. The Daoist tradition was to seek longevity with health and well-being. To live a full and active life and to die healthy requires action, not luck.

External Factor	Score
Wind	
Cold	
Damp	
Fire/Heat	
Dryness	
Summer Heat	
Pollution (specify)	

External factors

Consider the environment you live in. Consider the climate, any pollution that may be epidemic, and then complete the following five-point scale:

1. *I never experience this external factor.*
2. *I rarely experience this external factor.*
3. *I experience this external factor sometimes.*
4. *I quite often experience this external factor.*
5. *I very often experience this external factor.*

This will give an idea of the potential external factors that you are susceptible to, and by considering the information in this chapter you will get some idea of the kinds of problems that may arise if you do not look after yourself.

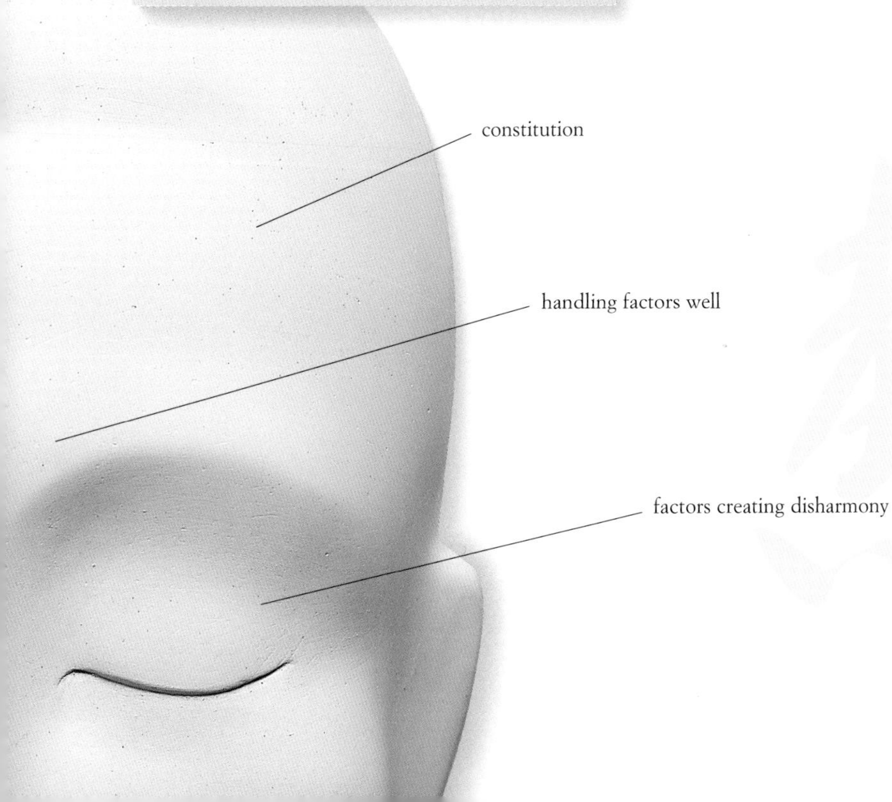

constitution

handling factors well

factors creating disharmony

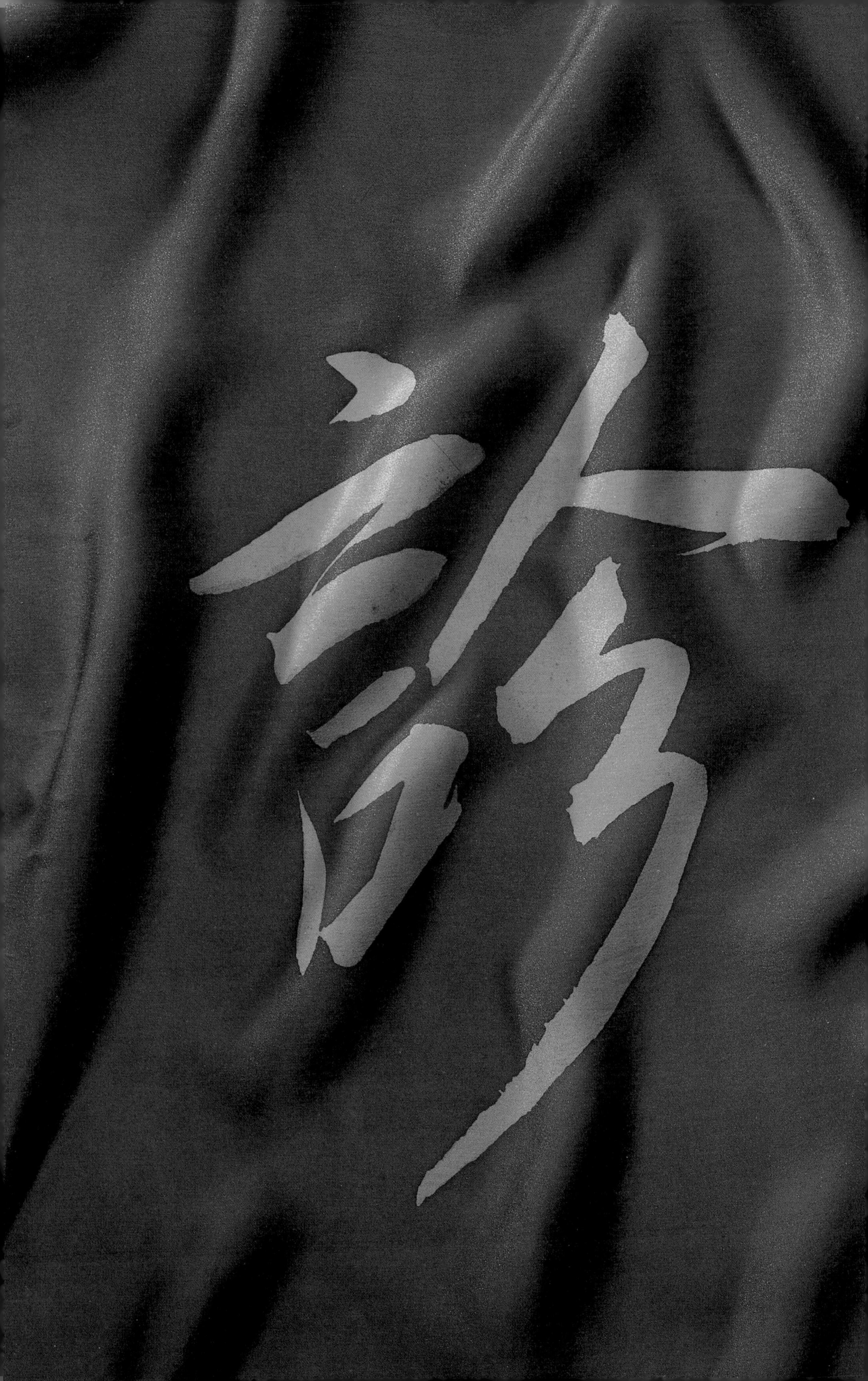

THE CHINESE APPROACH TO DIAGNOSIS

✦ ✦ ✦ ✦ ✦

診斷

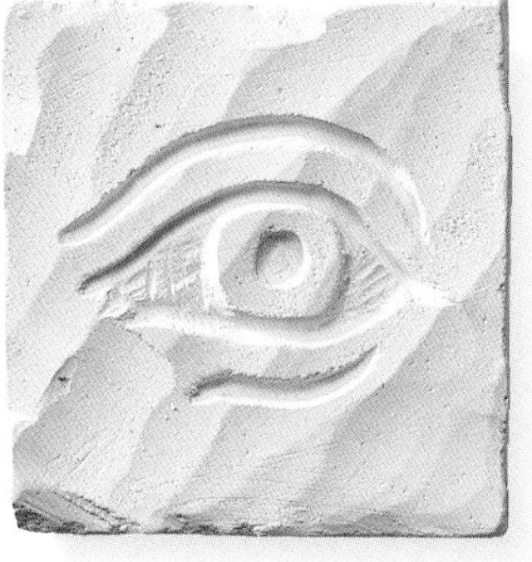

OBSERVING THE PATIENT

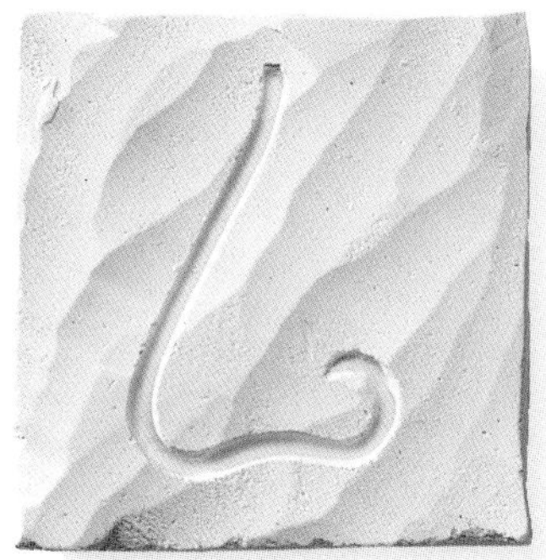

NOTING VOICE AND BREATHING

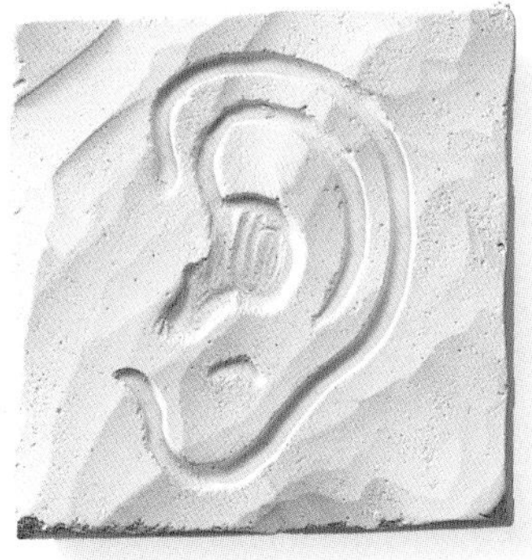

QUESTIONING THE PATIENT

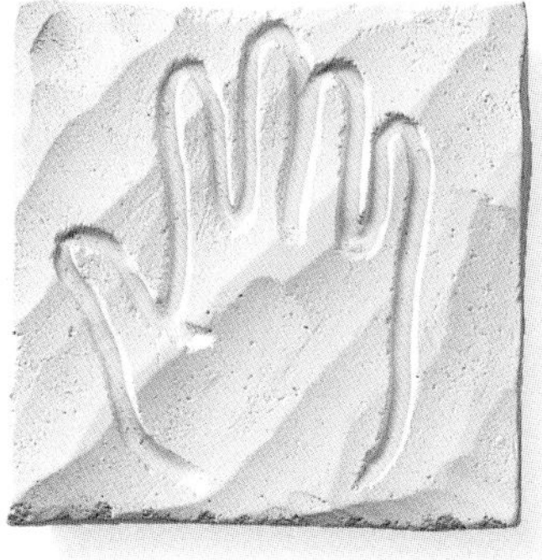

PALPATION AND PULSE-TAKING

DIAGNOSTIC TECHNIQUES

THE PRACTITIONER of Chinese medicine is confronted with the problem of trying to make sense of the myriad of processes going on within the individual. The need to have a systematic way of organizing all the information is of great importance if treatment plans and strategies are to be implemented successfully.

In this part of the book, some general approaches to diagnosis will be discussed, and several of the more commonly used frameworks for organizing such information will be considered.

The need to gather valid and comprehensive data is a sine qua non *of any assessment process, regardless of whether the problem is a burst pipe, a job applicant, a broken-down car, or an unwell person. Without this assessment it is impossible to formulate a hypothesis of what is going wrong and what to do about it. In Chinese medicine the diagnostic process is conducted in four areas – the four examinations.*

These four areas are ✦ LOOKING ✦ HEARING AND SMELLING ✦ QUESTIONING ✦ TOUCHING. Each area will reveal information that will contribute toward building a comprehensive whole. Invariably, in any diagnostic "story" there will be some contradictory indicators that may appear to stand in opposition to what other findings suggest. The balance of probability is likely to win out, and decisions will usually be made on the basis of the set of diagnostic indicators that "fit best."

LOOKING

THE FIRST thing that the practitioner of Chinese medicine will seek to do is to observe the patient and note anything about his or her physical appearance that may be of significance. To a large extent, this is something that we all do all the time with each other, for we make intuitive judgments about a person's health based on observed data. For example, "you look well today," "Are you a bit under the weather?" and so on. We observe general demeanor, face color, the condition of someone's hair, without really thinking about it. Chinese medicine seeks to do this in a more systematic way: here are some of the more important aspects of Looking.

PHYSICAL BODY APPEARANCE

A STRONG, healthy-looking body is likely to have a strong internal organ system and is less likely to suffer from a deficient condition than a weak and frail body. Very thin people may be prone to Blood and Yin deficiencies; obese people tend toward Qi deficiency and internal dampness. The way a person moves can provide useful information. Fast and jerky movements suggest an excess condition or Heat, whereas slow, deliberate movements suggest deficiency or cold.

Hair condition can give information about the Lung condition, and premature balding and greying indicate deficiencies of Blood and of Kidney Jing.

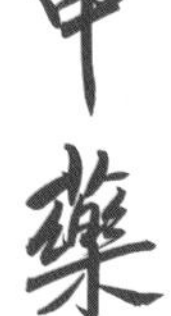

The color and the general appearance of the face and skin are also important. More significant aspects are

- Pale and lined face suggests chronic deficiency problems.
- Puffy, white face suggests Qi or possible Yang deficiency.
- Red face indicates some evidence of internal or external Heat.
- Bags under eyes suggest Kidney disharmony.
- Purple or blue lips can indicate a stagnation of Blood and may be related to a serious disharmony.

The condition of the skin can be important:

- Dry skin suggests Blood deficiency.
- Itchy skin suggests internal Liver Wind.
- Swollen skin (edema) can indicate Qi stagnation or a deficiency of Kidney Yang.

TONGUE

OBSERVATION OF the tongue is a central plank of Chinese medicine. It is not possible here to describe this most important aspect of "Looking" in great detail, but some general points can be made. The "geography" of the tongue is considered important. Various areas relate to the condition of specific internal organs of the body, and by observing the tongue condition in each of the areas, information is gathered regarding the condition of the relevant organ.

BELOW

The tongue is an invaluable diagnostic guide and is examined for its colouring and general condition.

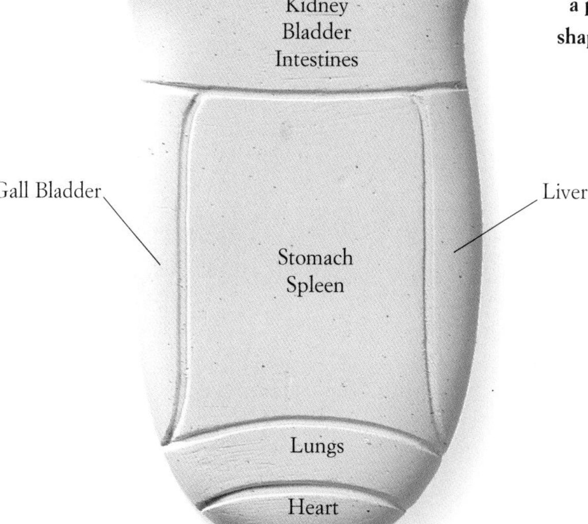

LEFT

Each area of the tongue represents a part of the body, and abnormal shape or color in any area points to a particular inner problem.

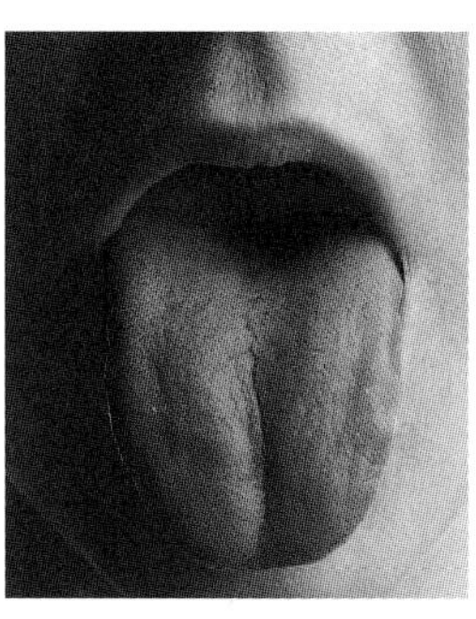

Pale red tongue
Normal

Pale tongue
Deficient condition

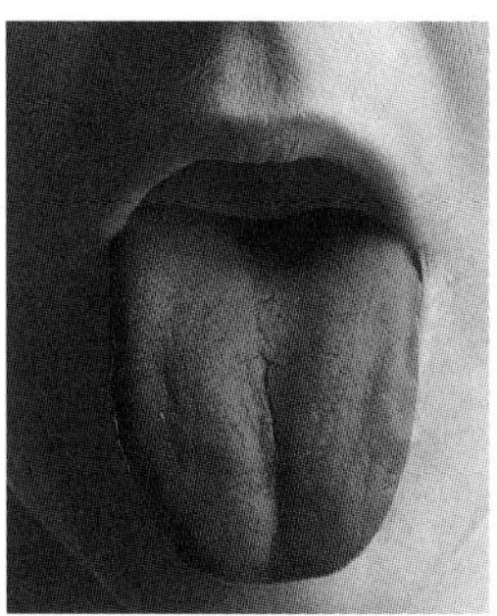

Red tongue
Internal heat

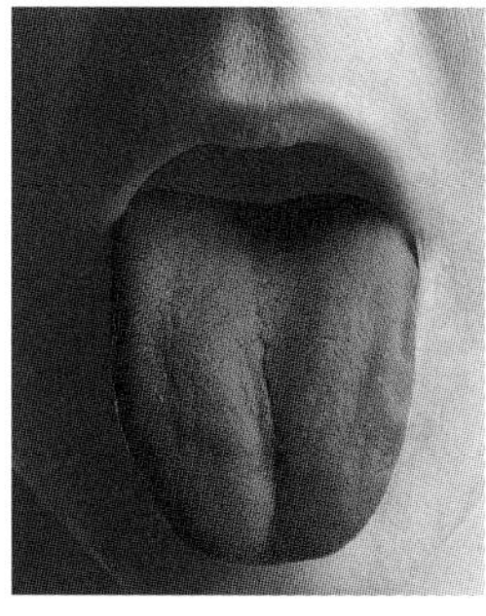

Purple tongue
Stagnant blood

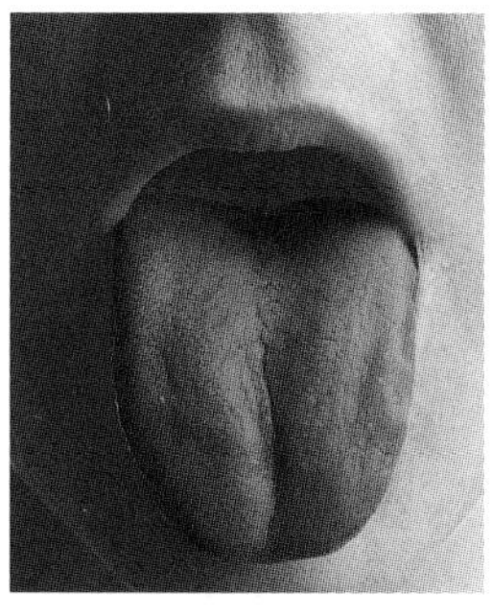

Blue/black tongue
Internal cold

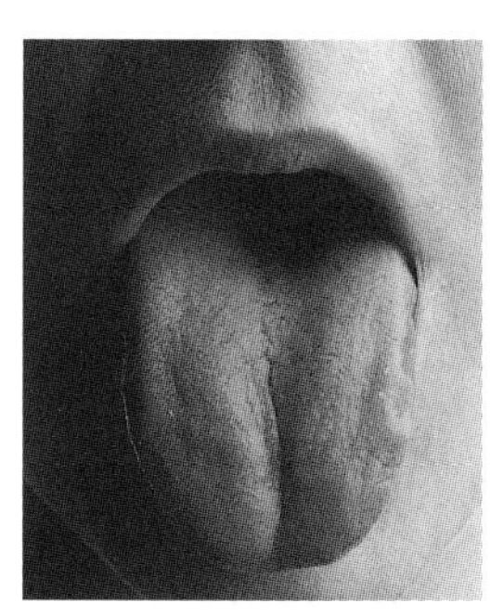

Thin tongue
Deficient condition

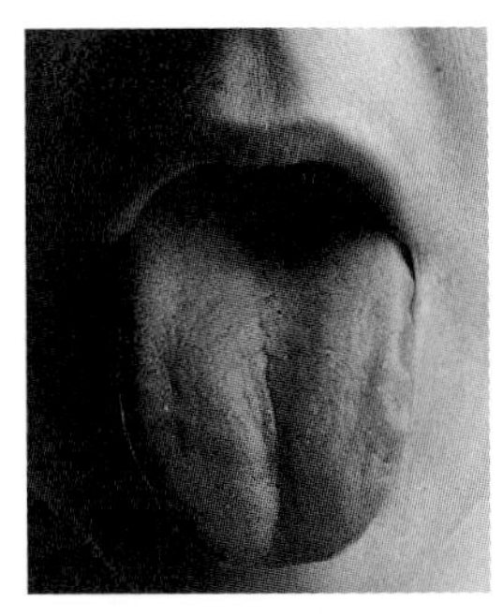

Swollen tongue
Damp present

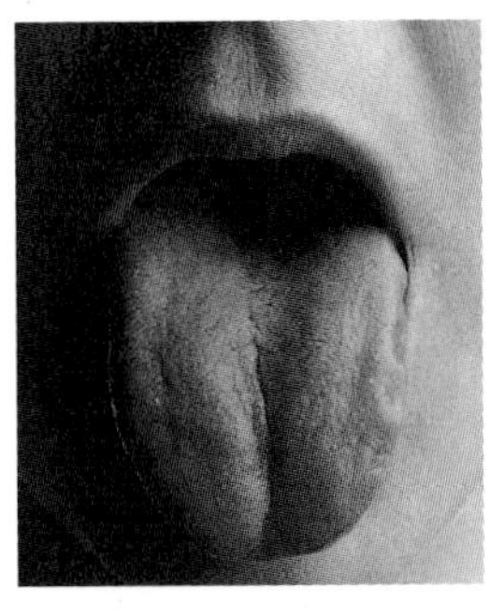

Stiff or deviated tongue
Wind present

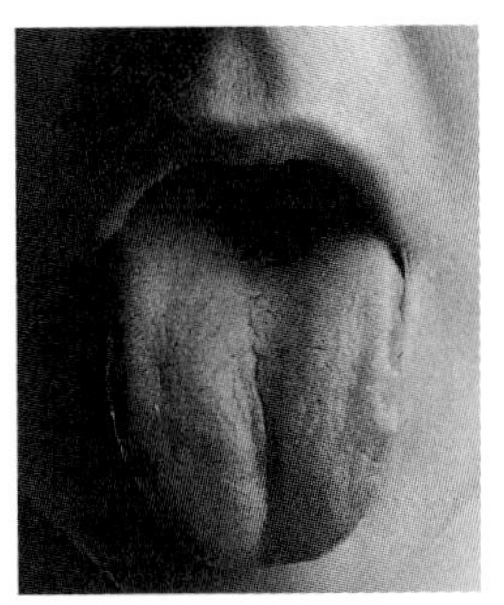

Quivering tongue
Qi deficiency

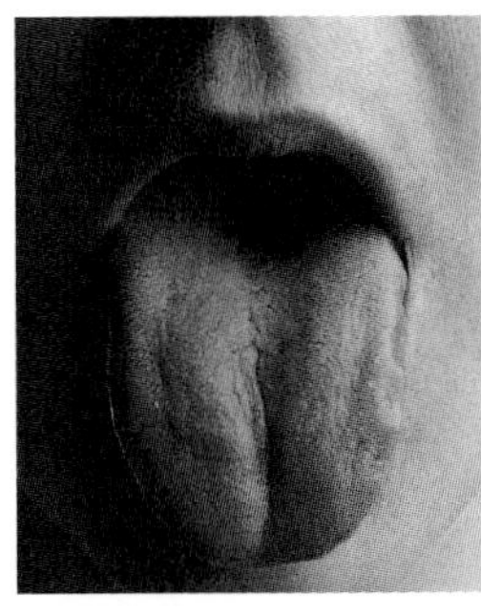

Short horizontal cracks
Qi deficiency

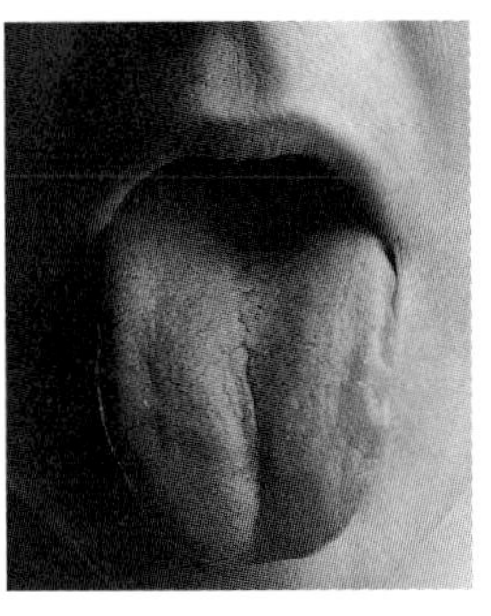

Toothmarks at side
Spleen Qi deficiency

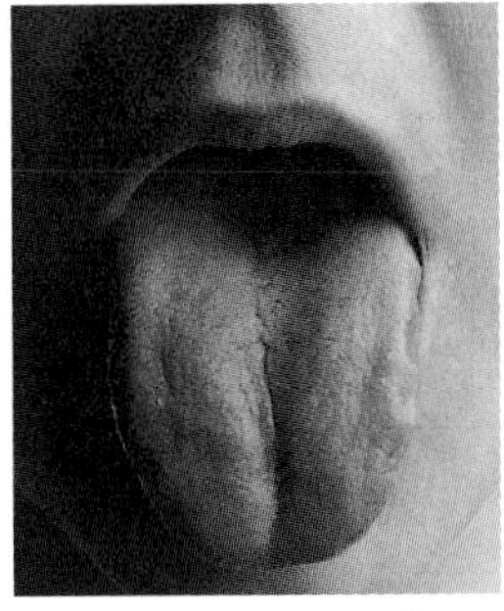

Shallow midline crack (not to tip)
Stomach deficiency

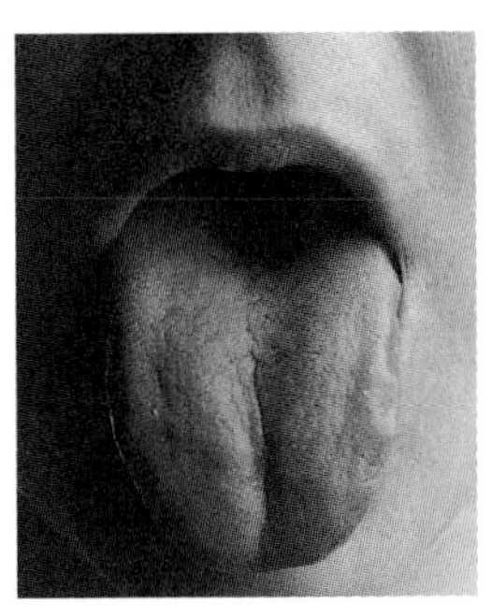

Long, deep midline crack (to tip)
Heart condition

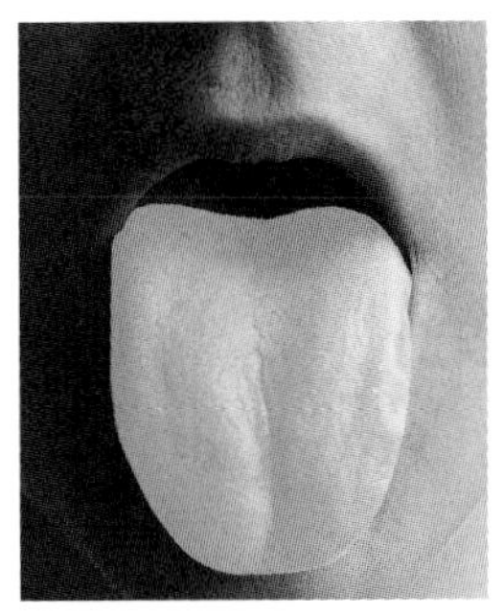

Thin white coating
Normal

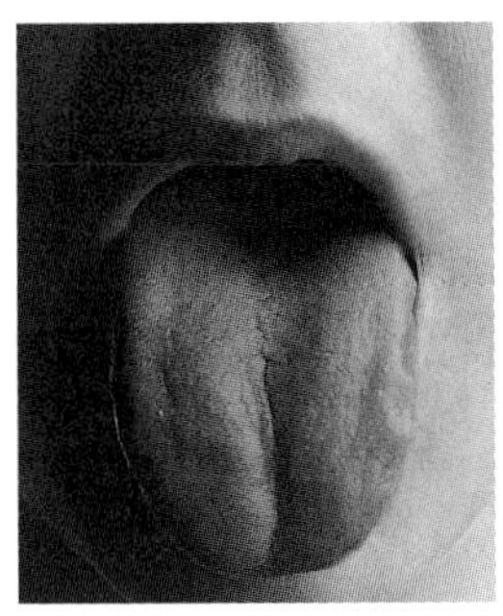

Thick coat
Pathogenic influence

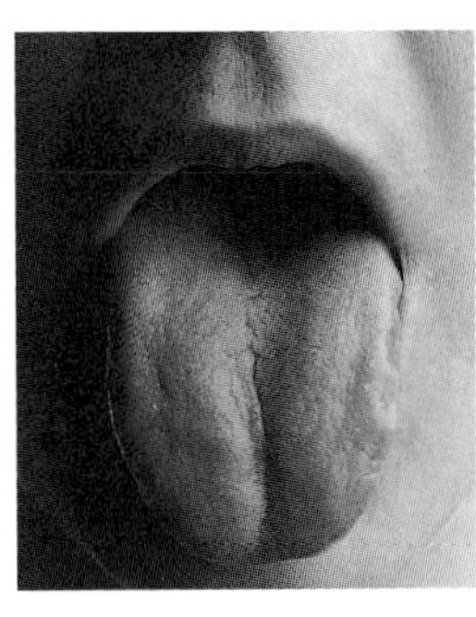

No coat/tongue peeled
Yin deficiency

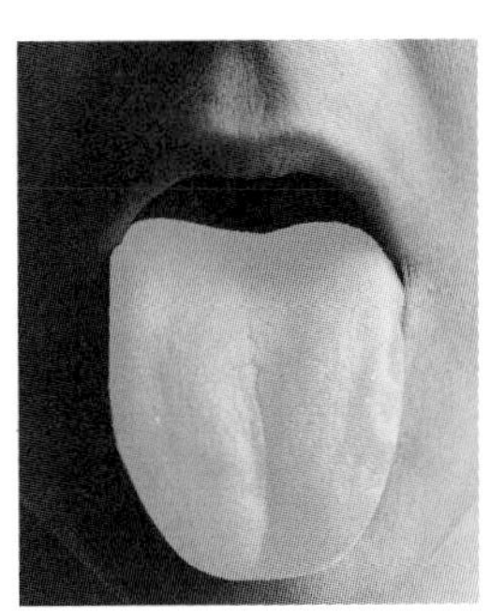

White coat
Cold present (normal when thin)

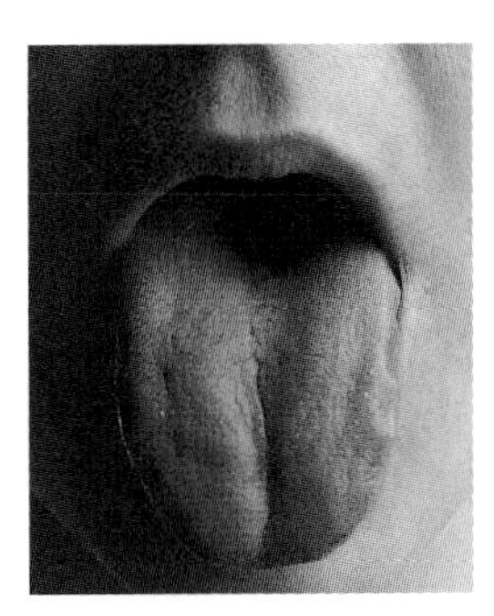

Yellow coat
Heat present

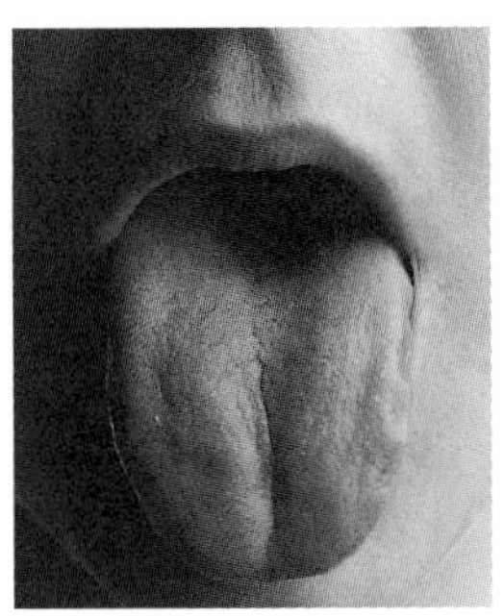

Slightly moist
Normal

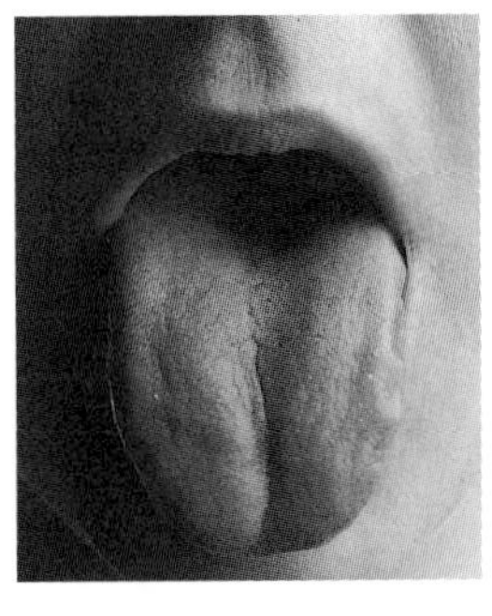

Wet tongue
Damp present

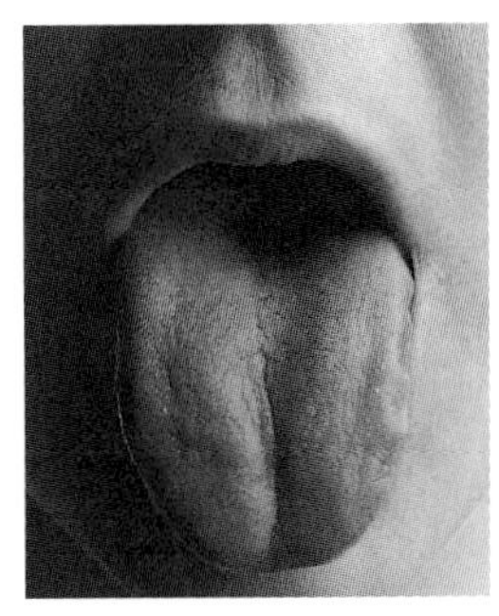

Sticky coat
Phlegm present

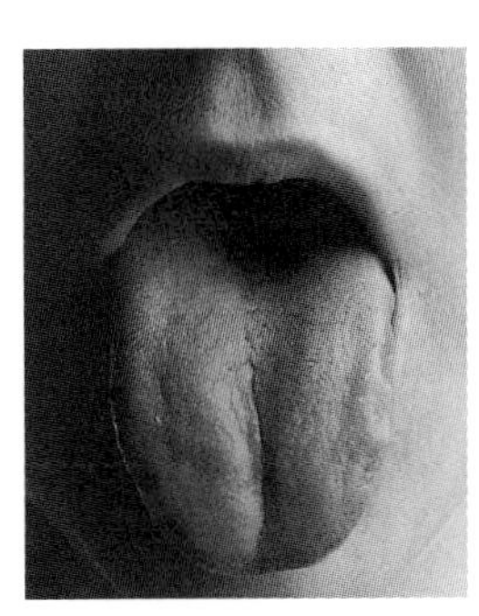

Dry tongue
Heat present

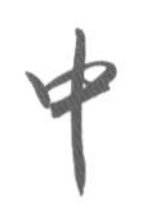

HEARING AND SMELLING

LISTENING TO the patient's voice can be useful. A loud, penetrating voice tends to suggest an excess condition, whereas a quiet voice is more indicative of a deficient condition. Talking too much can sometimes be a sign of Heat, whereas on the other hand an unwillingness to talk suggests the presence of Cold.

In a similar manner, the sound of the person's breathing can suggest an excess or a deficient condition.

The extent to which practitioners engage actively in smelling their patients is likely to be limited – especially in Western cultures, but some general points can be made. The presence of a strong, unpleasant smell tends to suggest the presence of Heat, whereas no smell at all usually suggests cold. If the urine and feces are foul-smelling this suggests the presence of Heat and possibly also of Damp.

QUESTIONING

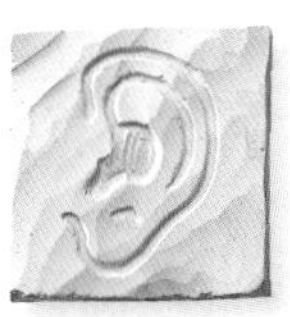

A LOT of information is gathered by asking the patient a series of questions and considering the answers with respect to the principles of Chinese medicine. There are various aspects that are usually covered in the course of a diagnostic interview. At the first consultation patients may be surprised at the length of the interview – and at the apparent irrelevance of many of the consultant's questions! Symptoms that may not seem at all related to the patient's complaint and lifestyle in general, all give clues to the cause of the problem and the type of treatment needed.

BELOW
The quality of a patient's voice, as well as his or her answers to the doctor's questions, and even bodily odors, can suggest a particular disharmony.

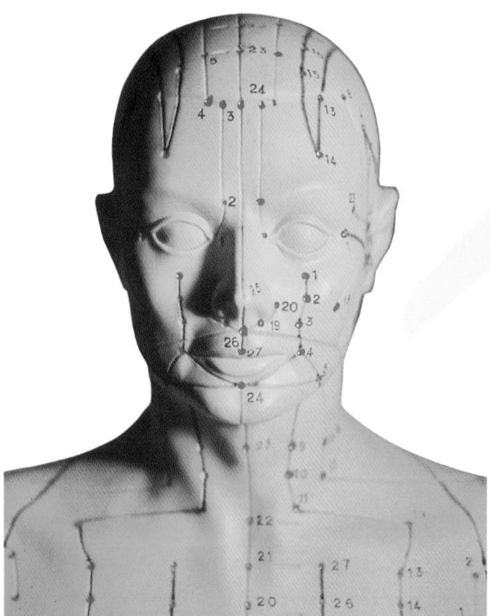

EARS

THE KIDNEYS are said to open into the ear. Thus the ears are related to the Kidneys in Chinese medicine, and problems with hearing may indicate a Kidney disharmony. The ears rely on Kidney Jing for their nourishment, and earache, tinnitus, or poor hearing could indicate that insufficient Kidney Jing is reaching them. This explains why such problems are notably a feature of old age, when Jing generally becomes weaker. Tinnitus can also be evidence of a Kidney or Liver disharmony. High pitch suggests Liver disharmony. Low pitch suggests Kidney disharmony.

KIDNEYS

LIVER

EYES

THE LIVER is said to open into the eyes, and eye conditions often indicate the health of the Liver. A deficiency of Liver Blood can cause eye problems, while bright, clear eyes indicate healthy Liver, and also Heart – to which the Liver is closely related. Pain in the eyes can indicate Heart or Liver disharmony or an external Wind invasion.

"Floaters" and blurring of vision suggest Blood deficiency. (The Liver stores and regulates Blood.) Eye pressure and/or dryness could suggest Kidney disharmony, since such disharmony is often characterized by dry conditions.

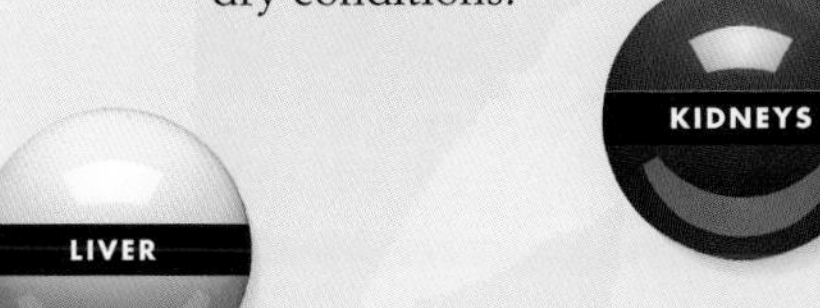

NOSE, THROAT, AND CHEST

THE LUNGS open into the nose and are the controllers of energy and breath, so their functioning is obviously related to the chest area and breathing. Problems of nose, throat, and chest therefore generally relate most directly to the Lungs, but also to the Heart, which influences the Lungs by governing the flow of the Blood.

Pain in the chest may suggest stagnant Blood or Wind-Heat invasion if it is associated with coughing and offensive yellow phlegm. Chronic nasal blockage and stuffiness suggests Damp and phlegm.

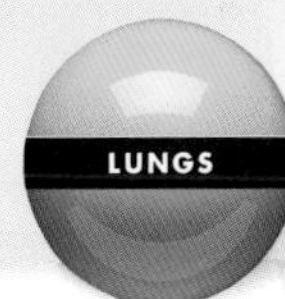

TRUNK AND ABDOMEN

THE LIKELY cause of any pain or discomfort in the trunk or abdomen depends partly on the exact location of the problem. Several of the Zang organs may be involved.

Pain or discomfort in the hypochondrium area, located just below the ribs at either side, often relates to Liver and Gall Bladder conditions.

Problems in the area of the epigastrium (the pit of the Stomach) generally relate to the Stomach and Spleen.

Problems located in the lower abdomen may indicate disharmony of the Bladder or Kidneys.

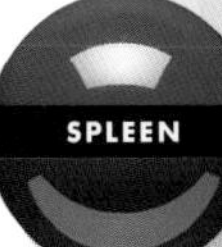

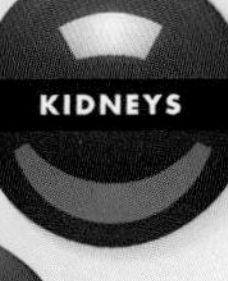

HEAD

IN CHINESE medicine the head is the confluence of all the Yang channels.

If there is an excess of Yang energy coming to the head, this can lead to problems such as headaches and dizziness. If there is a deficiency of Yang, then this can lead to lightheadedness or possibly unconsciousness.

A detailed differential description relating to channels and Zangfu involvement goes beyond the scope of this book, but suffice it to say that detailed information regarding disharmonies in the head area is very important in Chinese medicine.

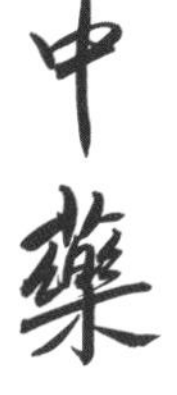

DIGESTION

THE PATIENT'S account of any problems or idiosyncracies involving digestion are often a good guide to the condition of the Spleen and the Stomach, even if they do not seem to the patient to be linked to the main problem. To take extreme examples, lack of appetite suggests Spleen deficiency, whereas constant hunger suggests Stomach Heat.

Other features can be linked also to other organs. For example, a taste in the mouth can point to a variety of possible disharmonies, usually of the Spleen and Stomach, but also of the Kidneys and the Liver.

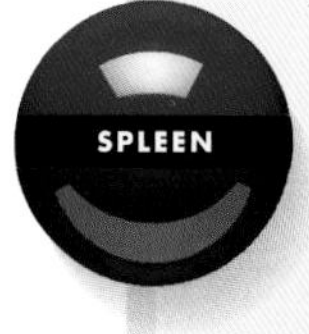

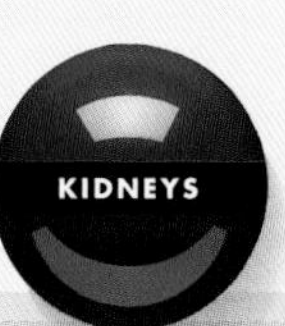

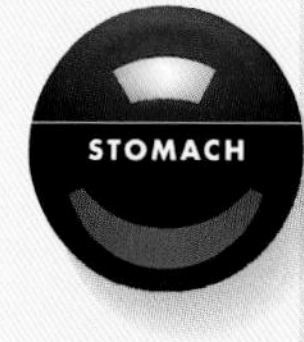

BOWELS

THE NATURE of bowel movements is an important indicator of possible disharmonies in the body, and acquiring detailed and accurate information about bowel movements is very important in Chinese medicine.

The main organs involved are Spleen and Stomach. Deficiencies of their functioning and Cold or Damp excesses all affect this aspect of the digestive system. Kidneys and Liver disharmonies may also be indicated.

Constipation may suggest Heat, Cold, Blood deficiency, or a Liver-related disharmony. Diarrhea may suggest Heat, Spleen, Kidney, or Liver disharmonies.

KIDNEYS

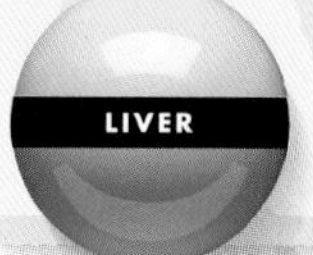

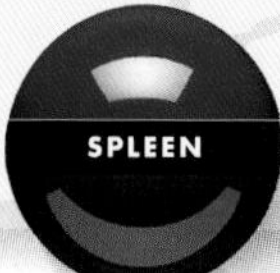

DRINK AND FLUIDS

THE PATIENT'S thirst or lack of thirst, the type of liquid desired, and even the manner of drinking are all relevant to a diagnosis. The important thing for the physician to consider is the type and amount of fluids taken in. Generally:

A preference for drinking cold liquids suggests a Heat pattern, and a preference for drinking warm liquids suggests a Cold pattern.

No thirst suggests a Spleen disharmony with Cold. Thirst but lacking a desire to drink suggests Damp-Heat. Sipping slowly usually suggests Yin deficiency.

BLADDER

FEATURES CONNECTED with urine are also of considerable importance and can be interpreted by the physician as part of the pattern of disharmonies. In particular, the color of the urine is observed. If clear, it suggests Cold, and if dark, it suggests Heat; Damp is suggested by cloudy urine.

In addition, the way in which urine is passed is a useful indicator: difficult urination suggests a Kidney or Bladder disharmony, and frequent urination suggests deficiency of Kidney Qi.

Extremes in the amount of urine passed suggests a Kidney disharmony.

Pain on urination suggests stagnation or Heat; pain after urination suggests a deficiency problem.

KIDNEYS

SLEEP AND ENERGY PATTERNS

THE PATTERN of the patient's sleep and energy are pointers toward the health of the Qi, Blood, and the Yin of the body. Patients may sleep restlessly, be unable to sleep, sleep at inappropriate times, or be unable to keep awake. This may be related to diet and lifestyle and may indicate Zangfu deficiencies or disharmonies.

The nature of any insomnia experienced suggests a particular pattern of disharmonies: not getting to sleep easily relates to Blood deficiency; continually waking and sleeping indicates a Kidney disharmony; dream-disturbed sleep suggests either a Liver or Heart disharmony. Falling asleep during the day or general lethargy and low energy suggests a Spleen disharmony, or possibly a Kidney disharmony if the problem is very severe.

SWEAT

THE CHARACTERISTICS of any pattern of sweating, as described by the patient, can be very helpful in discriminating disharmonies. This can be further corroborated at the next stage of the diagnosis (palpation), when the practitioner feels the condition of the patient's skin.

There are various important factors, and these include especially the area of the body affected, the time of day, and the types of sweat. The Heart Blood can be involved in any abnormal patterns of sweating – smelly, nervous sweat particularly indicates the Heart.

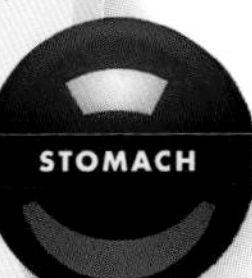

Sweating in the area of the head only suggests Stomach heat, and sweating in soles/palms/chest ("Five Palm Sweat") suggests Yin deficiency. As to time of day, daytime sweat suggests Yang deficiency; night sweats suggest Yin deficiency.

PAIN

AS WE all know, there are many different types of pain, and the patient may feel pain over an extended period or in short sudden bursts. It is always important to ascertain the location, duration, and nature of any pain that the patient may be suffering. Again, a description of the full differential diagnostic features of pain goes beyond our discussions here, but some important aspects can be indicated.

Pain that is acute, sharp, and specific usually indicates an Excess condition. It may be caused by invasion by external factors such as Wind, Cold, Heat, or Damp; interior Cold or Heat; stagnation of Qi, Blood, or Phlegm due to an external injury or a Zangfu disharmony.

Pain that is dull, achy, more chronic, and more generalized usually indicates a deficiency condition. It may be caused by Qi or Blood deficiency.

For all pain experienced, the location of the pain will give pointers to the affected channels and can be of importance for both exterior and interior disharmonies.

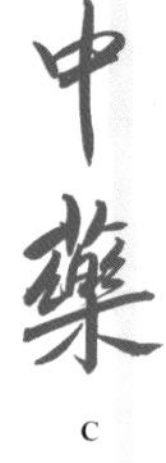

CLIMATIC FACTORS

THIS AREA relates to climatic factors to which the patient may be subject, and to the way in which the individual responds to Heat, Cold, Damp, and Wind. Responses can differ greatly between individuals, and this can be a good guide to an understanding of any internal disharmonies in the patient.

Dislike of Cold, with liking for Heat, suggests a Cold pattern, or a Yang deficiency (particularly common in older people), while dislike of Heat and liking for Cold suggests a Heat pattern, or a Yin deficiency.

Adverse reaction to Damp suggests that the patient has a tendency to suffer from internal Dampness, and dislike of Wind may be indicative of a Liver disharmony, particularly in relation to Liver Wind.

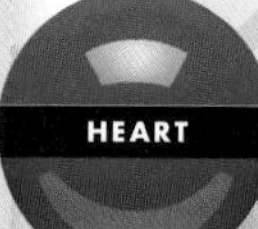

EMOTIONAL FEATURES

IT IS always important to try to ascertain any disharmonies that may be associated with the individual's emotional state.

The seven emotions are central in Chinese medicine to the concept of how disharmonies occur, and an understanding of how the patient responds emotionally can indicate any potential area of disharmony and the Zangfu system that may be involved.

In particular, anxiety may suggest Heart pattern and disturbed Shen; depression may suggest Lung or Heart disharmony; anger/frustration may suggest a Liver disharmony; poor concentration may suggest a Spleen disharmony; fear may suggest a Kidney disharmony.

LIFESTYLE FEATURES

THIS IS the area in which Chinese medicine and modern Western medicine have much in common. Most medical opinion stresses the importance of regular exercise and of balanced diet, with only a moderate consumption of alcohol; but Chinese medicine takes these matters a step further, in the light of its philosophical underpinnings.

The Chinese practitioner questions the patient closely on lifestyle areas and asks about diet, consumption of alcohol, any drugs or medication taken (prescribed or illegal), smoking, exercise patterns, family background and relationships, occupations, and hobbies. This builds up a picture to explain the nature of the disharmonies leading to the patient's complaints.

GYNECOLOGICAL FEATURES

TO GAIN an accurate diagnostic picture with women patients, it is important to explore the patterns of menstruation and any symptoms accompanying it. This is a detailed area in itself, which is beyond the scope of this book.

General points to be explored include the regularity or otherwise of the menstrual cycle, the amount of blood lost during a period, the color and consistency of blood, and the nature of the flow, whether there is any menstrual pain, and whether the patient experiences any other symptoms, such as bloating, headaches, food cravings, mood swings, or similar symptoms, either before or during a period. Any other vaginal problems (such as leucorrhea) would also be relevant.

TOUCHING

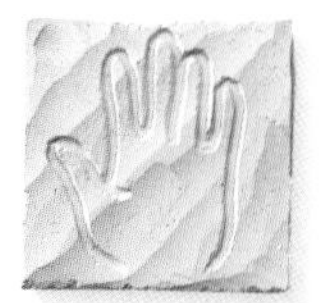

THE LAST aspect of the Four Examinations involves the practitioner working "hands-on" with the patient. There are two aspects of touching that need to be considered: palpation of the body and taking the pulse. Pulse-taking is such an important aspect of Chinese medicine that a whole mystique has built up around it, raising it to the level of an art form rather than an aspect of diagnosis. We shall consider both aspects of touching, looking at palpation first.

PALPATION

Palpation refers to the systematic feeling of the surface of the body in order to discover any external or internal disharmonies. There are three main aspects to be observed.

It should also be borne in mind that many acupuncture points are naturally tender when they are palpated strongly, so this may not indicate any disharmony. Any such palpation information can only be considered in conjunction with all other aspects of a diagnostic picture.

BODY TEMPERATURE

It can be useful to correlate the patient's report of whether he or she feels hot or cold by feeling the skin, generally.

- If the skin feels cold, then this suggests a Cold disharmony.
- If the skin is hot to the touch, then this may suggest an invasion by external Heat.
- If the skin begins to feel hot after being held for a while, then this may indicate internal Heat, possibly due to Yin deficiency.

BODY MOISTURE

Again, it can be useful to correlate the patient's report of sweating and moisture by direct feeling of the skin.

- Moist skin may suggest a Lung disharmony.
- Dry skin may suggest a deficiency of Blood or Body Fluids.

PAIN

An important indicator of areas of stagnation can be gained by palpating along the meridians looking for possible tender spots – "Ashi" points as they are called in Chinese medicine. They may indicate a local channel problem or may be indicative of a more deep-seated Zangfu disharmony.

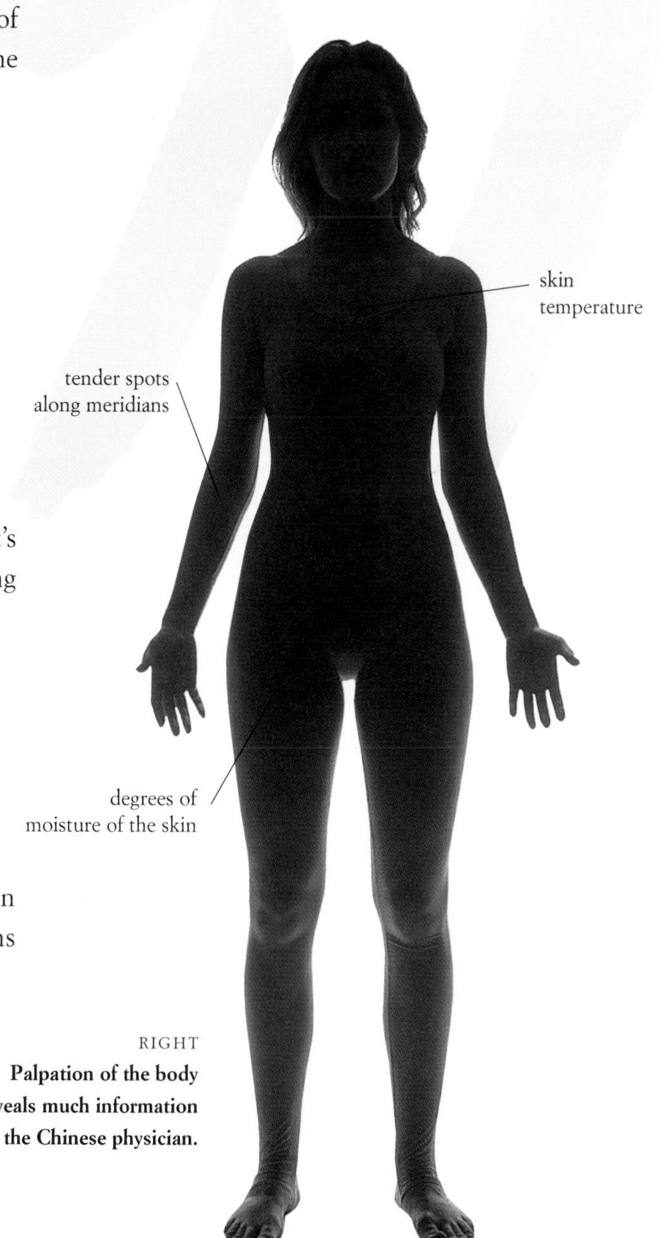

RIGHT
Palpation of the body reveals much information to the Chinese physician.

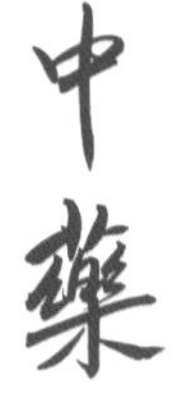

PULSE

THE TAKING of the pulse is considered to be of prime diagnostic importance in Chinese medicine. The emphasis is on the quality of the pulse in various positions on the wrist. It is recognized that there are about twenty-eight different pulse qualities that can be felt on three different positions and at three different depths on the wrist of each hand – each with its own subtle nuance of interpretation.

Clearly, conveying a complete and full understanding of the nature and significance of pulses in Chinese medicine is beyond the scope of this book. Any fledgling practitioner of Chinese medicine soon learns that feeling and understanding pulses is something more of an art, requiring practical experience under the guidance of a qualified physician.

With that important preamble in mind, we will explore some of the basic aspects of the pulse in Chinese medicine.

PULSE POSITION

There are three positions near each wrist on the radial artery. Each position relates to a specific aspect of the Zang organs. These positions are shown diagramatically below.

PULSE DEPTH

The depth at which the pulse is felt is also considered important. There are three levels, each requiring slightly increased pressure. These levels are the superficial level near the skin, the middle level, and the deep level close to the bone.

POSITION	LEFT WRIST	RIGHT WRIST	ENERGY
First	*Heart*	*Lung*	*Qi*
Second	*Liver*	*Spleen*	*Blood*
Third	*Kidney Yin*	*Kidney Yang*	*Yin*

LEFT
The pulse is taken at three depths and in three positions.

PULSE RATE

As in Western medicine, the speed of the pulse is taken and compared with the average of about 68–75 beats per minute.

PULSE WIDTH

The width of the pulse between fingers is noted.

PULSE STRENGTH

An important indicator of whether a disharmony is an excess or a deficiency can be gained from judging the strength of the pulse.

PULSE QUALITY

There is a variety of qualities of the "feel" of the pulse, and these are considered indicators of a particular disharmony pattern.

PULSE RHYTHM

The consistency of the pulse flow and the nature of any inconsistency are considered important.

The major features of the most common pulses are shown opposite. Again, it should be remembered that this is offered as a summary of a topic that is considerably more complex. There are other less common pulse qualities that could also be described, but the table gives a breakdown of those most commonly observed. It should also be noted that an individual's pulse can exhibit a variety of qualities in different positions and depths, and a full diagnosis may involve having to consider the qualities observed in relation to the appropriate organ defined by the position.

There are stories of Chinese physicians who can diagnose the whole pattern of an individual's disharmony from feeling the pulses. For most practitioners the pulse is taken as one, albeit very important, piece in the overall jigsaw that makes up the Chinese medical diagnosis.

PULSE CHARACTERISTICS

PULSE	CHARACTERISTIC	SIGNIFICANCE
floating or superficial	more apparent at surface; lacking at middle and deep levels	*invasion by external factor – Cold, Wind, etc.*
deep	more apparent at deep level; lacking at surface and superficial levels	*internal disharmony*
rapid	fast pulse, significantly above average	*internal Heat*
slow	slow pulse, significantly below average	*internal Cold*
thready/thin	feels like a very fine thread under the fingers; quite distinct	*Blood deficiency*
large/big	feels very broad but distinct under the fingers	*excess condition*
empty	feels similar to a large pulse; but lacks the distinctness	*Blood and Qi deficiency*
full	feels similar to a large pulse very powerful at all levels	*excess condition*
wiry	feels taut and distinct beneath fingers; like guitar string	*Liver disharmony*
slippery	"slips" along under the fingers; like a viscous fluid	*internal Damp; Spleen disharmony*
choppy	feels uneven; like fingers bobbing on surface of sea	*Blood deficiency*
tight	similar to wiry pulse but feels like a vibrating cord	*excess condition; stagnation*
irregular/ knotted	slow; may skip a beat on an intermittent basis	*Heart Blood disharmony*
intermittent	skips beat regularly	*Heart disharmony (serious)*

Yin	Considered an amalgam of Interior, Cold, and Deficiency characteristics
Yang	Considered an amalgam of Exterior, Heat, and Excess characteristics
Interior	Whole body symptoms; chronic problems; Zangfu system affected
Exterior	Sudden onset; acute disorder; invasion by external pathogenic influences – Heat, Cold, Damp, and so on; channel problems; floating pulse; head and neck symptoms rather than whole body
Cold	Pale; aversion to cold; slow, deliberate movements; heat helps problem; introverted; clear urine; tendency to diarrhea; pale tongue, whitish coat; slow pulse
Heat	Reddish complexion; fever; rapid movement and speech; dislike of heat; cold helps problem; thirst; dark urine; tendency to constipation; reddish tongue; yellow coat; fast pulse
Deficiency	Tiredness and lethargy; weak, insipid movement; weak breathing; quiet voice; pressure can relieve discomfort; poor appetite; pale tongue; empty pulse
Excess	Heavy movement; loud voice and breathing; pressure exacerbates discomfort; thick tongue coat; large pulse

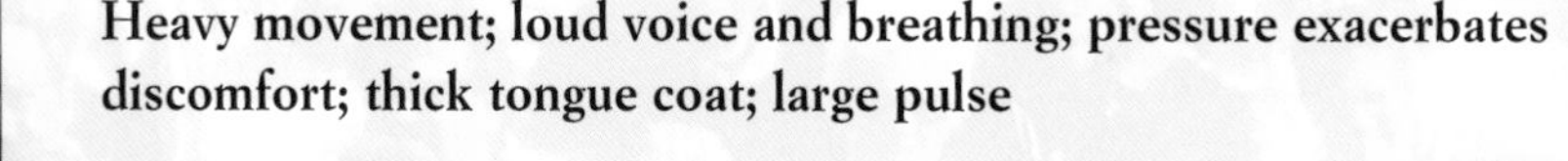

PATTERNS OF DISHARMONY

HAVING GATHERED together a very comprehensive set of information during the diagnostic process, the practitioner of Chinese medicine requires a way of organizing it in order to acquire a clear overall understanding of the energetics and disharmonies observed.

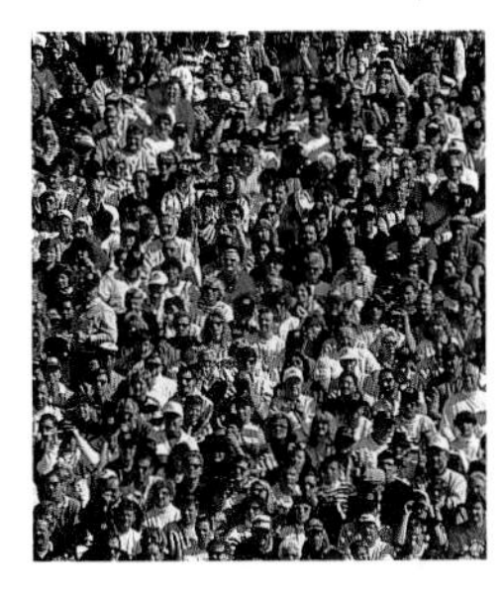

ABOVE
A mass of symptoms can be interpreted to read as a pattern.

There are several different organizational patterns that can be applied in Chinese medicine. Those most commonly used are the Eight Principles applied to the Zangfu system, the Five-Element patterns, and, especially with relatively simple external conditions, Channel patterns.

In this part of the book we will look at the Eight-Principle patterns and at how they can be applied to the Zangfu system in order to describe more accurately the nature of internal disharmonies. Each of the four aspects of diagnosis reveals for each of four pairs of principles which of the pair applies to the patient, and so a whole picture is formed.

DIAGNOSTIC PATTERNS

Eight-Principle patterns
Zangfu patterns
Five-Element patterns
Channel patterns
Six-Stage patterns
Four-Level patterns

A number of acupuncturists will use the Five-Element system to organize their diagnosis, but this system will not be described in any detail in this book. The Eight-Principles approach as applied to the Zangfu system tends to be the dominant model used in China and increasingly in the West.

THE EIGHT PRINCIPLES

THE EIGHT-PRINCIPLES approach of diagnosing in terms of bipolar qualities is in keeping with the philosophy of Yin and Yang. These Eight Principles consist of four mutually interdependent pairs of characteristics: Yin and Yang, Internal and External, Cold and Hot, Deficiency and Excess. To be strictly accurate, this system considers Yin and Yang to be superordinate qualities under which the other three pairs are subsumed (see right). Groups of general characteristics are associated with each of the Eight Principles.

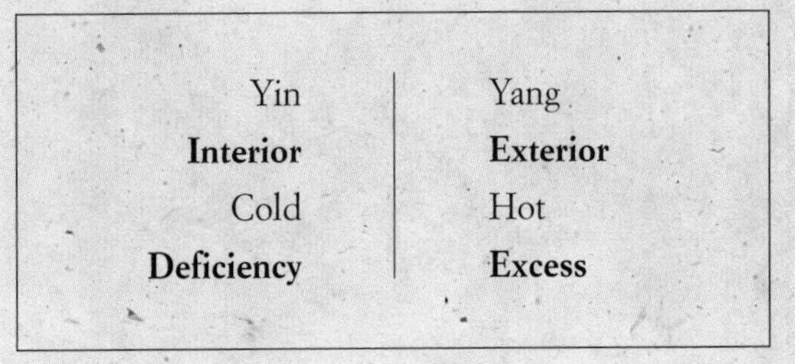

Yin	Yang
Interior	**Exterior**
Cold	Hot
Deficiency	**Excess**

LEFT
Characteristics associated with the Eight Principles.

DIAGNOSTIC PATTERNS

THE PHILOSOPHY of Chinese medicine offers many alternative perspectives from which to diagnose and treat the disharmonies revealed by physical and mental complaints. The Eight-Principle patterns simply provide a systematic way in which to organize a lot of information about a very dynamic energy system – the human body. There is always a combination of changing patterns.

For example, a patient may present evidence of a Wind-Cold invasion, which is an Exterior/Excess pattern, with Cold predominating. If this is not treated, the Wind-Cold will turn to Wind-Heat (the Yin aspect turning to Yang), which is an Exterior/Excess pattern, with Heat predominant. The Exterior condition could then become internal, probably affecting the Lungs, and this could weaken the Lungs, resulting in a Qi deficiency. Thus, the problem will become an Internal/Deficient pattern, with once more the Yin aspect becoming dominant over the Yang.

Although there are combinations of patterns that are quite commonly seen, these are always fluid and changeable over time. It is therefore vital that the practitioner of Chinese medicine uses the Eight-Principle pattern in a flexible way to track the changing matrix of energetic balances and imbalances.

Some of the more commonly observed pattern combinations are given on pages 104–105. In each case the pattern of symptoms will reflect the features of the combination, subsumed under the overall perspective of whether the pattern is predominantly Yin or Yang. It should be remembered that in any given individal it is perfectly possible for combinations of apparently opposite patterns to coexist. When a treatment program is planned and implemented it has to be applied with an eye constantly on the complex, and at times contradictory, nature of change in the energy patterns of the body.

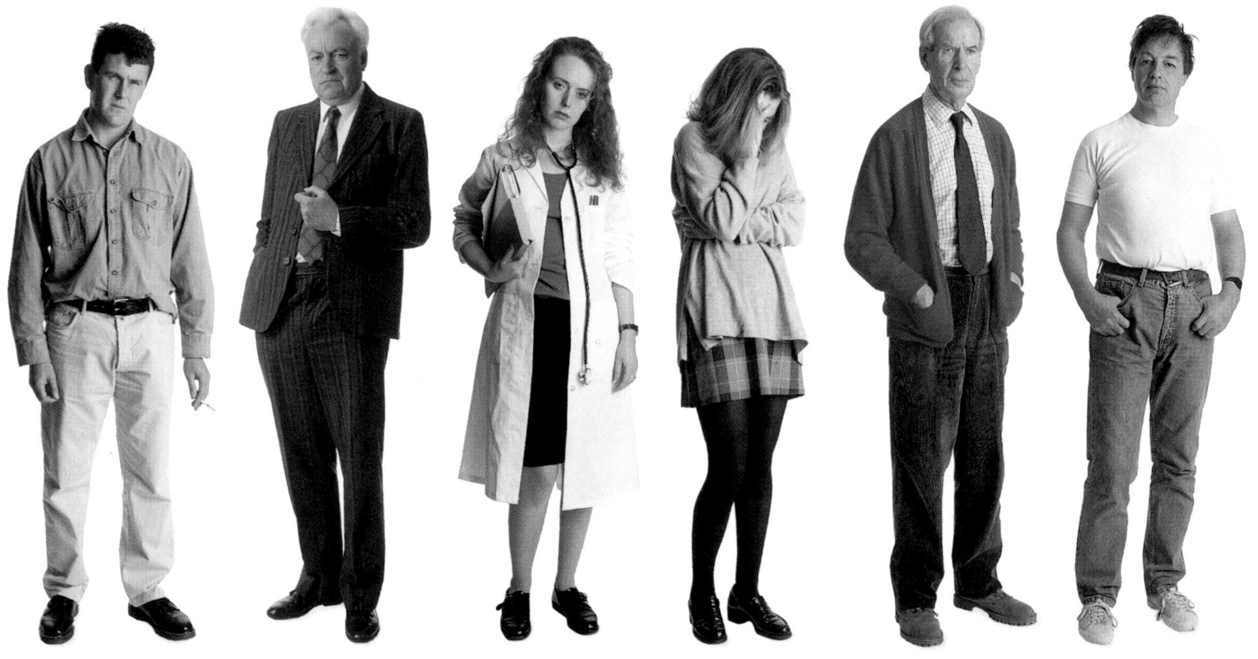

ABOVE

Each individual has a particular pattern of disharmonies, although certain combinations are commonly observed.

COMMON DISHARMONIES

THE INTERACTION of external pathogenic factors and internal emotional and dietary patterns can lead to the development of a complex series of interactive disharmonies in the Zangfu system. External causes – Wind, Cold, Heat, Summer Heat, and Damp – can enter the channels on the surface of the body and externally affect the Lungs, the most "external" of the Zangfu. But prolonged exposure to these factors can result in their penetrating more deeply: for example, Cold and Damp can ultimately penetrate to the Kidneys. Anger and frustration, internal causal factors, can cause stagnation of the Liver Qi.

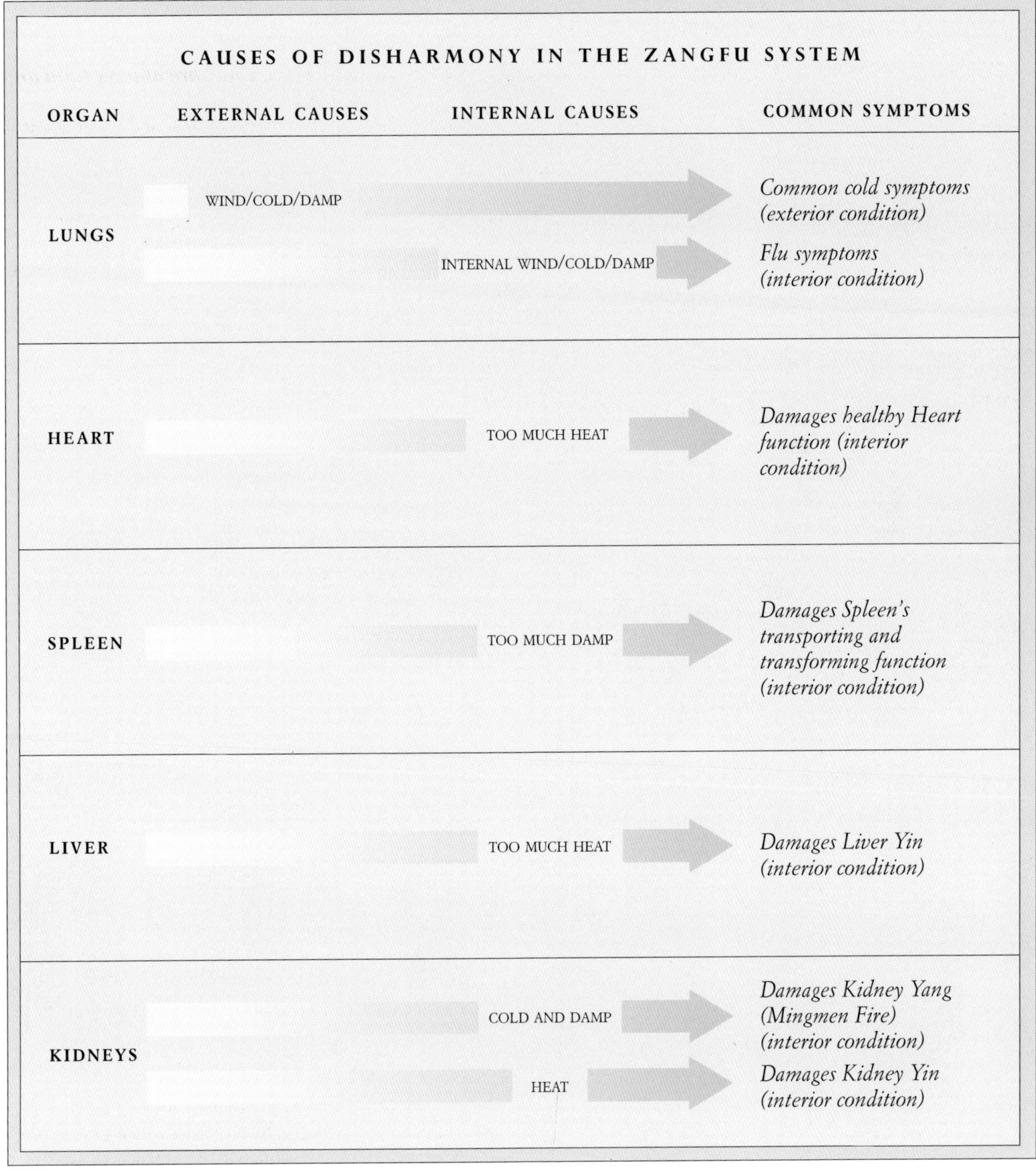

CAUSES OF DISHARMONY IN THE ZANGFU SYSTEM

ORGAN	EXTERNAL CAUSES	INTERNAL CAUSES	COMMON SYMPTOMS
LUNGS	WIND/COLD/DAMP		*Common cold symptoms (exterior condition)*
		INTERNAL WIND/COLD/DAMP	*Flu symptoms (interior condition)*
HEART		TOO MUCH HEAT	*Damages healthy Heart function (interior condition)*
SPLEEN		TOO MUCH DAMP	*Damages Spleen's transporting and transforming function (interior condition)*
LIVER		TOO MUCH HEAT	*Damages Liver Yin (interior condition)*
KIDNEYS		COLD AND DAMP	*Damages Kidney Yang (Mingmen Fire) (interior condition)*
		HEAT	*Damages Kidney Yin (interior condition)*

EXTERIOR COLD (EXCESS)

THIS IS a combination of a Yang and a Yin pattern, and consequently the two forces will mediate each other. The resultant combined symptoms will not be too extreme.

Tony wakes up feeling slightly shivery with his body aching. His nose is running with a clear, thin discharge. He decides that bed is the best place for him that day!

In this simple example, the pattern is excess in nature, but in some instances there may be an element of Wei Qi deficiency and a more exterior/deficient pattern may occur. This is more likely to be a situation where the symptoms are perhaps more chronic but less severe. If, for example, Tony had a tendency toward deficiency then he might feel as if these symptoms were continually coming and going and occasionally flaring up. This might be the kind of individual who could be described as generally "under the weather" and susceptible to all minor ailments. Thus, even in a combined pattern that is fairly clear, there may be other patterns that are contributing to the overall picture, and these should be looked at to give a rounded view.

ABOVE
The first symptoms of a cold.

EXTERIOR HEAT (EXCESS)

THIS IS a combination of two Yang patterns and the result will be a strong Yang pattern. The symptoms are likely to be much more extreme with Yang features predominant.

Despite staying in bed for the day, Tony begins to develop a rasping sore throat and he has an elevated temperature. He is sweating and bringing up thick, yellow phlegm. His pulse is rapid. He feels lousy and remains in bed.

As with the first element, the likelihood of the Wind-Cold developing into Wind-Heat may also be a function of the individual's underlying deficiency pattern.

ABOVE
The patient becomes feverish.

EXCESS COLD

THIS IS a combination of a Yin and Yang pattern that will mediate the overall pattern. If pain is present, the excess pattern will result in this being intense and very sensitive to the touch.

Derek has been raiding his mother's freezer, and he ate a whole tub of ice cream. He is complaining of severe cramping pain in his abdomen and has been to the toilet with acute diarrhea. His mother's sympathies are stretched to the limit!

It is likely that the intense cold of the ice cream has invaded the Stomach and Spleen setting up an excess Cold pattern. Derek should recover fairly quickly and it's to be hoped he won't raid the freezer again in a hurry!

ABOVE
Heat leads to the desire for cold.

DEFICIENT COLD

THIS IS a combination of two Yin patterns and the resultant pattern will present as strongly Yin in nature. In clinical practice this is often seen as a feature of chronic Yang deficiency, usually affecting the Spleen or the Kidneys, creating a relative excess of Yin in the body. It can also occur in Heart and Lung patterns.

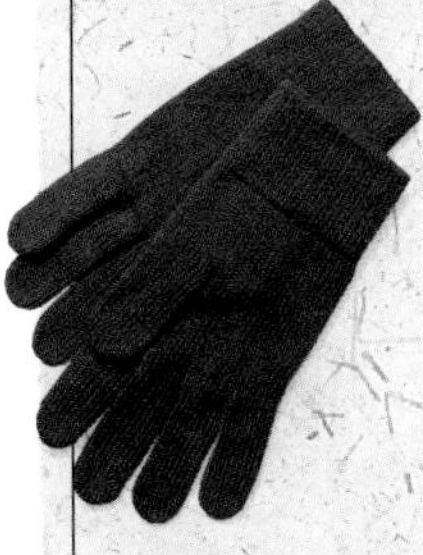

ABOVE
Yang deficiency causes Cold.

Margaret is 79 and lives alone on her pension. She is constantly complaining of being cold, even in mild weather, and has little or no energy to do anything. She eats and drinks very little and suffers from chronic diarrhea, especially first thing in the morning. Her ankles are swollen and her back is constantly cold and aching.

This is a classic example of the Kidney Yang energy becoming deficient as a feature of the aging process and further exacerbated by Margaret's poor diet and lack of heating at home. In extreme cases in old age, the deficiency of Yang energy leads to hypothermia.

EXCESS HEAT

BOTH THE patterns here are Yang in nature, so the resultant combination pattern will be markedly Yang in presentation. They will generally present classic Heat signs and extremely dominant behaviors.

Bill did not suffer fools gladly and would get very frustrated and angry when things were not working out the way he planned. He was subject to episodes of extreme temper, where he would get very red in the face and invariably complain of thumping headaches. Bill was on medication for high blood pressure, and his doctor had warned him that if he didn't slow down a bit he would end up having a stroke.

Bill's anger and frustration were causing his Liver Qi to stagnate. This creates internal Heat in the Liver that builds up and rises to the head as Liver Fire on occasions. Bill died of a massive stroke at the age of 51.

ABOVE
Excess of Heat has classic behavior manifestations.

DEFICIENT HEAT

THIS IS a combination of a Yin pattern and a Yang pattern, and the two will relatively mediate one another in the combined pattern. This pattern is most commonly seen as a result of a deficiency in Yin energy, leading to a relative excess of Yang. The pattern is often referred to as "Empty Heat" and is characterized by "Five-Palm sweats," night sweats, and a general mental agitation.

Pauline has been going through the menopause and is having tremendous problems with hot flushes and night sweats. She complains of a constant, nagging low back pain and she is continually feeling "on edge," as if she is going to bite everyone's head off for no good reason. She is tearful and depressed at times and her sleep pattern is poor.

A feature in menopause is the deficiency of Kidney Yin that results in the "empty heat" symptoms that Pauline is experiencing. The Empty Heat is invading the Heart and disturbing the Shen, causing the restlessness and the emotional symptoms.

RIGHT
Night sweats and disturbed sleep.

SELF-REFLECTION

HERE ARE some simple examples to start you thinking about the Eight-Principle patterns. In each instance, think about the information that you are given about the disharmony and decide whether you think that the problem is predominantly: exterior in nature or interior in nature, hot in nature or cold in nature, deficient in nature or excess in nature.

In the light of this, then make a judgment as to whether you think the disharmony is predominantly Yin in nature or predominantly Yang in nature.

1 You have been out at an evening football match. The weather is cold and wet and you were standing in a part of the ground where there is little cover. The next morning you wake up feeling shivery, with a slight fever. You are sneezing and have a thin, clear discharge and a muzzy head.

ANSWER *In this instance the problem is one of an excess of Cold invading the exterior of the body – although Cold is essentially Yin in nature, the sudden onset of an exterior excess factor suggests a predominantly Yang energy.*

ABOVE
Disharmonies can have great complexity.

2 You are feeling very tired and lethargic. Your face is pale, your skin is dry, and your hair feels dry and lacks body. You have felt progressively worse over the last few months and now you are feeling light-headed and you notice that your fingers feel a bit tingly.

ANSWER *In this instance there is clearly a long-term problem that is leading to an interior pattern of deficiency. There is insufficient information to suggest Heat or Cold, and by the same token it is unclear whether the energetic disharmony is essentially Yin or Yang in nature.*

3 Your doctor tells you that you have a problem of high blood pressure and that you are going to have to slow down a bit. You find this very difficult, and when you get frustrated at work or at home you get very red in the face, feel very hot and bothered and usually end up with a thumping headache.

ANSWER *In this instance there seems to be evidence of Heat that is being generated from an interior disharmony. The sudden onset of these attacks suggests an excess condition that rapidly builds up inside. The problem of the high blood pressure suggests a chronic condition that has built up over a long period of time and is probably the result of an underlying deficiency problem. It is possible that there are both Yin and Yang aspects in this instance.*

Consider how you have done with these little scenarios. As you can see, the diagnosis in real life is rarely quite as simple and straightforward as a choice between one thing and another.

Starting to think of examples in terms of these Eight-Principle patterns enables you to see how a practitioner of Chinese medicine begins to analyze what is going on with the patient's disharmonies.

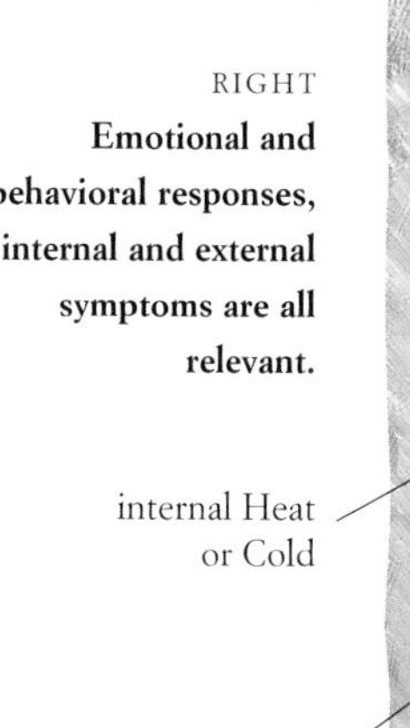

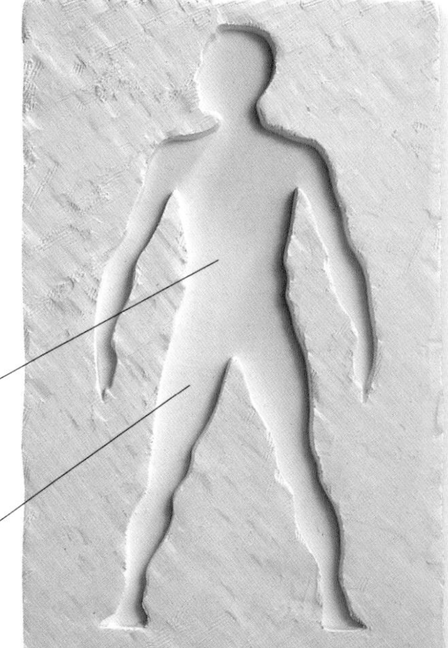

RIGHT
Emotional and behavioral responses, internal and external symptoms are all relevant.

ZANGFU PATTERNS

*W*HEN PRACTITIONERS *of Chinese medicine use the Eight-Principle patterns as a guide to understanding the nature of the patient's disharmony, they will normally map the patterns onto particular Zangfu systems. Thus, for example, they will be able to pinpoint a case of deficiency or excess that predominantly affects the Spleen system, and so on. So the diagnosis is built up by marrying the observations made in terms of the Eight Principles with a knowledge of the functions of particular Zangfu systems. In reality, a range of disharmonies is likely to coexist affecting different Zangfu systems in different ways, but in order to illustrate the nature of the general process it may be useful to look at how a set of signs and symptoms are organized to illustrate a disharmony in just one Zangfu system at a time. Each of the following case histories demonstrates a particular Zangfu pattern. For each one, we will examine what might be going on in the body to produce such symptoms, and we will figure out what might have caused the problem in the first place. We can then assess what sort of treatment Chinese medicine can offer. All the treatments described will be discussed in much greater detail on pages 125–161.*

ACUPUNCTURE
page 131

MOXABUSTION
page 142

CUPPING
page 145

ACUPRESSURE
page 149

SELF-HELP ACUPRESSURE
page 150

CHINESE HERBALISM
page 163

QIGONG
page 189

SELF-HELP PROTOCOLS
page 192

TAIJI AND TAIJIQUAN
page 206

LIFESTYLE
page 211

ZANG ORGAN PATTERNS

THE ZANG organs are considered to dominate in the Zangfu systems, and the practitioner will often look first at the possible Zang organ disharmonies for diagnosis and treatment. A collection of symptoms can be diagnosed together, but it is unhelpful to see this as a "syndrome" that has a name and becomes a "thing" that the patient is suffering from. The Chinese physician is always mindful that the illness is a dynamic process: seeing it as a "pattern" is much more helpful. Some symptoms are fairly obviously linked to the relevant Zang organ (shortness of breath to Lungs; stabbing chest pain to Heart) and others less obviously so (irritability and depression to Liver; edema or swelling caused by fluid retention to Kidneys), even though the connection is recognized in Western as well as in Chinese medicine.

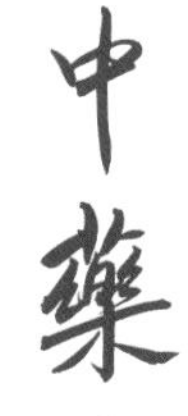

THE LUNGS

THE FUNCTIONS of the Lung system in Chinese medicine include governing the formation of Qi in our bodies, dispersing and descending Qi throughout the body, regulating the water passage (through the link with the large intestine), and supporting the Kidneys.

So, consider someone with the following signs and symptoms and let us follow through an analysis of the disharmony, starting from an understanding of the Eight-Principle patterns and of the function of the Lungs.

John finds himself short of breath, especially when he has been exerting himself, and when he talks you notice that his voice quality is weak and somewhat insipid. He has a chronic cough, very often bringing up some watery sputum, and he sweats easily – especially during the day.

John complains of having no energy at all and of feeling lethargic all the time. He looks very pale and appears to be tired. His tongue is pale, with a slight white coat, and his pulse is deep and somewhat empty.

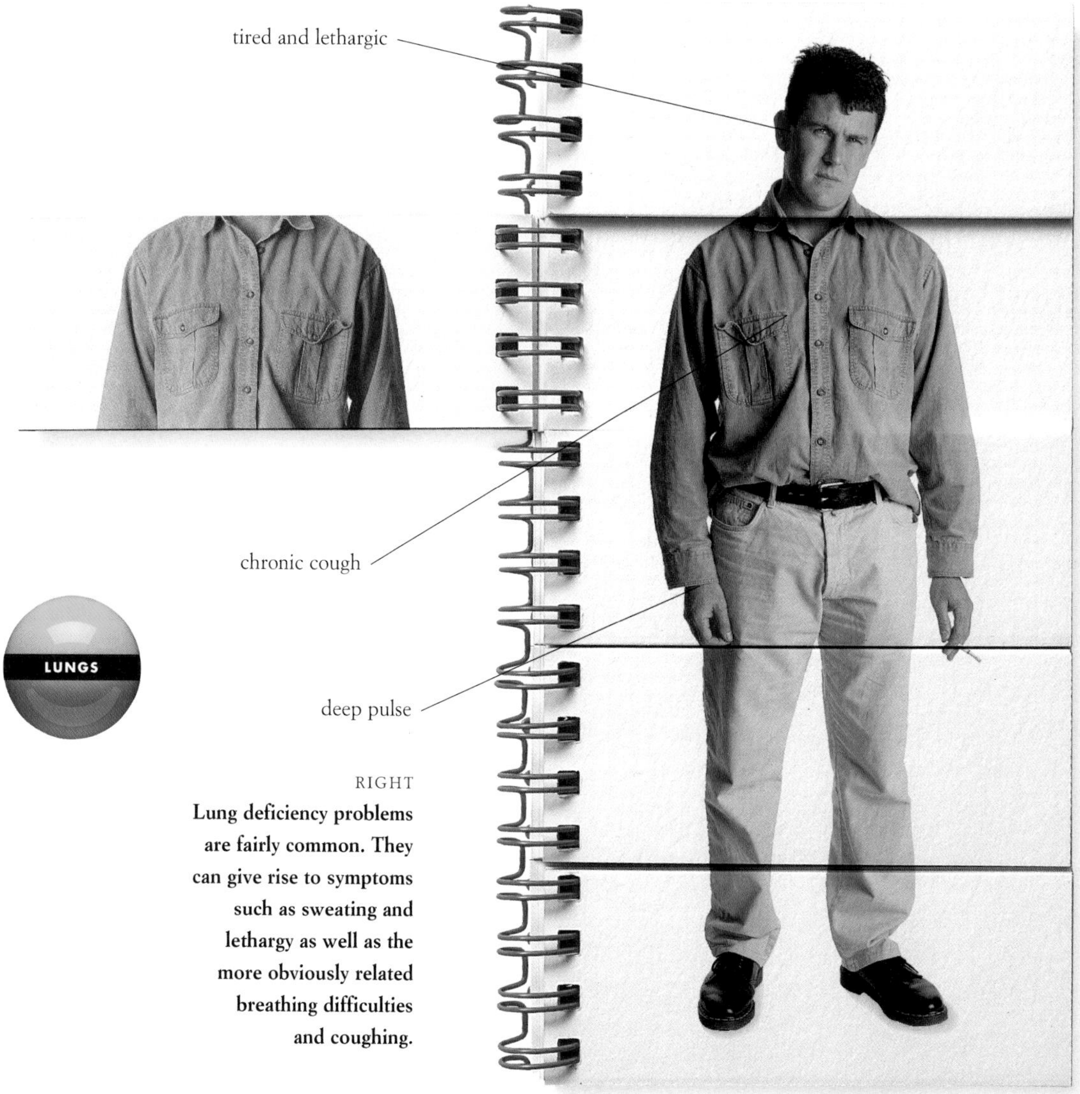

RIGHT
Lung deficiency problems are fairly common. They can give rise to symptoms such as sweating and lethargy as well as the more obviously related breathing difficulties and coughing.

What is going on with John?

From the information given, it is clear that John's problem is one of deficiency rather than excess. As the problem has been going on for a long time, it has become an internal disharmony, which in this instance is resulting in problems with the Lung functions.

When Qi is deficient the Lungs will fail to govern respiration, and this results in the shortness of breath and the weak voice. The deficient Lung Qi will not descend adequately, and the chronic cough develops. Also, because the Lungs are failing in their function of governing the flow of water, water sputum is formed, and this rises up with the chronic cough. The Lungs have the function of spreading the defensive Qi (Wei Qi) throughout the body, and when there is a deficiency pattern here, then this allows for Body Fluids to be easily lost, hence the sweating on minimal exertion. It will also mean that John is likely to be very susceptible to external pathogenic factors and that he may regularly go down with minor ailments; since the Qi is deficient, these are never fully resolved. The net result is that John's energy system will become steadily depleted, leading to tiredness and chronic lethargy.

These signs and symptoms can be seen as an example of a Zang pattern disharmony: the manifestation of Lung Qi deficiency.

What might have caused John's problem?

There is a variety of factors that may be contributing to John's Lung Qi deficiency. There may well be a Pre-Heaven or congenital weakness that would make the Lungs generally vulnerable. Also, being the outermost of the "internal" Zang organ systems, the Lungs are most directly susceptible to invasion by external pathogenic factors – of which the most specific are Wind/Cold/Damp. If the body is not strong enough to eliminate fully the external invading influences then the Lungs can be injured, leading with time to Qi deficiency. Once this cycle becomes established, it evolves into a vicious circle that further depletes the Wei Qi, leads to further invasions by Cold/Wind/Damp, and this further exacerbates the problem.

If John works in a mainly sedentary occupation, sitting crouched over a desk all day, this can restrict the flow of Qi to the Lungs, and lead to deficient Lung Qi. If he smokes or has antibiotics prescribed for chest infections, this will also lead to deficiency of Lung Qi.

What can Chinese medicine do to help John?

The main principle of treatment will be to tonify the Lung Qi, and for this acupuncture, moxabustion, or herbal formulae may be prescribed. It would also be important to advise John on dealing with habits that may exacerbate the problem and cultivating habits to improve it. If relevant, stopping smoking would be essential, and it might be helpful to suggest that John take a class in Qigong exercises, which can slowly strengthen the Qi of the chest.

Other Lung Patterns

There are other Lung disharmony patterns that are often observed. These include

- *Lung Yin deficiency*
- *Lung Dryness*
- *Wind-Cold invades Lungs*
- *Lung-Heat invades Lungs*
- *Wind-Damp invades Lungs*
- *Phlegm-Heat obstructs Lungs*
- *Phlegm-Damp obstructs Lungs*
- *Phlegm Fluids obstruct Lungs.*

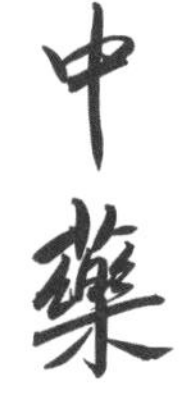

THE HEART

IN CHINESE medicine the Heart is seen as governing the Blood, controlling the blood vessels and housing the Shen, or, perhaps more helpfully, our moods and emotions.

To illustrate how a typical Heart disharmony may manifest itself in terms of the Eight-Principle patterns, consider the following case example. This shows the symptoms of a Heart problem that is caused by emotion as well as by physical exertion combined with lack of any form of beneficial exercise.

Dave is a 50-year-old company executive. He is complaining of palpitations and a stabbing pain in his chest, which radiates to the inner aspect of his left arm.

The symptoms get worse upon physical exertion and also when he gets emotionally wound up – which happens a lot, both at home and in the work setting. Sometimes he experiences shortness of breath. His hands tend to get cold and are quite clammy to the touch. His tongue is purple, with a few dark spots. His pulse is tight and wiry.

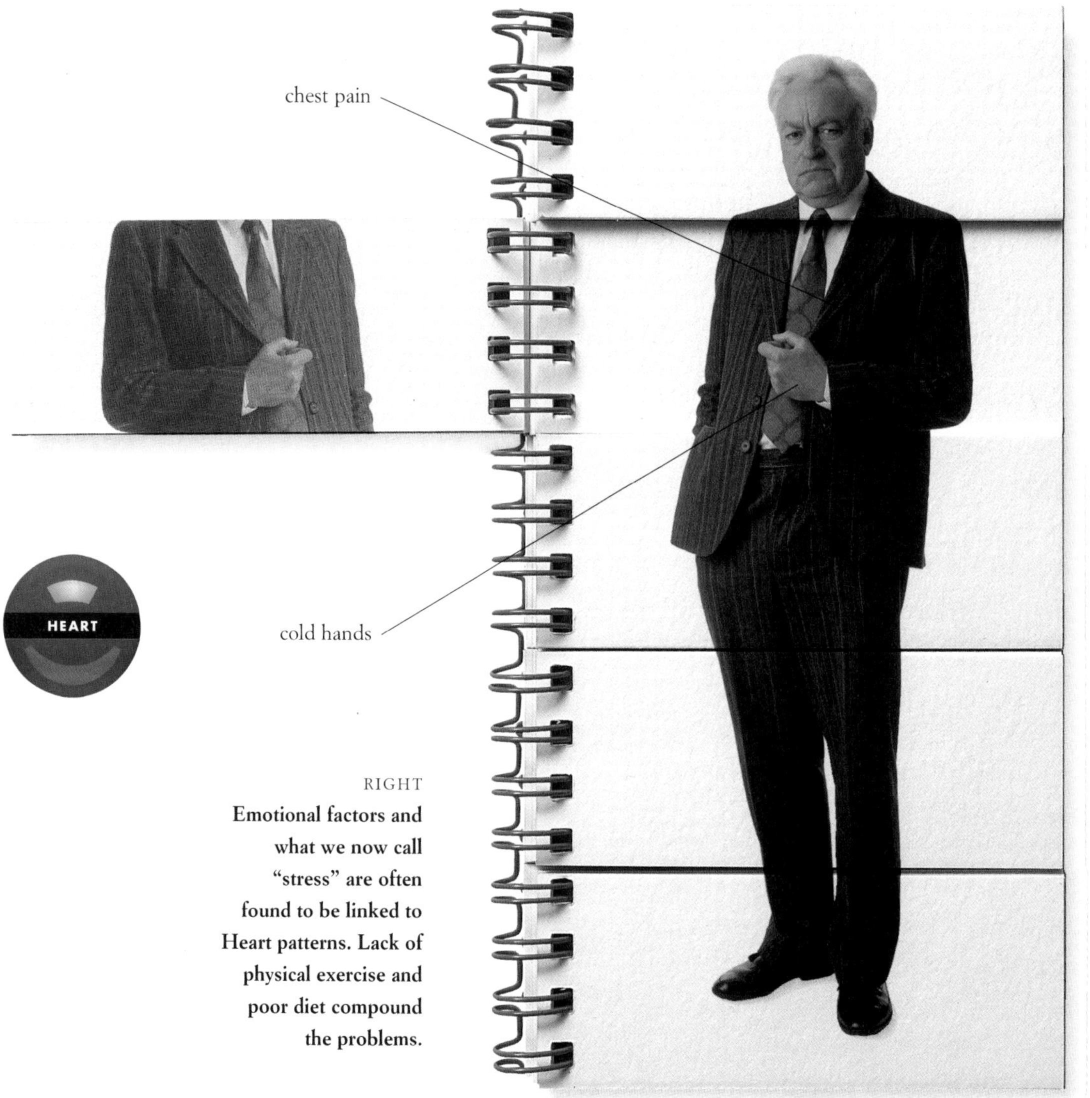

RIGHT
Emotional factors and what we now call "stress" are often found to be linked to Heart patterns. Lack of physical exercise and poor diet compound the problems.

What is wrong with Dave?

The symptoms that Dave is experiencing are the classic ones of the condition known to Western medicine as angina pectoris. This is often the precursor to or consequence of a life-threatening event such as a heart attack. But how is such a condition to be regarded in terms of Chinese medicine?

In this instance, the Heart Yang is deficient and this results in the Heart's function of governing the Blood being impaired. When the Yang energy is insufficient to move the Blood thoroughly, there will be a stagnation of Blood flow – leading to the classic symptoms described. A stagnation is seen as a local internal excess pattern here, caused by the initial deficiency. Since the Yang energy is deficient, this will lead to experiencing Cold – especially in the extremities. There is also evidence that the Heart is not adequately housing the Shen, given the tendency to emotional upset that is referred to.

In summary, Dave's problem is an example of a combined deficiency and excess pattern affecting the internal Heart Zang, with some Cold signs also being present.

These signs and symptoms are classic examples of a Zang pattern disharmony: Stagnation of Heart Blood.

What might have caused Dave's problem?

It is likely that stress and a sedentary lifestyle will play a significant part in this type of problem. Over time, emotional upset can deplete the Heart Qi, and this in turn can lead to Heart Blood and Heart Yang deficiency. In Chinese medicine it is often said that anxiety is "stored in the chest," and ultimately the deficient Yang will lead to stagnation of Blood in the chest area. The stagnation causes the pain, so classic of the angina attack, and the radiation down the arm usually follows the path of the Heart and/or the Pericardium channel.

It is evident that a sedentary lifestyle that is lacking physical exercise will also tend to deplete the Qi, and this leads to further exacerbation of the Heart problem.

Can Chinese medicine help Dave?

The treatment principle in terms of Chinese medicine will depend upon whether Dave is suffering a severe attack of stagnation pain or whether the condition is less acute.

In the first case, the focus will be on moving the stagnant Blood and promoting circulation in the chest. In this instance, acupuncture and herbal prescriptions may be used. In the less acute stage these treatments can be supplemented with moxabustion in order to help tonify the deficient Heart Yang. Qigong exercises will be helpful, and a sensible regime of diet and exercise would also be suggested.

Note: In a life-threatening situation involving Heart problems – for example, a full-scale narrowing of the coronary arteries (myocardial infarction) – conventional Western emergency approaches would be most appropriate, although the use of acupuncture may be helpful as a first-aid emergency treatment.

Other Heart Patterns

There are several other Heart patterns that are commonly observed, including

- *Heart Qi deficiency.*
- *Heart Yang deficiency*
- *Collapse of Heart Yang*
- *Heart Blood deficiency*
- *Heart Yin deficiency*
- *Heart Fire blazing*
- *Phlegm Fire agitating the Heart.*
- *Phlegm misting the Heart.*

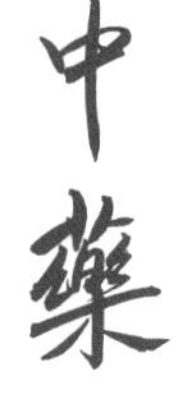

THE SPLEEN

THE MOST important functions of the Spleen are those of transportation and transformation. The Spleen is essential in the extraction and transformation of vital Qi from food and drink, and in distributing this nourishing Qi throughout the body. When the Spleen function is impaired a variety of disharmonies can commonly be seen.

The following case gives an example, enabling us to see, from the perspective of the Eight-Principle patterns, how the Spleen function can be impaired.

Ellen has been feeling very tired and lethargic for some time. She complains of a sensation of fullness in her chest and bloating in her lower abdomen. She is a final-year medical student and she is having to study hard for her examinations, but she is finding that she has a very short concentration span. She admits that her diet has been poor over the last few months. Her tongue is pinkish, with scallop marks around the side and a slightly greasy coating; there are also some cracks across its body. Her pulse is somewhat empty and slippery in character.

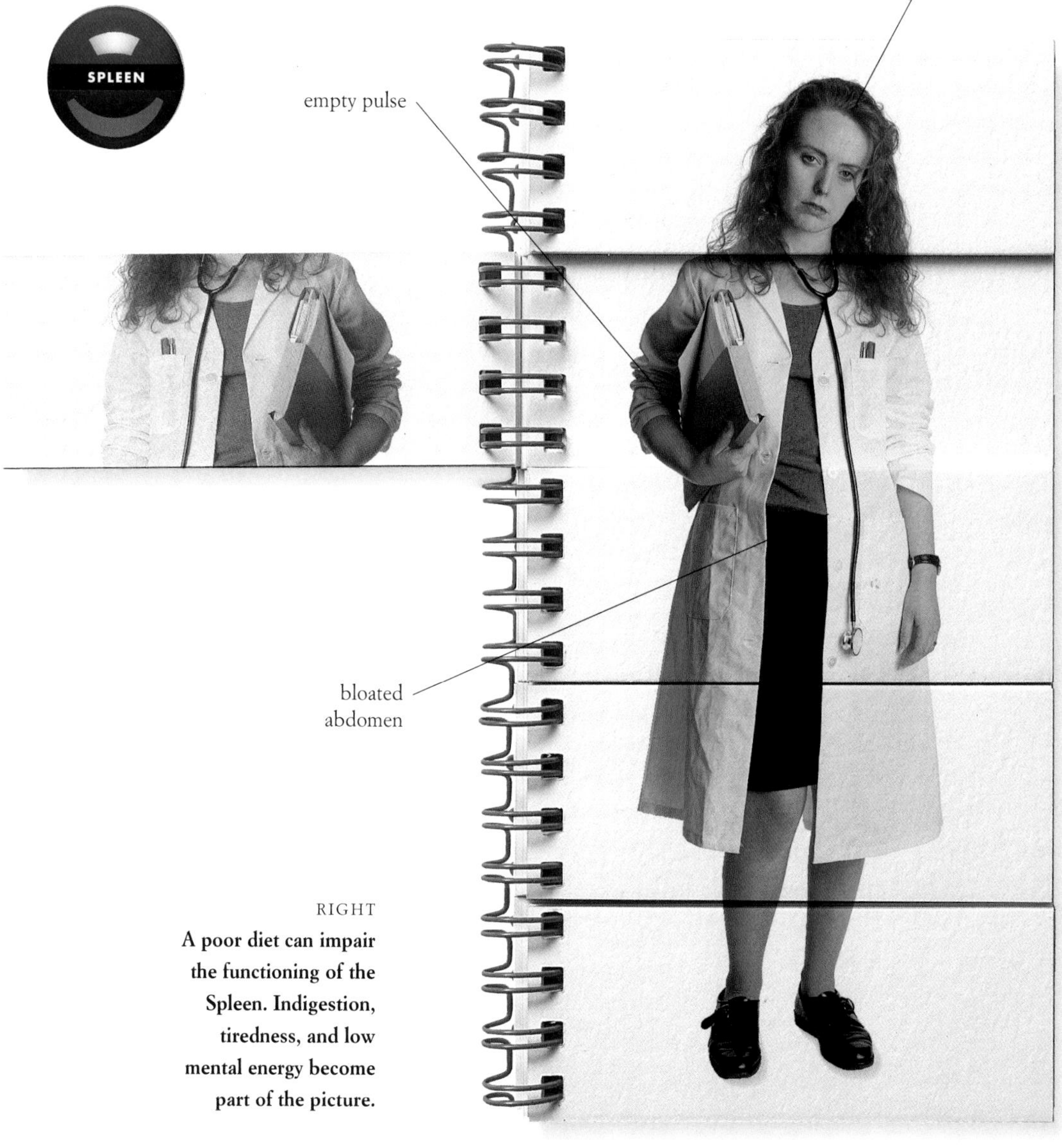

RIGHT

A poor diet can impair the functioning of the Spleen. Indigestion, tiredness, and low mental energy become part of the picture.

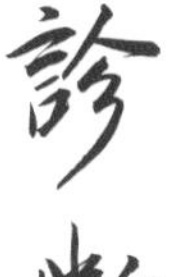

What is Ellen's problem?

The whole pattern is very much one of Deficiency. Ellen has been thinking and studying too much without being careful to get appropriate rest, and, in addition, her diet has been poor. It is likely that these factors have combined to impair Ellen's Spleen function. The Spleen's ability to transfer and transport the damp and greasy food is limited, leading to the feeling of abdominal distension. This may also result in loose stools if it carries on over a long period of time. The greasy coating on the tongue, the slippery pulse, and the stuffiness in the chest suggest that Ellen is retaining Dampness, which further impairs Spleen function. The Spleen fails to send food Qi to the Lungs and this affects the overall Qi of the body, hence Ellen is feeling very tired and lethargic.

Ellen's pattern of disharmony is an example of deficiency of Spleen Qi.

What is the cause of Ellen's problem?

As we have seen, it is likely that the combination of irregular meals and poor diet, along with engaging in too much mental activity, is behind the impairment of Ellen's Spleen function. It is also perhaps exacerbated in Ellen's case by a lack of physical exercise.

Can Chinese medicine help Ellen?

The main treatment principle in this instance will be to clear Damp and tonify the Spleen Qi. Acupuncture with moxabustion may be used, and herbal preparations may also be given. It would also be very important to encourage Ellen to adopt a balanced and regular dietary regime, and to balance her mental exertions with enough rest and regular physical activity. It would also be important for Ellen to avoid too much in the way of energetically damp and cold foods.

In China, students often seek out treatment to strengthen their Spleen in the run-up to important examinations, when they know they are going to be engaged in a lot of mental activity.

Other Spleen Patterns

There are other patterns of Spleen disharmony that may regularly be observed in clinical practice. These include

- *Spleen Yang deficiency*
- *Spleen Qi sinking*
- *Spleen failing to control the Blood*
- *Cold-Damp invading the Spleen*
- *Damp-Heat invading the Spleen.*

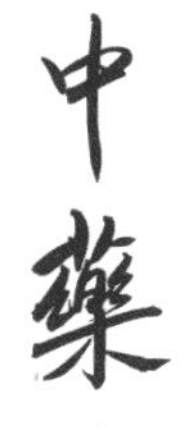

THE LIVER

IN CHINESE medicine the Liver is the Zang organ responsible for promoting the smooth flow of Qi and Blood throughout the body. If Qi flow is impaired for any reason, virtually any of the body systems is susceptible to problems.

Andrea comes to the clinic complaining of very bad premenstrual tension. In the week before her period she experiences abdominal bloating and breast tenderness, and she can be very moody and emotional – tending to fly off the handle at the smallest of things. She reports that she has had a very acrimonious argument with her boyfriend, which has left her feeling very upset. Also she is feeling angry and frustrated in her work because she feels that she has been unfairly passed over for promotion. Her tongue is unremarkable and her pulse is very wiry.

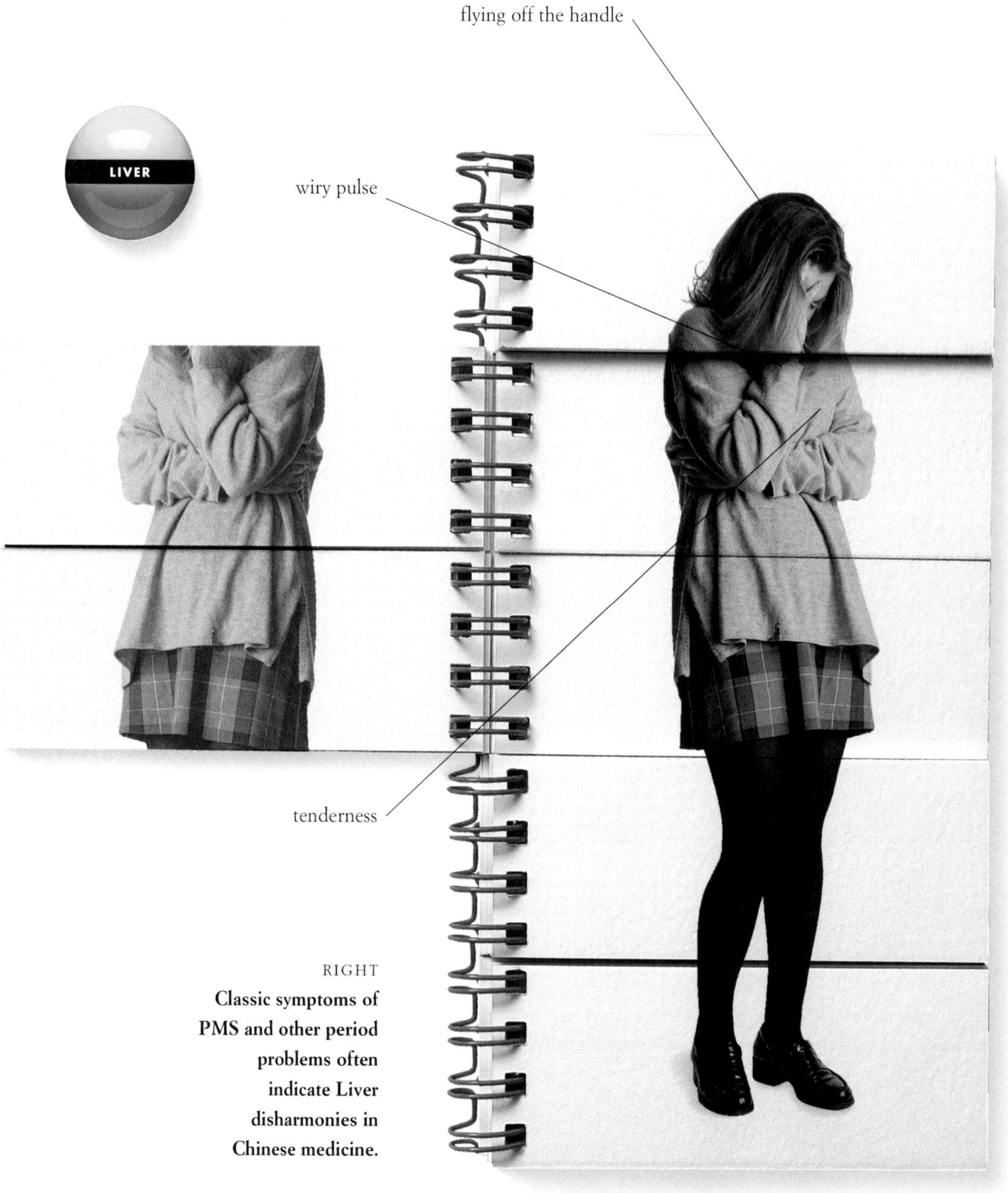

RIGHT
Classic symptoms of PMS and other period problems often indicate Liver disharmonies in Chinese medicine.

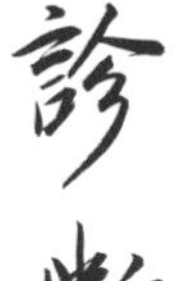

What is happening to Andrea?

ANDREA IS exhibiting all the features of an excess condition in which the Liver's ability to promote the smooth flow of Qi is being seriously impaired. The bloating and the breast tenderness suggest that the Qi is stagnating and not flowing smoothly, and the tendency to emotional outbursts indicates a sudden and uncontrolled shifting of Qi that presents chiefly as an emotional reaction rather than as a physical one.

The situation is somewhat analogous to a pressure cooker that reaches a point of high pressure where it has literally to "blow off" its excess energy in the form of steam.

This collection of signs and symptoms suggests an excess pattern of stagnant Liver Qi.

What is behind Andrea's problem?

WITHOUT A doubt, the major contributory factor relates to Andrea's emotional turmoils. There is clear evidence of anger and resentment in both her private and her professional life. The Zang organ associated with Anger is the Liver, and when Anger is not dealt with appropriately it will build up and impair the spreading function of the Liver. Thus, the Liver Qi stagnates, leading to the symptoms that Andrea reports.

These problems are especially noticeable at the time preceding Andrea's menstrual period, as this is the part of the cycle where the Qi is required forcibly to move the menstrual Blood.

Can Chinese medicine help Andrea's problem?

THE FIRST thing that needs to be said is that Chinese medicine cannot remove the sources of anger, frustration, and resentment in Andrea's life. If she cannot effectively resolve these issues then it is likely that the problem will recur. However, that said, there is no doubt that both acupuncture and herbal remedies can significantly help to move stagnant Liver Qi. In addition, acupressure massage can also be of benefit.

Other Liver Patterns

Other Liver disharmony patterns that can be observed in clinical practice, include

- *Liver Blood and Yin deficiency*
- *Stagnation of Liver Blood*
- *Liver Fire blazing upward*
- *Liver Yang rising*
- *Liver Wind*
- *Cold stagnating in the Liver channel*
- *Damp-Heat in the Liver and Gall Bladder.*

THE KIDNEYS

THE KIDNEYS are very important in Chinese medicine. They are seen as the fundamental root of the Yin and Yang energy of the whole body. When there is a Kidney disharmony, this will inevitably lead to further disharmonies in the other Zangfu systems. Not only do the kidneys maintain the essential warmth of the body, but they also dominate our reproductive processes, regulate fluid balance in the lower Jiao, and support the Lungs in ensuring healthy breathing.

Consider the following case example, which in many ways is typical of older people.

Tom, who is is 66 years old, is complaining that he can never get warm, even when the weather is quite mild. He feels cold especially in his low back area and around his knees. He is slow and stiff in his movements and has a very pale complexion.

Tom has always been a very active man, but now he finds that he has very little energy for anything. He complains of passing a lot of urine and invariably has very loose stools – especially first thing in the morning. His tongue is pale and wet, his ankles are somewhat swollen, and also his pulse feels empty and a bit weak.

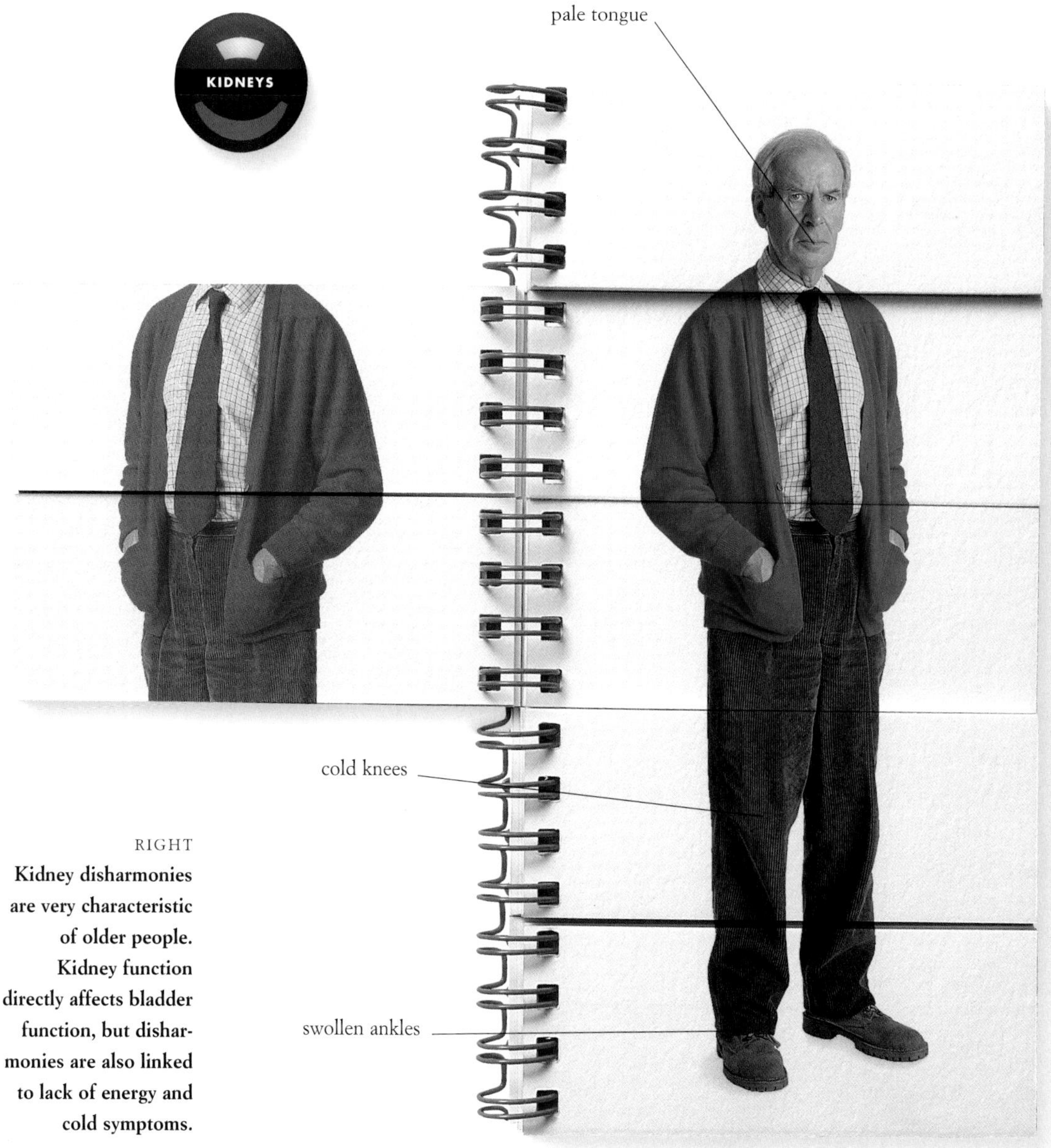

KIDNEYS

pale tongue

cold knees

swollen ankles

RIGHT
Kidney disharmonies are very characteristic of older people. Kidney function directly affects bladder function, but disharmonies are also linked to lack of energy and cold symptoms.

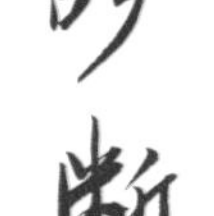

Isn't this what happens to everyone when they get old?

We may think that Tom's condition is a natural result of growing older, but it is interesting to see how it would be viewed from the perspective of Chinese medicine. As we age, our Kidney energy gradually depletes, and eventually there is insufficient Kidney Yang energy to generate "Mingmen Fire," the source of warmth in the whole body. The Kidneys also have a role in strengthening the bones, and any weakness is especially felt around the lower back area.

It is also the case that if the Kidney Yang energy is deficient, this will fail to move Body Fluids around the body, leading to clear, copious urine and the accumulation of fluids under the skin. Hence the problem of edema in the ankles.

There will also be insufficient Yang energy from the Kidneys to support the function of the Spleen, and thus the Spleen energy will tend to descend rather than rise, leading to the problem of loose stools. This is especially a problem early in the morning, when the natural rhythm of the universal energy cycle is at its point of maximum Yin and minimum Yang.

These physical signs and symptoms indicate that the likely explanation is that Tom is experiencing chronic deficiency of Kidney Yang.

What is likely to cause Tom's problem?

It is more than likely that in Tom's case this is a feature of general aging; however, the disharmony may be exacerbated by any long-term illness that depletes the body Qi. It is also believed that too much sexual activity throughout life will deplete the Kidney Qi, ultimately leading to Kidney Yang deficiency.

If there is a poor and inappropriate diet, this will also damage the Spleen, and, over time, internal Damp will accumulate. This will cause changes that will ultimately injure the Kidney Jang energy.

Can Chinese medicine help Tom's problem?

Chinese medicine cannot reverse the natural aging process, but with appropriate changes in lifestyle, it can help to ensure that this process is more one of natural maturation.

Tom would benefit from acupuncture, strong moxabustion to warm the Kidney Yang energy, and Yang-tonifying herbal preparations. In addition, advice could be given to eat warming and nourishing foods and to avoid external factors such as drafts and cold, damp environments.

Given an appropriate combination of these factors, there is every reason to expect that, even at his age, Tom's well-being and quality of life will significantly improve.

Other Kidney Patterns

Chinese medicine sees problems with the Kidneys as predominantly problems of deficiency, although there can be some excess difficulties as well. The more common Kidney disharmonies include

- *Kidney Yin deficiency*
- *Kidney Qi not firm*
- *Kidneys failing to grasp the Qi*
- *Kidney Jing deficiency*
- *Kidney Yin deficiency with Empty Fire*
- *Kidney Yang deficiency with Water overflowing the Lungs or Heart.*

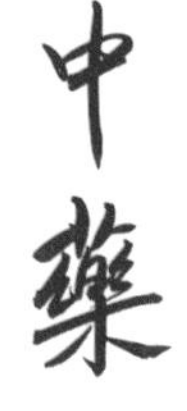

FU ORGAN PATTERNS

WE HAVE seen that the Fu organs are associated with the reception, separation, and distribution of substances. They are thus considered to have a mainly Yang aspect, since movement tends to characterize their function. Since each Fu organ is paired with its equivalent Zang organ, in many clinical contexts there is likely to be a dynamic relationship between any Zang disharmony and the associated Fu organ, and vice versa. Thus, for example, where there is a Liver disharmony this may also involve a Gall Bladder disharmony. However, there are several disharmonies that are seen as being chiefly related to the Fu systems.

THE STOMACH

Bob came to the clinic complaining of a severe burning sensation in his epigastric (upper abdomen) area, accompanied by sour acid regurgitation in his mouth. He said he felt hungry most of the time and he drank a lot of cold drinks. Questioning revealed that Bob's diet was dominated by fast foods – he especially liked curries and deep-fried foods.

He had halitosis (bad breath) and, when questioned, he revealed that his gums would bleed regularly, especially when he brushed his teeth. His tongue was red with a dry yellow coating and his pulse was rapid.

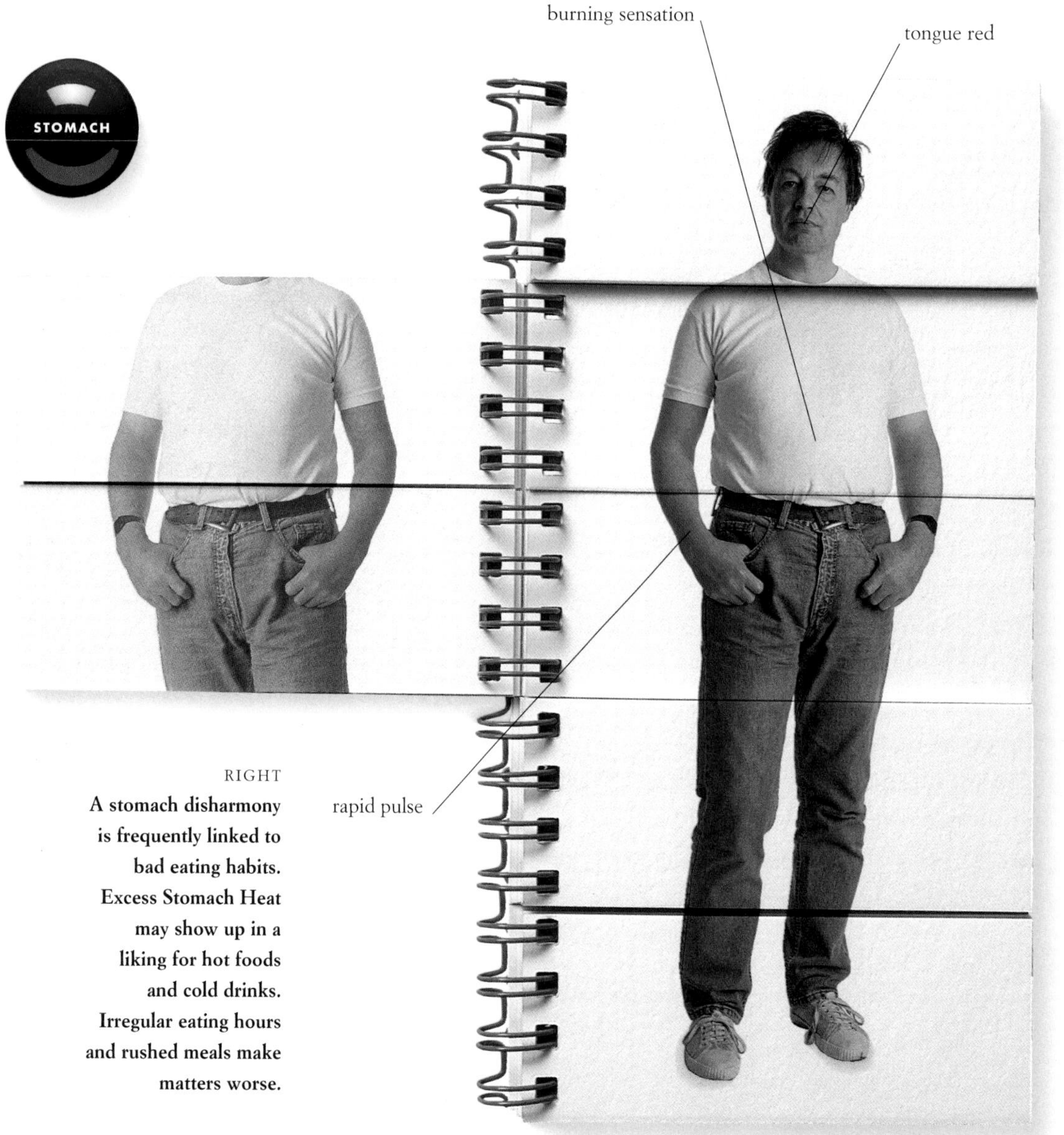

RIGHT
A stomach disharmony is frequently linked to bad eating habits. Excess Stomach Heat may show up in a liking for hot foods and cold drinks. Irregular eating hours and rushed meals make matters worse.

What is the matter with Bob?

Bob is showing evidence of an excess condition involving a lot of internal Heat. The Fu organ system that is affected is that of the Stomach. The Stomach receives the ingested food, and Heat is building up and consuming the Stomach fluids. This internal Heat interferes with the Stomach's natural function of causing the Qi to descend, and the result is that sour Stomach fluids are being regurgitated upward. In some instances this can cause nausea and vomiting as well. The Heat also rises along the line of the Stomach channel to the mouth, causing the bleeding gums. The dry, red tongue with the yellow coat, together with the rapid pulse, indicate the presence of pathological internal Heat.

Bob is suffering from an internal excess disharmony of the Fu system: Stomach Fire.

What has caused Bob's problem?

The major contributory factor to the Stomach Fire disharmony is undoubtedly Bob's dietary habits. A liking for energetically hot and greasy foods takes Heat directly into the Stomach. In addition to this, the lifestyle associated with Bob's eating habits is also very important. This includes factors such as the regularity of meals and the emotional state during eating.

It also involves the actual context for eating: does it happen in a rush while you are doing other things or are meals eaten quietly sitting at the table in a relaxed way?

It is more than likely with a disharmony such as this that there will be external pressures on the individual. These may be felt at work or may have to do with personal relationships, and they will bring a strong emotional component to bear on the situation. Equally, it is more than likely that there will also be a Spleen disharmony present in a situation like this. It is very possible that disharmonies of other Zangfu systems contribute to this as well.

What can Chinese medicine do to help Bob?

The important thing in a condition of a full Heat excess is to clear the excess as quickly as possible. Acupuncture can be used to clear Heat and to stimulate the Stomach's natural descending function; herbal prescriptions may also be given.

In addition to this direct treatment to clear the excess Heat and regulate the Stomach, Bob will have to look at his dietary habits as a matter of urgency. If he does not do this, then there is no doubt that the condition will recur and will possibly worsen, seriously damaging other Zangfu systems.

Bob's case is offered as one example of a disharmony more directly affecting the Fu system: there are a range of others. It is not necessary to deal with these in any more detail. The important thing to understand is that disharmonies do not simply confine themselves to the five major Yin organ systems of the Zang.

Other Fu patterns

There is a variety of patterns that are commonly seen in relation to the Fu organ system and they are very commonly linked to the paired Zang organ system. The practitioner will make these connections both in diagnosis and in treatment planning.

Stomach may be linked with the Spleen
Bladder may be linked with the Kidney
Large Intestine may be linked with the Lung
Small Intestine may be linked with Heat
Gall Bladder may be linked with the Liver

CONCLUSION

THE CASE histories we have looked at give a detailed insight into how the Principle patterns can be further refined to look at patterns of Zangfu disharmony. These are just a few examples to illustrate the kind of process that a practitioner of Chinese medicine will go through in looking at the range of signs and symptoms that the patient presents.

In addition to the whole spectrum of Fu disharmonies, there are several other typical combined patterns that have not been mentioned. In such combinations there are characteristic linkages between the disharmonies of certain organs. For example, Kidney and Lung Yin deficiency often occur together with a mutual reinforcement, one of the other.

It is also worth bearing in mind that any patient is going to present several disharmony patterns at the same time. The practitioner has to be able to identify the various patterns that are occurring, whether they are excess or deficient, and to plan a treatment program accordingly.

WHAT PATTERNS CAN YOU SEE?

It may be useful to end this part of the book by giving you, the reader, the opportunity to try to identify the patterns that may be present in a given case history. Remember, this book is not offering anything that remotely approaches a training guide to Chinese medicine, but perhaps it can begin to help you think in the way that a Chinese medical practitioner thinks.

Read the following typical case history carefully and try to decide what is going on. Make a note of any signs or symptoms that you can identify and allocate them to the categories of the Eight-Principle patterns:

Yin	Yang
Interior	**Exterior**
Cold	Heat
Deficiency	**Excess**

Decide whether you think the condition is predominantly Yin or Yang in nature. Finally, do you think the pattern that you identify can be associated with any Zangfu pattern?

Maria is a 32-year-old nurse. She is going through a very difficult divorce and is fighting over the custody of her two children with her estranged husband. In addition to this, she has recently been promoted at work, and she is under a lot of pressure there to fulfill the demands made on her by her new job.

She is complaining of feelings of abdominal distension, fullness in her chest, and a constriction in her throat. She says that she has absolutely no energy and her legs feel like lead. She finds it difficult to lift and work with her patients. Her symptoms get worse prior to her period, and she gets very moody and irritable with her children and work colleagues at this time.

She says that her diet is "OK," but she admits to being a bit obsessive about her weight and she eats a lot of salads at times and then binges on "junk food," especially when she is very tense. As she puts it, "Whenever I have to talk to my husband, my diet goes right out the window."

Her tongue is a normal pinkish color with slight toothmarks on the side. Her pulse is wiry.

Well, what do you think might be going on with Maria? Compare your ideas with my suggestions.

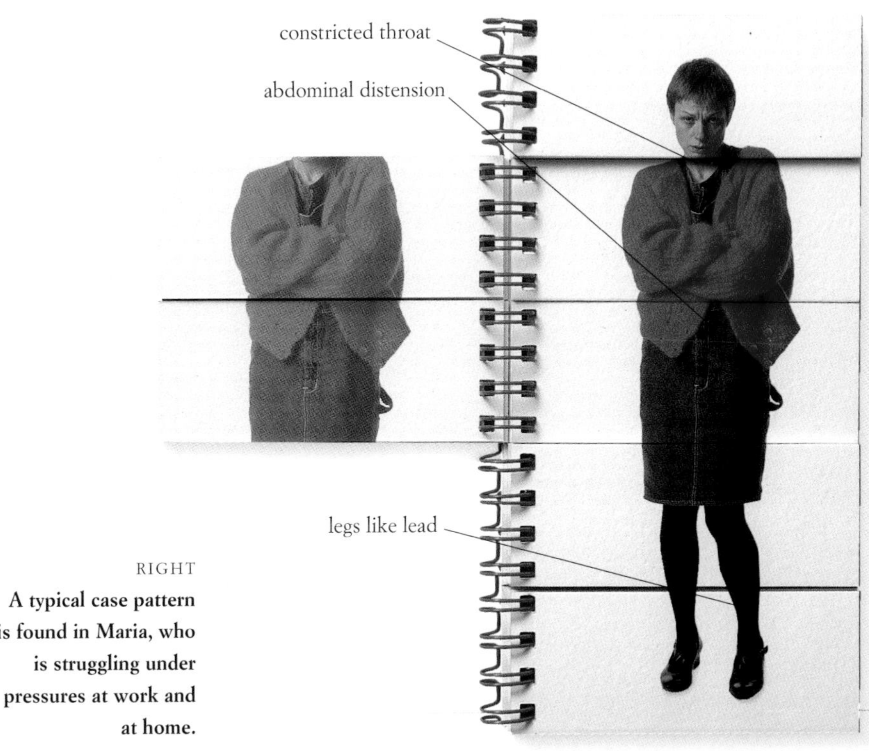

RIGHT
A typical case pattern is found in Maria, who is struggling under pressures at work and at home.

General considerations

In this case study there are various factors about the general situation that are worth singling out.

1. Maria is a nurse and is likely to be engaged in some quite heavy physical work.
2. She has a demanding position at work and is under a lot of pressure.
3. She is in an extremely stressful situation as a result of her marriage breakdown.
4. Her dietary patterns are not good.
5. Emotionally, she is very moody and irritable.

What is going on?

The major predisposing problem is probably one of stress, from work and from the family situation. This has caused her Liver Qi to become stagnant., as suggested by the pattern of emotional outbursts (worse before a period), the constricted throat, and the wiry pulse.

It is likely that the Liver disharmony has invaded the Spleen, in itself deficient because of irregular and inconsistent dietary habits. This will produce Qi-deficient symptoms such as a feeling of being bloated, with heavy legs and general lethargy. The slight toothmarking also suggests Spleen Qi deficiency. So the diagnosis would be: Liver Qi stagnation (excess pattern) and Spleen Qi deficiency (deficient pattern).

TREATMENT

The principle would be to promote the smooth flow of Liver Qi and to tonify the Spleen. Maria should adopt a more balanced dietary pattern and perhaps take counseling to help her through her marital breakup. As for Chinese medicine, acupuncture and/or herbal remedies would be appropriate.

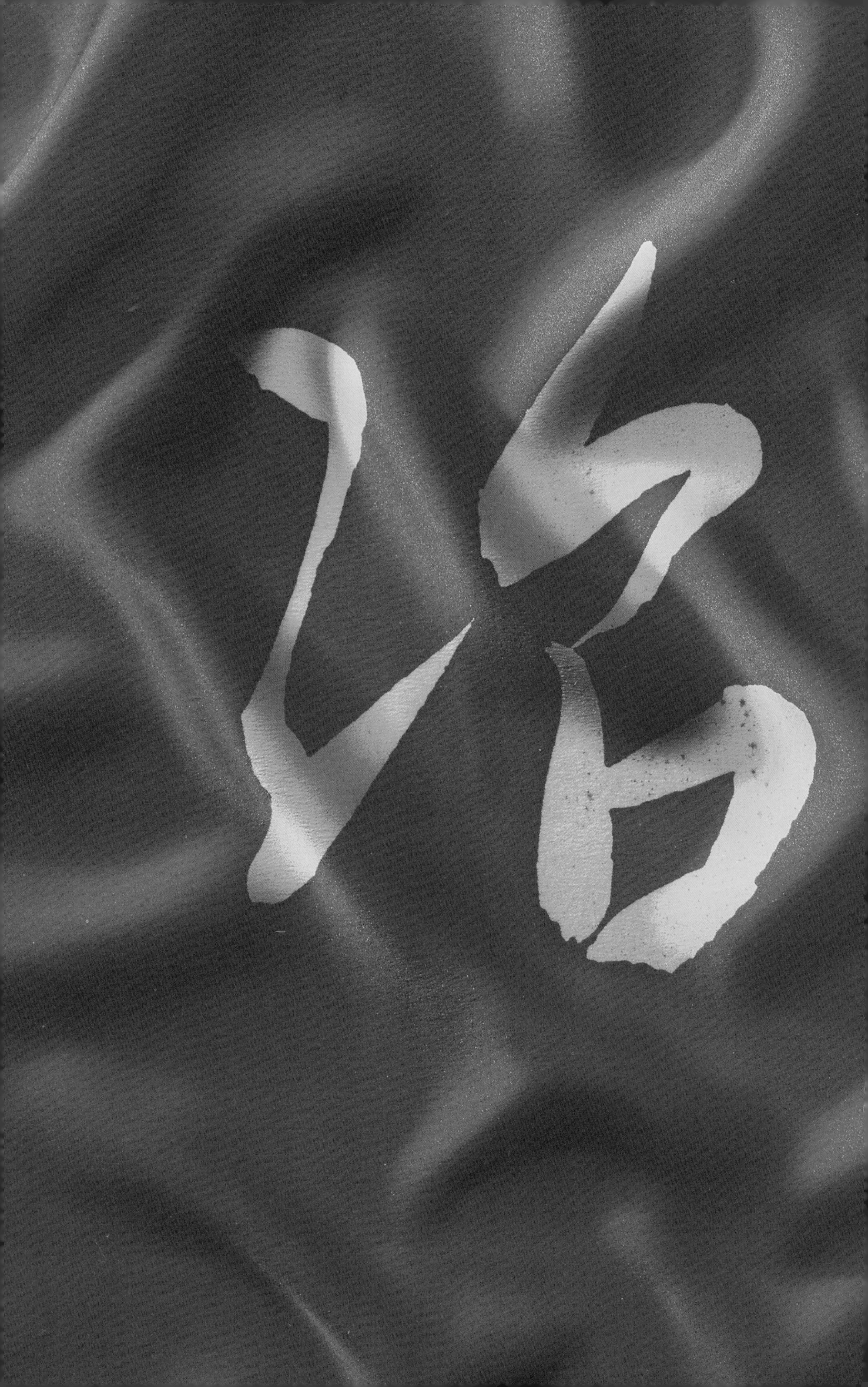

THE CHINESE APPROACH TO TREATMENT

治療

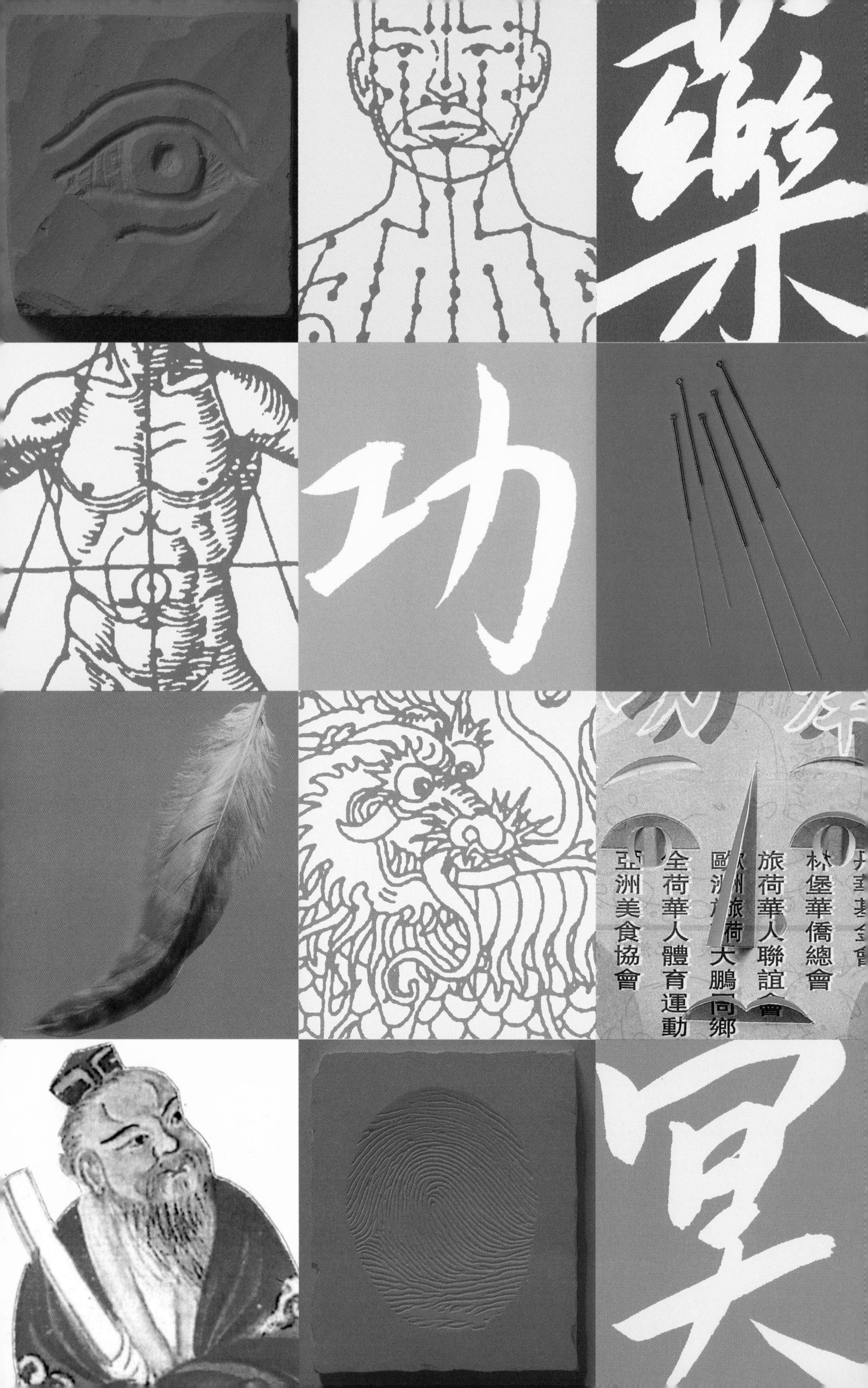
功
旅荷華人聯誼會
全荷華人體育運動
亞洲美食協會

THE MODALITIES

HAVING SET out the principles underlying the Chinese view of the human body and its dysfunctions, we can now look at the approaches (modalities) that have been developed to treat disharmonies and facilitate the individual's return to balance and good health. Acupuncture, herbal medicine, moxabustion, cupping, acupressure massage, Qigong, diet, and general approach to lifestyle factors (including Feng Shui) are discussed.

All medicine arises out of the need to avoid pain and keep illness and disability at bay, and the desire to lead a healthy and fulfilling life. Philosophies, theories, and principles must lead to forms of treatment that work.

As has been demonstrated in the earlier sections of this book, Chinese medicine has as rich a philosophical and theoretical background as can be found anywhere in human experience. But what has rooted it into the social fabric of generations of Chinese, is the fact that it has spawned practical treatment approaches that can relieve human suffering, from a minor irritation to a life-threatening situation, in a very real way.

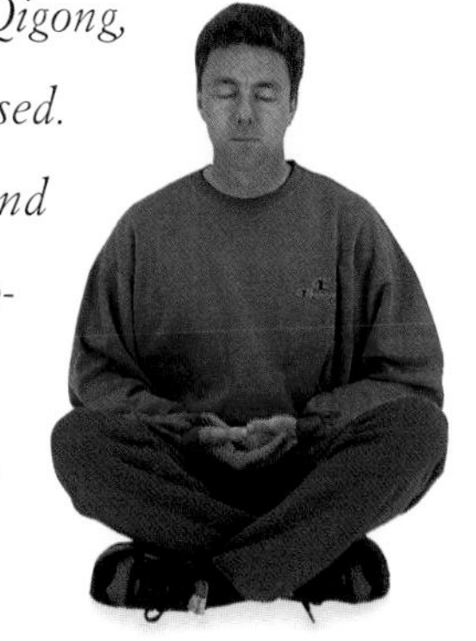

ABOVE
Therapeutic exercise to sustain and restore harmony has been advocated since at least the second century A.D.

This book aims to inform readers how Chinese medicine can help them, or their friends and loved ones, with their illnesses and health concerns. It does not teach "how to do" Chinese medicine. The emphasis is on demystifying the process, not on "do-it-yourself" tips. From earlier chapters it can be seen that Chinese medicine, although logical, elegant, subtle, and holistic, is certainly not simple. The book describes some exercises and techniques that can be tried at home and gives useful pieces of advice; but the overall message is quite clear – if you want to address specific problems with Chinese medicine, you need to seek out a fully qualified and experienced practitioner.

ABOVE
The herb Si Di Huang. Accounts of Chinese herbal medicine date from the third century BC.

For this reason, the discussions on the various modalities in the following sections aim simply to outline connections that can be made between the treatments in general and the underlying principles of Chinese medicine. However, acupuncture point locations and prescriptions are not given, there is no information on the herbs to use for particular disharmonies, no description of specific Qigong exercises, and so on. All use of treatment protocols in Chinese medicine requires appropriate professional training and can be gleaned in only a very superficial way from any book – no matter how thorough or well written.

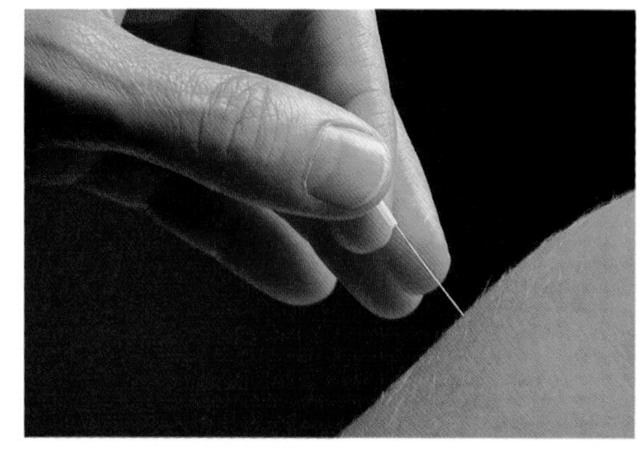

RIGHT
Treatment by acupuncture is described in the *Neijing*, an important Chinese medical text that dates from 200 B.C.

PRINCIPLES OF TREATMENT

REGARDLESS OF which treatment approach is decided upon, there are always common aims and objectives involved. The principles behind all forms of treatment derive from the Eight-Principle patterns, elaborated on in the discussions on the Zangfu disharmonies. A pressure cooker provides a useful analogy to help in understanding the aims behind any form of treatment.

When the cooker is operating efficiently, the pressure inside is maintained at an optimum level in order to cook the food. This is achieved by bringing the cooker up to the appropriate temperature and keeping it at this level by using a simple valve. The whole system is in dynamic equilibrium, and the energy is used to achieve the ends for which the system was designed. However, problems can arise.

EXCESS

If the valve blocks and the pressure inside the cooker rises beyond the optimum, the whole system becomes unstable. Unless some action is taken, the cooker will soon explode. It could be said that the cooker has experienced a condition of excess, which must be reduced in order to re-establish equilibrium.

DEFICIENCY

If the valve is faulty and pressure is leaking away from the cooker at a faster rate than it is building up, it will take forever to cook the food – or it may not cook at all if pressure is lost altogether. In this instance the cooker has experienced a condition of deficiency. The system needs to be tonified in order to build up the pressure to the optimum level necessary for equilibrium.

TREATMENT

When a condition of excess is apparent in the disharmony, it is necessary for the treatment to focus on reducing the excess and getting rid of the factors – whatever they may be – that brought about the excess in the first place. If a condition of deficiency is apparent in the disharmony, it is necessary for the treatment to focus on tonifying the deficiency and ensuring that the energy is

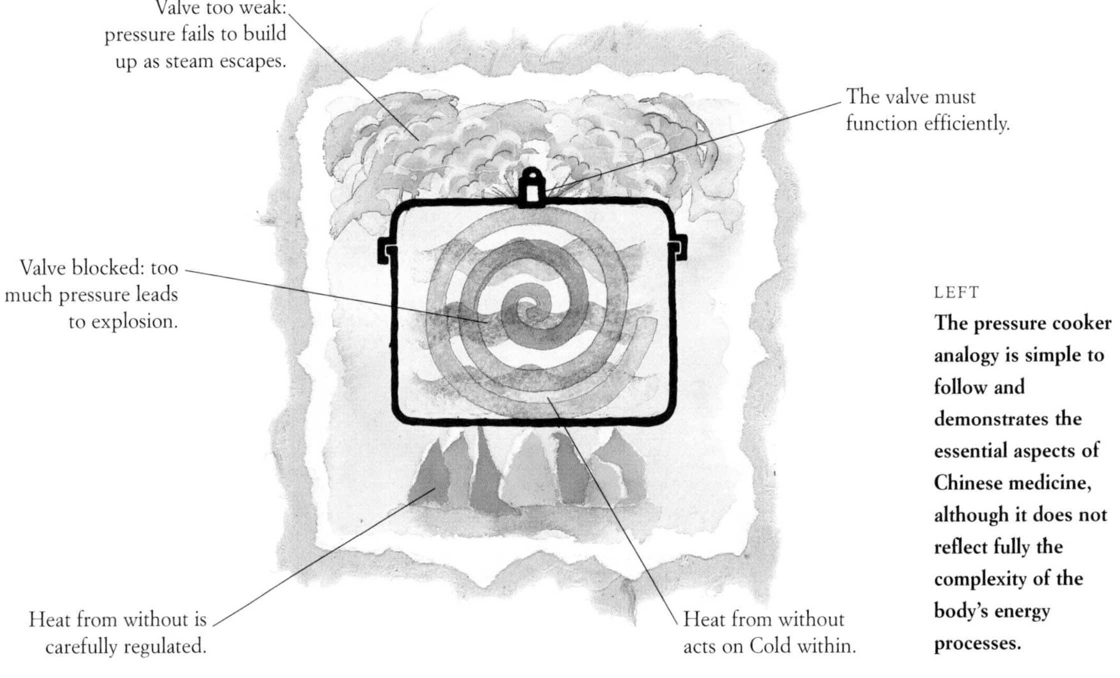

LEFT
The pressure cooker analogy is simple to follow and demonstrates the essential aspects of Chinese medicine, although it does not reflect fully the complexity of the body's energy processes.

PRINCIPLES OF HEAT AND COLD

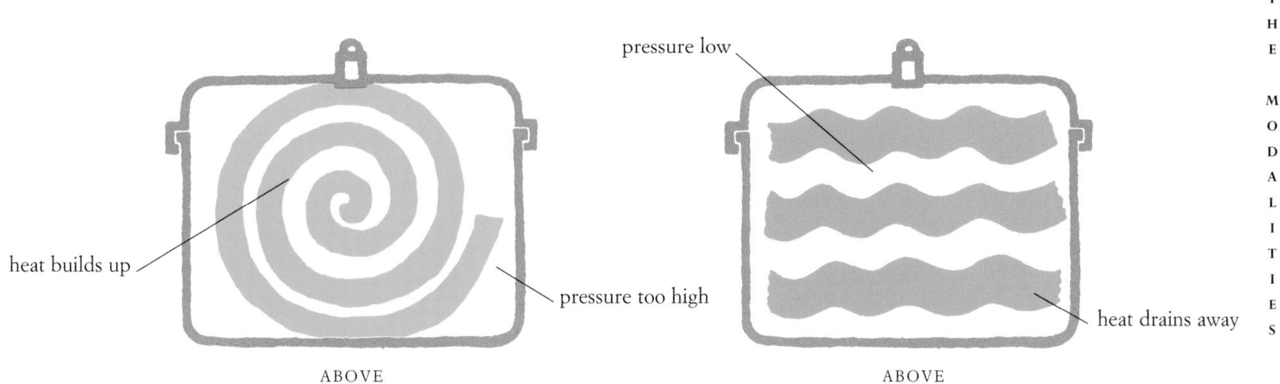

ABOVE
If there is too much Heat in the body, Heat needs to be expelled.

ABOVE
If there is too little Heat, the body must be warmed.

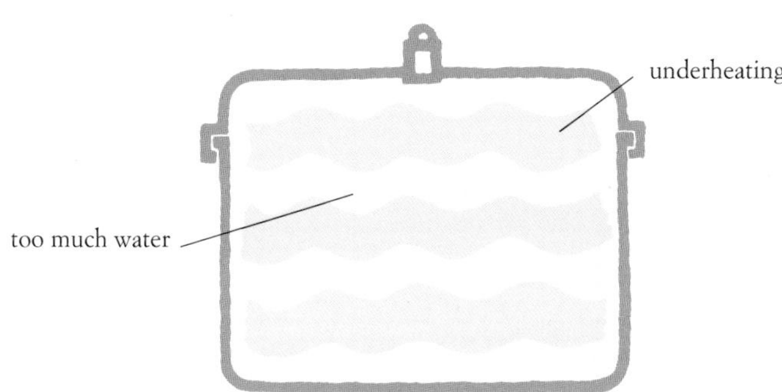

ABOVE
If there is too much water (Damp) in the body, this can turn to Phlegm under the action of internal Heat. Excess Damp needs to be drained (or resolved), just as excess water should be removed from the pressure cooker.

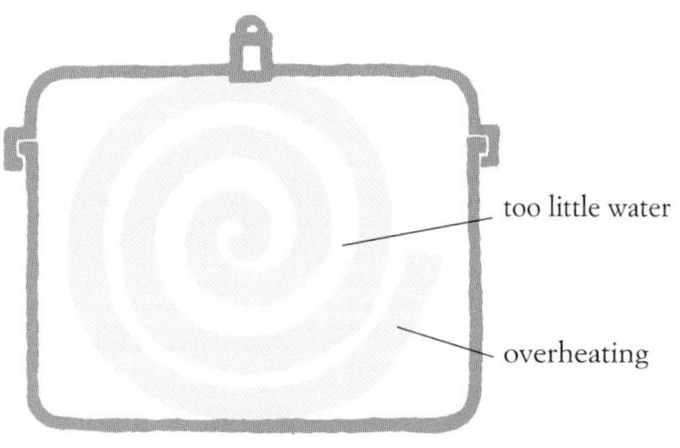

ABOVE
Insufficient Body Fluids make the body dry and flaky, as seen in dry skin conditions. The production of fluids must be promoted and Heat brought back into equilibrium (as in the pressure cooker water is added and heat adjusted).

maintained at the appropriate level to ensure health and well-being.

The pressure cooker analogy can also demonstrate the Principles of Heat and Cold. The cooker requires a certain amount of Heat to work efficiently – too much or too little causes problems. Similarly, the body requires an optimum level of Heat to function efficiently. Too much Heat leads to an excess, and too little Heat leads to a deficiency. If too much Cold is present, this also produces an excess – in much the same way that, if the cooker is exposed to extreme Cold, its fluids freeze, expand, and cause severe damage.

ESSENTIAL ASPECTS OF TREATMENT

- When a deficiency exists, the energy is tonified.
- When an excess exists, the energy is reduced.
- When too much Heat is present, it is expelled or cooled.
- When too much Cold is present, it is expelled or warmed.
- When Damp is present, it is resolved.
- When Phlegm is present, it is resolved.

PRINCIPLES OF DIAGNOSIS

ONE PROBLEM when seeking help from Chinese medicine is that there are very few practitioners or practices offering all the modalities. For example, a growing number of practitioners are trained and qualified in acupuncture, but a much small number are also trained in Chinese herbal medicine. Whereas in mainstream medicine there is a well-developed network of specialisms and systems for the referral of patients, in Chinese medicine individuals have to make their own decisions as to where to seek help. It is essential to consult a fully qualified practitioner – not only are you putting yourself in his or her hands, but you are also more than likely seeking the help of a modality of medicine that is new and strange to you.

To find out which modality of Chinese medicine is most appropriate for you, it is invariably necessary to seek advice from a professional. However, the following hierarchical approach offers some general principles.

You are quite well but wish to use the principles and approaches of Chinese medicine to stay fit and healthy.
✦ Consider dietary advice and general lifestyle principles. ✦ Consider going to a Qigong or Taiji class. ✦ General acupressure massage to relax and tonify may be appropriate.

You have a minor ache or pain, possibly following an injury or simple accident. The problem is acute and superficial – usually at the channel level.
✦ Acupressure massage may be helpful. ✦ Self-help acupoint stimulation with finger pressure may be appropriate. ✦ Qigong exercise may help.

You have a minor problem, but it is not clearing.
✦ Consult a professional practitioner – acupuncture is often most effective with stubborn stagnation problems in the channels and collaterals. ✦ The use of acupressure and moxabustion may be suggested. These can sometimes be used as part of a self-help regime (subject to the advice of the practitioner).

You are feeling quite unwell – either an acute short-term problem or a more long-term chronic problem.
✦ Consult a professional practitioner of acupuncture and/or herbal medicine without delay.

You are not feeling that unwell, but your life is generally out of balance and you feel vulnerable, often in a way that is hard to pin down.
✦ Consult a professional practitioner to clarify the nature of any pattern of disharmony that may be present. ✦ Consider calling in a Feng Shui practitioner to analyze the energetic dynamics of your house and/or workplace – the contextual energetics can often upset your own biological energetics.

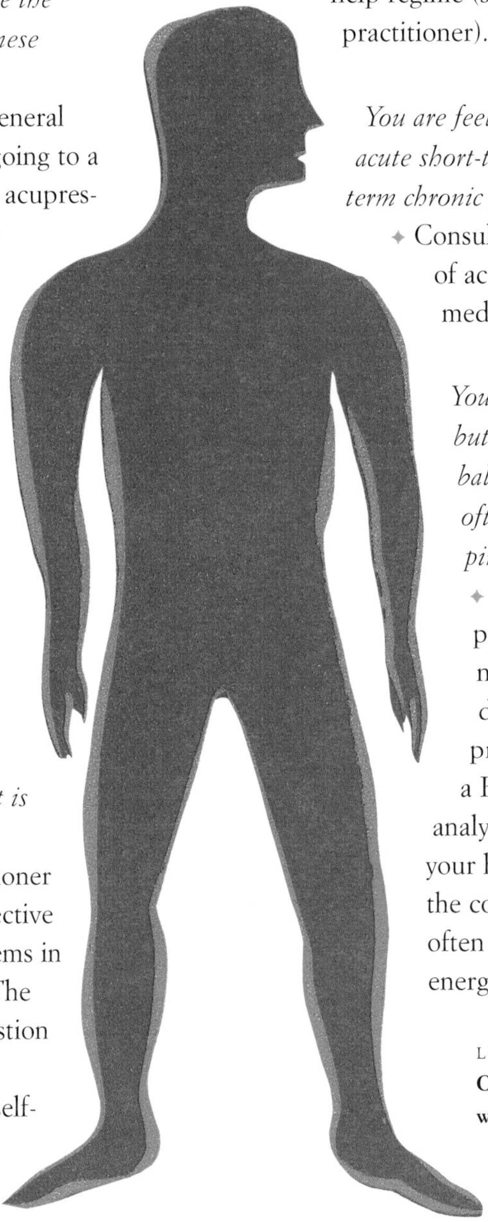

LEFT
Chinese medicine offers many ways of keeping you well.

PREVENTION

THE IDEAL for any system of medicine is to prevent illness and disharmony from developing in the first place. In this regard, the modalities of Chinese medicine may well have something to offer those people who are concerned about how best to look after themselves and how to stay fit and healthy.

Generally speaking, acupuncture and herbal medicine remain the preserve of the professional practitioner, and both modalities are more likely to be used once a disharmony is apparent. It is, however, possible to use both also in a preventive role.

HERBAL MEDICINE

Certain patent herbal formulae can be used to keep the Qi and Blood tonified, thus keeping the body's energetic system working effectively. But no product based on Chinese herbs can provide a complete elixir of good health. Also, certain remedies, when taken on their own, can be positively counter-productive – gingseng (Ren Shen), for example. The best advice is to always consult a herbal practitioner before taking herbal preparations of any kind – even if you are simply looking to stay healthy.

ACUPUNCTURE

Acupuncture too can be used in a preventive way. An over-worked brain can damage the Spleen and lead to Qi deficiency. Since acupuncture can be used to keep the Spleen tonified, it is therefore useful in situations requiring intense mental activity – when one is studying for an exam, for example.

RIGHT
In the hands of an experienced professional, each modality can help to tone the body to prevent disease.

LIFESTYLE PRACTICES

In terms of maintaining good health, Chinese medicine is of most benefit in the area of general lifestyle practices. Much of the advice regarding diet, habits, and exercise is not wholly unique to Chinese medicine; it represents good common sense in any context, although some of the ideas regarding healthy dietary patterns may challenge certain "sacred cows" (for example, eating a lot of cold, raw foods such as salads can be considered positively bad from the perspective of Chinese medicine).

Learning Qigong or Taiji can be a very effective way of maintaining good health, but it is important to find an experienced and reputable teacher. A Feng Shui consultation on your home and/or workplace can lead to changes that will enhance many aspects of your life, but, again, it is important to get advice from a reliable and professional practitioner.

The practices of Chinese medicine can become an integral part of a healthy lifestyle. In the following chapters you can consider what relevance they may have in your life.

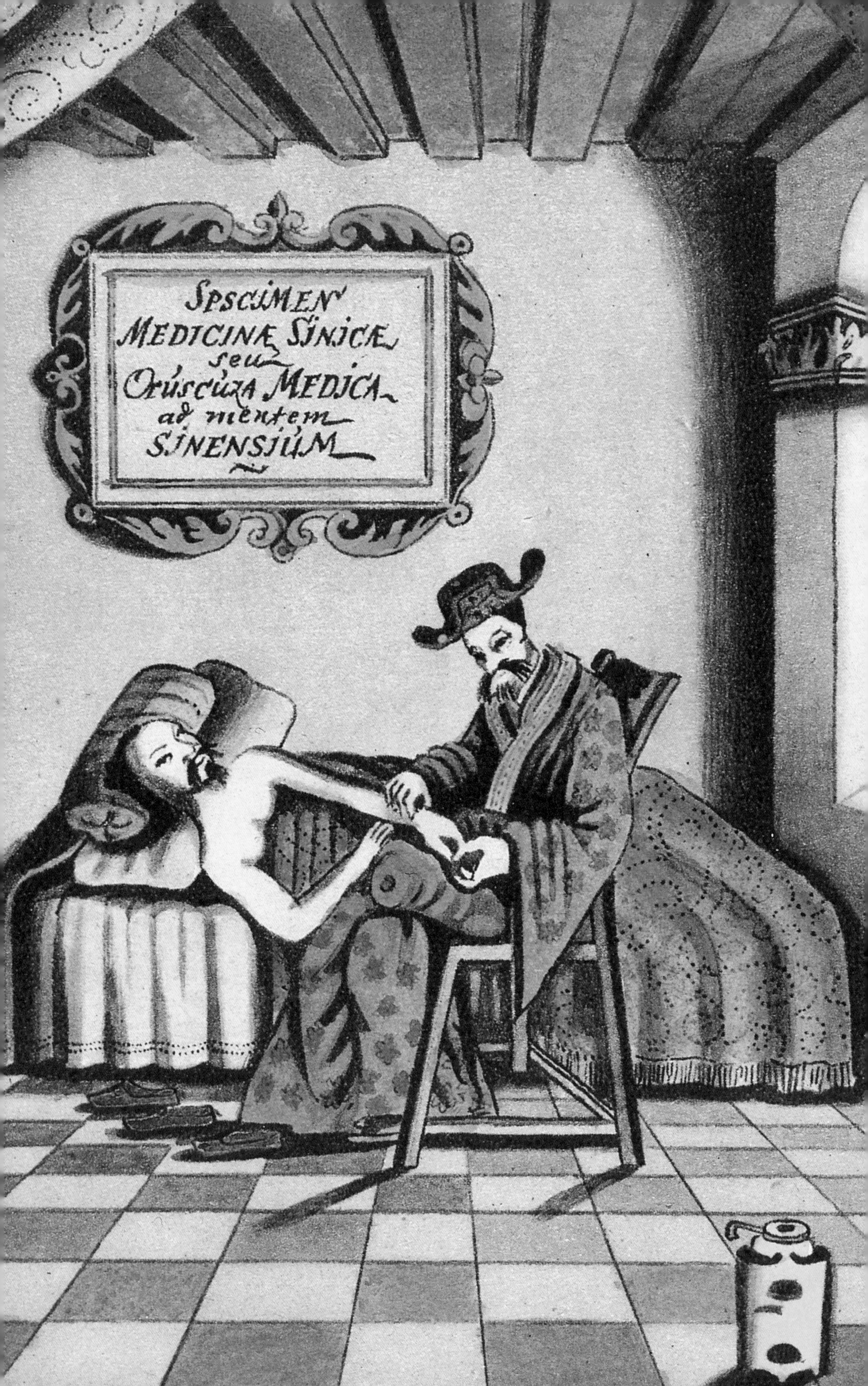
SPECIMEN
MEDICINÆ SINICÆ
seu
OPUSCULA MEDICA
ad mentem
SINENSIUM

ACUPUNCTURE

THE IMAGE *of the body being pierced by fine needles in an apparently random way is perhaps the stereotypical view of Chinese medicine. At face value, it must be difficult to imagine how this kind of treatment can benefit particular problems. For most people in the West, Chinese medicine will start and end with this image – somewhat arcane and bizarre, and something to be doubted or feared. But the Chinese have been using and refining the techniques of acupuncture for more than 3,000 years, with consistent and remarkable effect.*

It should be remembered that acupuncture has evolved as an essentially empirical science – in other words, it is founded on a body of knowledge that has been developed from the on-going and systematic observation of the effect of needling specific points and areas of the body. Initially, crude needles, made from sharpened stones, animal bones, or bamboo, were used "to remove obstructions from the channels and regulate the flow of Blood and Qi." This quote, from some point between 200 B.C. *and* A.D. *100, indicates that the theory of acupuncture has been in place for centuries. Over time, the initial practice of inserting "needles" into "ashi" points (where pain is experienced) was systematically developed: the energetic model of Qi, Jing, Blood, and Fluids was articulated, and the energy flows were mapped as the meridians of the body. Specific points were identified and their actions recorded. Even now, the theory of acupuncture continues to be developed and refined.*

In terms of clinical practice, acupuncture today is a far cry from the early developments, but fundamentally the theories and principles remain the same.

ABOVE
Acupuncture "needles" in earlier times were far from being the refined instruments used today.

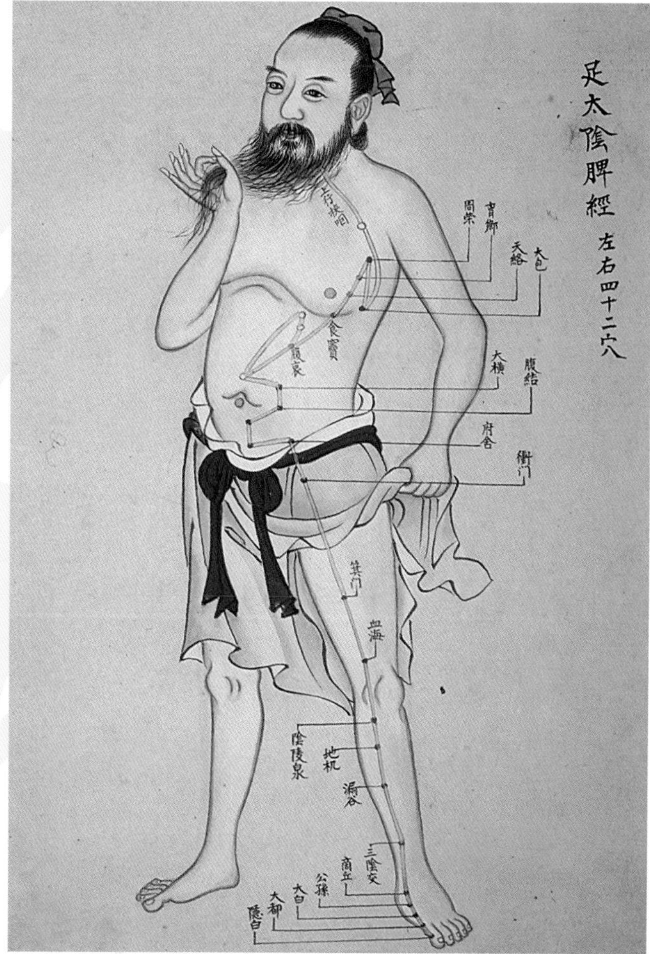

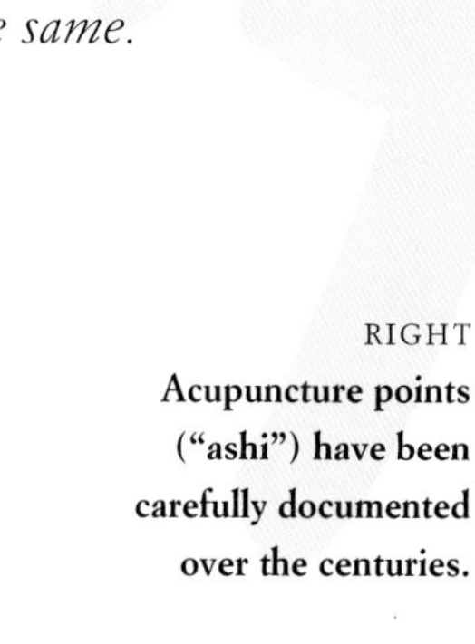

RIGHT
Acupuncture points ("ashi") have been carefully documented over the centuries.

LEFT
Acupuncture has always been preceded by a lengthy diagnosis.

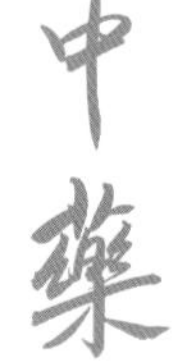

HOW ACUPUNCTURE CAN HELP

IN CHINESE medicine, a disharmony can result from a variety of factors, including

- *a deficiency or an excess of the Yin and/or Yang energy of the body*
- *an invasion by an external pathogenic factor, which may remain superficially on the outside of the body or penetrate more deeply into the interior of the body*
- *a problem at the level of the channels or the collaterals, or affecting the functioning of the internal Zangfu system of the body*
- *Heat or Cold associated with the disharmony.*

The diagnosis of the patient's disharmony in terms of the Eight-Principle patterns leads to an understanding of what the treatment seeks to achieve. Acupuncture works by addressing the identified treatment principles. Thus, for example, when a pattern of deficiency is identified, acupuncture is used to tonify the appropriate energy system of the body. Since Chinese medicine sees all illness as a process of energetic disharmony – which acupuncture can help to reestablish – there are no disorders for which this form of treatment is inappropriate. The conditions that acupuncture can help, and how, are summarized in the following table.

There are very few situations where acupuncture is contraindicated. The following are the most common.

- Where the patient has a hemophilic condition.
- Where the patient is pregnant (certain points and needle manipulations are contraindicated in pregnancy).
- Where the patient has a severe psychotic condition or has recently taken drugs or alcohol. Although acupuncture would generally be contraindicated in these circumstances, it should be stressed that it can be very helpful in drug and alcohol rehabilitation regimes.

LEVEL OF PROBLEM	ACUPUNCTURE FUNCTION	COMMENTS
Channel problems (superficial)	Moves Qi, clears stagnation, and expells external pathogenic factors. Local and distal points may be used. Often very quick.	*A lot of pain problems on exterior of body and acute conditions are treated at this level.*
Zangfu disharmony (interior)	Choice of points dictated by pattern of disharmony and Zangfu system affected.	*Chronic and long-term problems, of both excess and deficiency, are treated, but treatment may be protracted.*
Combination	Can be used to treat various levels of problem at once. Priorities need to be set; an excess is usually treated before a deficiency.	*Often used in conjunction with other treatment options – herbs, for example.*

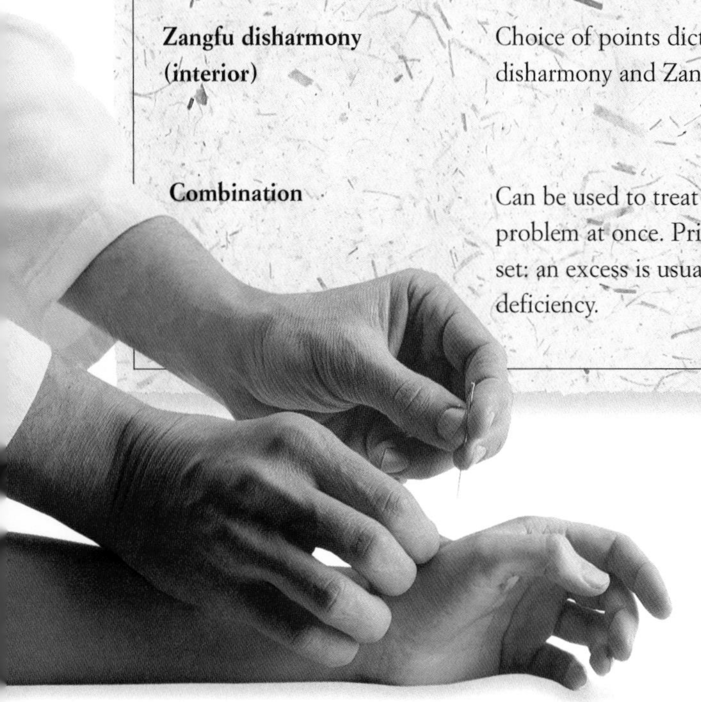

LEFT
Many conditions can be cured or at least ameliorated by acupuncture, administered by a qualified and experienced practitioner. A distal point (farthest from the site of the symptoms) is usually needled, as well as local points. A course of treatment is generally required, although results may sometimes be immediate and dramatic.

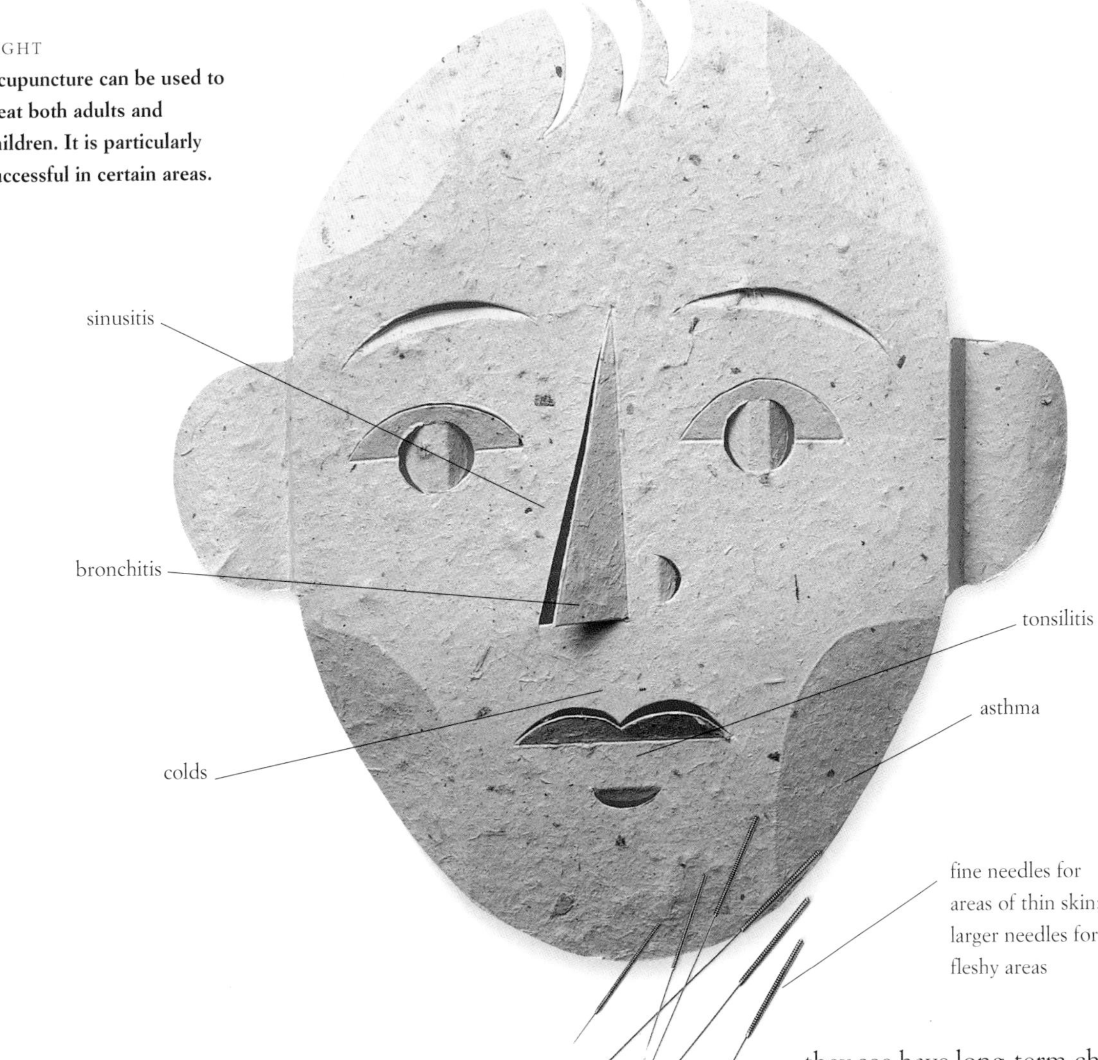

RIGHT
Acupuncture can be used to treat both adults and children. It is particularly successful in certain areas.

There are no contraindications for the use of acupuncture in the treatment of patients with HIV-related disorders, although rigorous hygiene protocols must be adhered to. Given the energetic nature of most HIV-related disorders, acupuncture can be very helpful to patients suffering from Aids since it can address a particular disharmony in a very specific manner – often more effectively than drugs. Acupuncture cannot offer a cure for Aids, but it can be most helpful in supporting the management of a variety of symptoms connected with it.

There are some conditions – psoriasis and eczema, for example – where acupuncture may have limited success on its own, but for these it can be effective alongside other treatments, especially herbal remedies.

In the West, the problem for many practitioners of acupuncture is that most people they see have long-term chronic conditions. For these patients acupuncture is very often a last resort, and in such situations progress is likely to be slow, with a large number of treatments being required. This, of course, is not always the case; sometimes acupuncture can produce rapid and dramatic results. Also, as Chinese medicine becomes more established in the West, a growing number of patients are choosing this as their first option for healthcare, and the range of conditions being successfully treated with acupuncture is growing all the time.

The rule of thumb for patients considering acupuncture is to assume that it will be able to help their condition – whatever it is. Thereafter, provided they consult an appropriately trained and experienced practitioner, they will be able to discuss in detail what acupuncture can do for their specific problem.

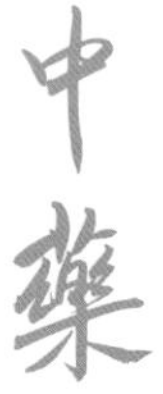

TOOLS AND TECHNIQUES

NEEDLES

Early needles were developed from sharpened stones, bamboo, and animal bones; and over the centuries, techniques have been refined to produce very fine steel needles. Initially, needles were sterilized and reused, and this practice remains the norm in China today. Sterilization standards are now very exacting, and practitioners in the West must follow rigorous guidelines. If a practitioner reuses needles, patients should satisfy themselves as to the standards of sterilization procedures. (Because of HIV and related disorders, neither patients nor practitioners can afford to be anything other than scrupulous in terms of needle cleanliness.)

ABOVE
Needles are always kept in totally sterile packs.

By far the most common practice in the West nowadays is the use of disposable needles – manufactured and packed under sterile conditions in foil-backed blister packs or in packs with guide tubes. Different manufacturers adopt slightly different packaging approaches, but the principle – one-time use followed by disposal – remains consistent. The used needles are stored safely in a "sharps" box and subsequently incinerated to dispose of them.

Needles are available in varying lengths and thicknesses. The choice of

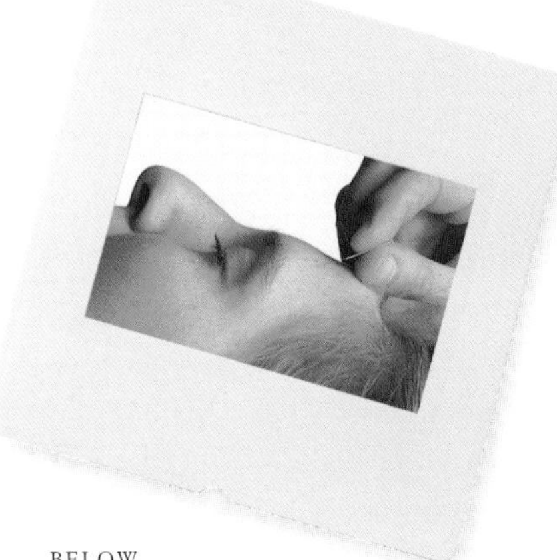

BELOW
Bony areas such as the forehead are needled superficially, with the needle at an angle.

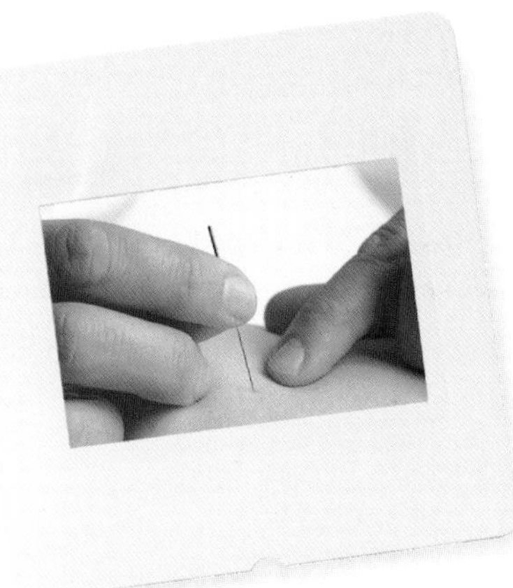

BELOW
Needles are usually inserted upright in fleshy areas such as the buttocks.

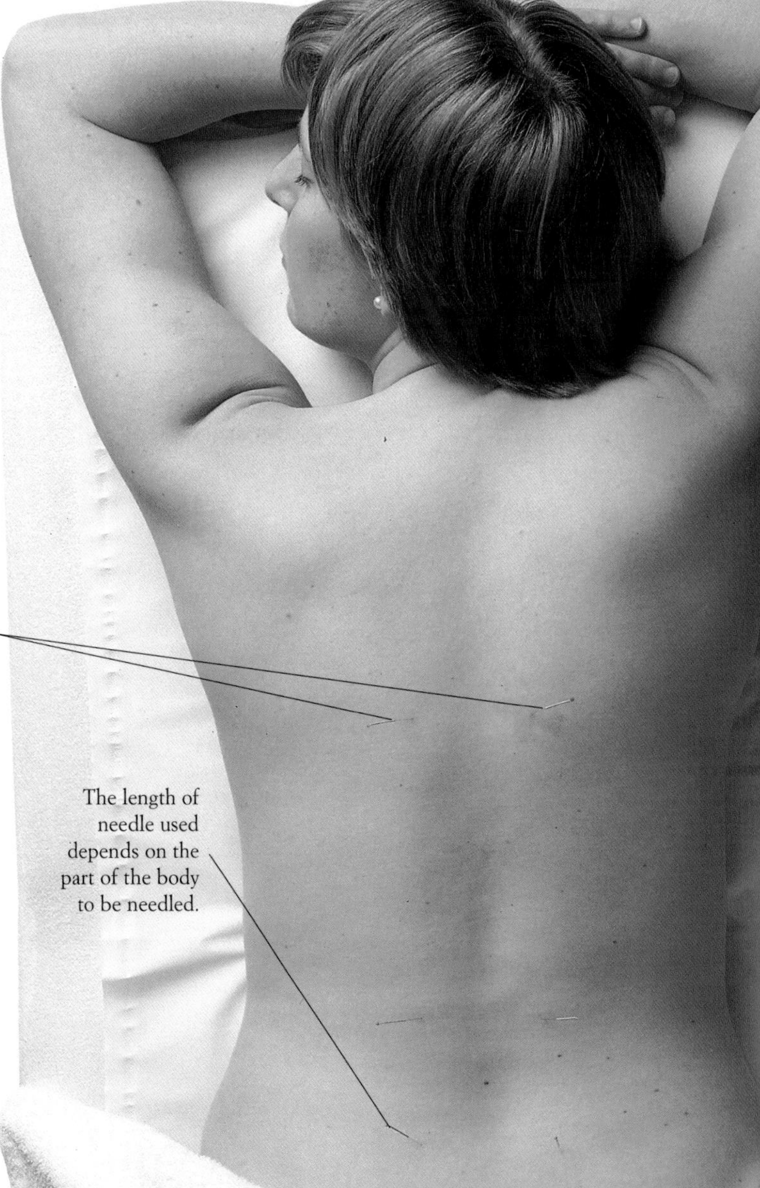

needle to be used is left to the clinical judgment of the practitioner but is usually governed by the point being needled and the effect the practitioner is seeking in terms of needle technique. The most commonly used needles are between half an inch and three inches in length. Longer needles may be used on occasion; for example, very long and extremely thin needles are sometimes used to follow the line of the meridians around the scalp, just underneath the skin.

Very sharp "pricking" needles are used to draw small quantities of blood from certain acupuncture points; for example, blood can be drawn from the point on the Lung channel at the outside edge of the thumbnail in order to expel excess Heat in the Lungs – a very effective treatment for a sore throat caused by an invasion by Wind-Cold that has turned to Wind-Heat. The "plum blossom" needle consists of a small hammer head on a flexible handle. Up to twelve small, sharp needles on the head are used to tap gently on the skin to stimulate the flow of Qi and Blood in the local area. This usually produces a redness of the skin and on occasions can cause superficial local bleeding. Such techniques are clinically indicated in a variety of different conditions, and the practitioner uses professional judgment as to the appropriateness of the technique after discussion with the patient.

Auricular acupuncture involves needling points in the ear that correspond to different parts of, and Zangfu systems in, the body. The ear points may be needled with conventional needles, but in some cases the needles are retained in the ear points over an extended period (a week or more) and specialized "press" needles are used for this. These very small needles are retained in place with a small patch of adhesive bandage. In some instances the press needles are replaced by small seeds that are held in place against the ear point on the adhesive bandage to act as a form of mild acupressure upon the relevant point.

LEFT
This patient with low back pain has needles inserted at ashi points on the back to disperse stagnant energy in the muscles.

ACUPUNCTURE NEEDLES

A variety of needles is used for acupuncture today, depending on the area of the body to be needled and the therapeutic effect desired.

STAINLESS STEEL

These needles range in size from a quarter of an inch to two inches (7mm–50mm).

COPPER-COIL HANDLED

The moxa is burned on the end of these needles.

PRISMATIC

This needle is used for letting blood.

AURICULAR

Press needles for auricular acupuncture

"PLUM BLOSSOM"

"Plum blossom" (pictured right) needle for tapping

FEATURED MATERIALS BY COURTESY OF THE ACUMEDIC CENTRE, LONDON

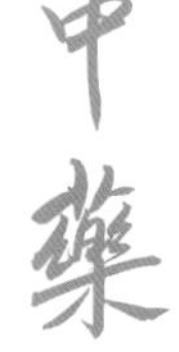

Needling techniques

The patient might imagine that once a needle is inserted into the appropriate point, nothing else happens until it is later removed.

However, this is far from the case. The subtlety and skill of the acupuncture practitioner involve far more than simply locating the right point on the body; the needle must then be correctly inserted and manipulated to enhance the desired therapeutic effect. In all instances, the practitioner is seeking to access the patient's Qi flow with the needle. The sensation of accessing the Qi is called "deqi" – literally, "acquiring the Qi" – and can be sensed by both patient and practitioner. The patient may experience deqi as a tingling or a numb sensation. On occasions, the sensation will spread along the line of the channel. It is very difficult to describe the experience: it differs quite markedly from the sensation experienced when being given an injection, for example.

However, once experienced, deqi is never forgotten, and the patient can become quite instrumental in advising the practitioner on when the needle has reached the correct point. The experienced and sensitive practitioner can also develop a subjective sense of when deqi is achieved that cannot be analyzed.

Practitioners who follow the Five-Element approach often needle very superficially and remove the needle as soon as deqi is attained. Practitioners of the Traditional Chinese Medicine (TCM) approach – the most common practice in China and the West – needle to a much deeper level to achieve deqi and then retain the needles in the point for anything from ten minutes to an hour, depending on the condition and the treatment effect required. The average time is about twenty minutes.

As noted previously there are conditions where the Qi is deficient, and conditions where the Qi has become excess. If a deficient condition is identified, the treatment needs to emphasize tonification; and with an excess condition, it needs to emphasize reduction.

Three main needling techniques are regularly adopted:

- *the reinforcing technique – when there is the intention to reinforce a deficiency*
- *the reducing technique – when there is the intention to reduce an excess*
- *the even technique – when there is no particular reason to overly reinforce or reduce.*

The techniques themselves involve lifting and thrusting the needle in the point, rotating the needle in a specific manner once deqi has been achieved, and sometimes flicking or stroking

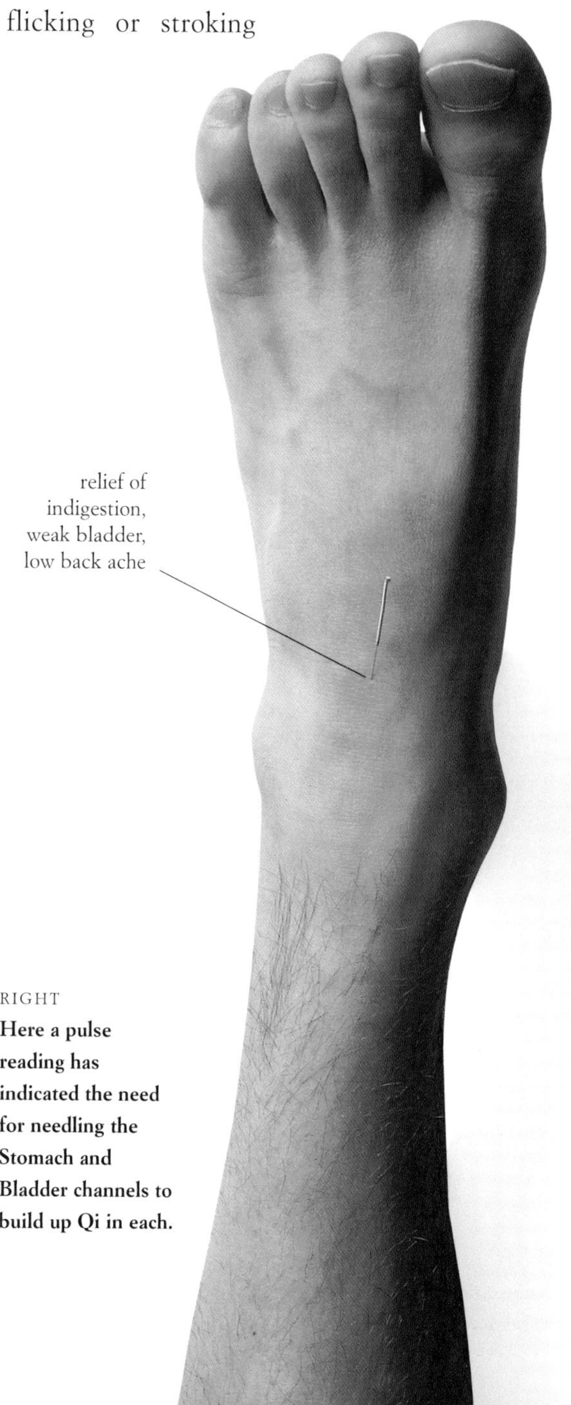

RIGHT
Here a pulse reading has indicated the need for needling the Stomach and Bladder channels to build up Qi in each.

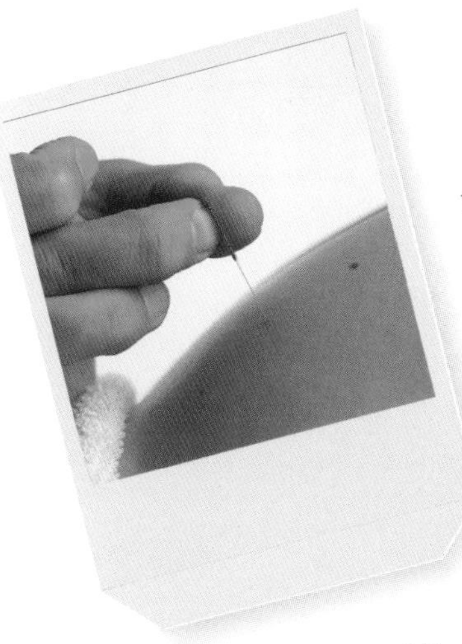

ABOVE
The needle may be lightly flicked to enhance the quality of Qi.

the handle of the needle with the finger. The specific technique adopted is often a matter of personal choice or preference on the part of the practitioner and is invariably developed idiosyncratically with experience. Other more complex needling techniques are used in very specific circumstances, some of which can be very complex and involved.

Depending on the therapeutic principles followed, the practitioner may use different needling techniques on different points; but at all times the mental intent of the practitioner is just as important as the physical manipulation of the needle. It is said in Chinese medicine that the Qi follows the mind intent, and if the mind is distracted or inattentive, the Qi will be scattered.

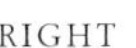

Thus, it must be emphasized that the true practitioner will always be very aware of what he or she is seeking to achieve with every needle that is inserted – an efficient needling technique cannot compensate for an unfocused mind with no clear intent of what is required.

The manner in which a needle is inserted is dictated by the area of the body to be needled. In large fleshy areas – the buttocks and certain parts of the trunk – needling may be quite deep and the manipulation of the needles quite vigorous. On the face, where the skin is tight, needling is much more superficial and can often run transversely under the skin and above the bone. Needle manipulation in such instances tends in general to be less robust. Other factors that influence needling include the following:

- The morphology of the individual – large bodies that are well endowed with fleshy areas are treated slightly differently than thin, wiry bodies where there is a minimum of spare flesh.
- Old and/or very weak patients – needling techniques tend to be less vigorous than on younger and stronger patients.
- Babies and very young children – these patients generally have very sensitive energy systems, and for them needling can be quite specialized. It often involves the brief puncturing of the appropriate point and immediate removal of the needle once deqi is achieved. Pediatric acupuncture is a specialized area, and practitioners usually require some additional training to work effectively with very young children.

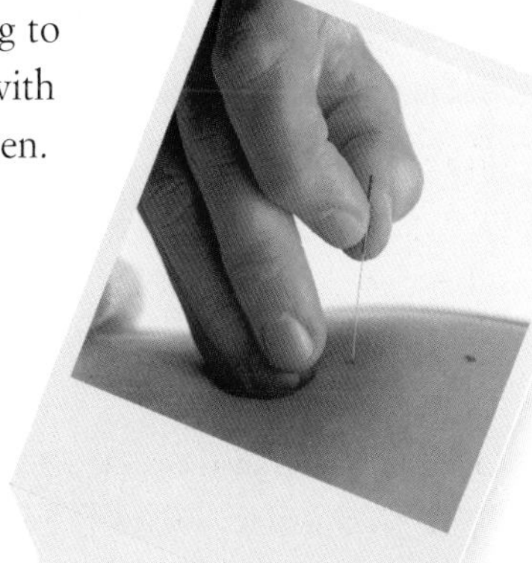

RIGHT
Vigorously rotating the needle stirs up stagnant Qi.

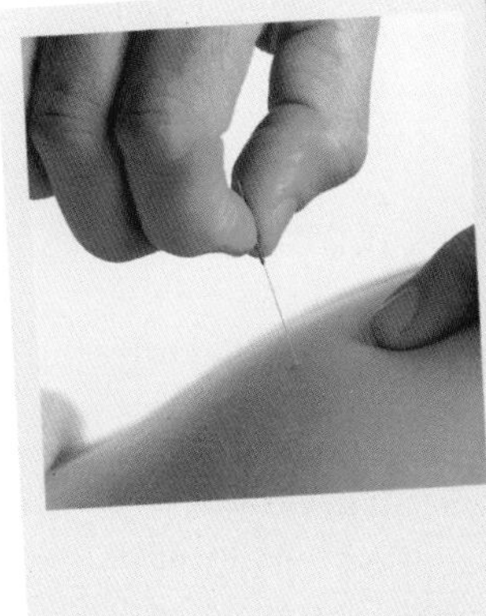

RIGHT
Manipulating the needle can reinforce Qi in the meridian.

THEORY AND PRACTICE

Although the meridians themselves are not thought of as physically identifiable, their existence is proved by observation of the effect of stimulating various pressure points. The theory and practice of acupuncture developed hand in hand as practitioners observed the effects of different kinds of needling in different specific areas of the body.

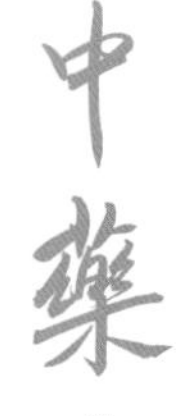

WHAT HAPPENS IN AN ACUPUNCTURE SESSION?

MOST PATIENTS are naturally anxious and uncertain when they first decide to try acupuncture. In order to allay some of these fears, the following pages describe a typical acupuncture session. There will of course be variations between practitioners, but certain generic elements will be common to all of them.

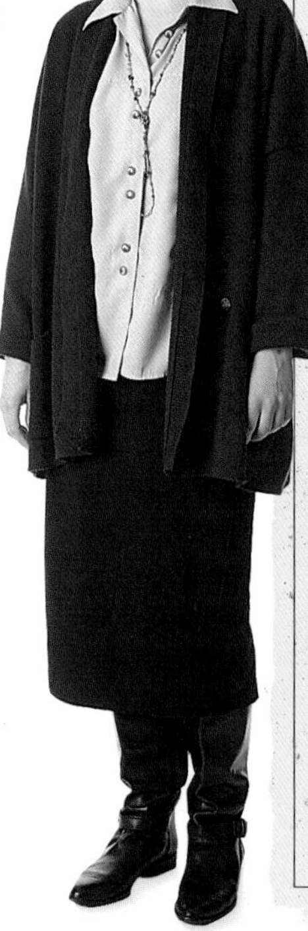

RIGHT
Before the first treatment, the patient may feel a little ill at ease.

IS ACUPUNCTURE SAFE?

A common anxiety expressed by new patients is whether it is safe to have the body punctured by needles. This is understandable.

The answer would have to be that if the practitioner does not know what he or she is doing, it is possible to inflict injury with an acupuncture needle. However, any fully trained and experienced practitioner knows how to use needles safely and effectively, and how to avoid any potential danger areas. Particular care needs to be exercised over the lung area on the upper back, where the direct vertical insertion of a needle could cause a pneumothorax (lung puncture). However, with the correct needling techniques there is no danger of this whatsoever. The importance of seeking an appropriately trained practitioner cannot be overstated. In the hands of such practitioners, acupuncture is a very safe and effective form of therapy.

THE DIAGNOSTIC INTERVIEW

ACUPUNCTURE IS no different from any other form of human interaction in which a therapeutic process takes place: an important prerequisite for successful treatment is the establishment of a rapport between practitioner and patient. Since acupuncture is a process whereby the energetics of the practitioner interact with those of the patient through the medium of the needles, the importance of a trusting, open, and confidential relationship cannot be overestimated.

Acupuncture treatment is not simply a mechanical process in which one person sticks steel needles into another. In essence, it is a combined physical, psychological, and spiritual process, and should be respected as such.

The practitioner starts by recording basic biographical information and asking the patient to describe in his or her own way the problem over which help is being sought. The practitioner must then organize this information in a coherent manner within the framework of Chinese medicine. As we have described, this is achieved by undertaking the four examinations:

✦ *looking* ✦ *hearing and smelling* ✦ *questioning* ✦ *touching.*

The information revealed by each of these four areas is then synthesized into a comprehensive picture. "Looking" involves observing all aspects of the patient's physical appearance and demeanor, including the very important observation of the tongue. "Hearing and Smelling" can reveal important clues as to whether a problem is one of excess or deficiency, although it is fair to say that there is a limit to the extent that Western practitioners actively smell their patients! Even Chinese medicine must adapt itself to the cultural norms and mores that pertain in the West. "Questioning" allows the practitioner to explore a whole range of issues that will build up a fuller picture of the patient's disharmony. Finally, "Touching" enables the practitioner to identify painful areas through palpation, to sense body temperature and skin condition, and, most important, to take the patient's pulses.

At the end of the diagnostic interview, which may take anything from thirty minutes to an hour, the practitioner has a mass of information that can be organized in terms of the Eight-Principle patterns of Yin/Yang, Interior/Exterior, Cold/Hot, Deficiency/Excess. This information enables him or her to identify the nature of the disharmony, and any Zangfu systems that are directly affected. In most cases the patterns will be complex interactions, and judgment is required in order to identify major and minor disharmonies, and to set priorities in terms of a subsequent treatment plan. Since it is highly unlikely that all the components of the diagnostic interview will unambiguously point in the same direction, the practitioner must look for a "best fit" model from the information that has been gathered.

Contractual discussion

Once the practitioner has completed the interview, he or she will have formulated a diagnosis and have a treatment strategy in mind. At this point it is important that information is shared between the practitioner and the patient.

The practitioner will normally take care to explain the nature of the problem, and the suggested treatment, as clearly as possible, in terms that the patient can understand. There is an obligation on the practitioner to make his or her understanding of the disharmony accessible to the patient, and the patient should expect and accept no less.

In all but a few cases, it is very unlikely that one acupuncture treatment will completely resolve a problem. More than likely, especially for long-standing, chronic conditions, a series of treatments, spread over several weeks or months, will be necessary. The practitioner should make it clear to the patient in what way acupuncture can be expected to help with the

LEFT
Before determining the treatment, the acupuncturist interviews the patient to form a complete picture of the case. The pulses are carefully taken and the patient's tongue is examined.

problem; and the patient should be told how many treatments are likely to be required, and over what length of time. Certain factors – such as how the patient responds to acupuncture – will determine the rate of progress and the number of treatments required, but, obviously, cannot be known prior to treatment commencing. Most practitioners suggest that five or ten treatments, say, are agreed to initially, after which progress will be reviewed and a further agreement reached in the light of what has occurred. The main point is that, at all stages of the process, patients should be clear about what they have or have not agreed to in terms of a treatment program. Some patients may insist on an agreement being signed with the practitioner, but this is rare. A mutual clarity of purpose is important not only in professional and ethical terms but also in terms of setting the treatment agenda at a subtle level of energetic interaction between patient and practitioner.

WHAT DOES IT FEEL LIKE TO HAVE ACUPUNCTURE?

THE POSITION for treatment is dictated by the needling to be used and by other clinical considerations. A treatment couch is generally used, and the patient will normally lie down on the back, front, or side. But in some instances it may be appropriate for the patient to sit on a chair. Sometimes the patient may have to move position in the middle of a treatment in order that different points can be needled.

When the acupuncturist inserts the needle, he or she is initially looking to locate the Qi in the meridian. When the Qi is accessed (deqi), a sensation is normally felt, both by the patient and by the practitioner. This feeling can vary from a dull, aching pain to a tingling "shock." The local area needled may begin to feel heavy, and the sensation of the needling may travel along the line of the meridian. The effect can thus spread beyond the local area. Some people are more responsive to needling than others and may experience the sensations and discomfort to a much greater degree. However, responsiveness to needling is not in itself indicative that acupuncture is working well, and patients who experience little or no sensation should not feel that acupuncture is not working. Depending on the treatment principle, the acupuncturist may or may not offer further stimulation to the needle once it is in place. This may cause the needling sensation to be reexperienced.

The needles are usually retained for a few minutes to over an hour, but twenty minutes is the average.

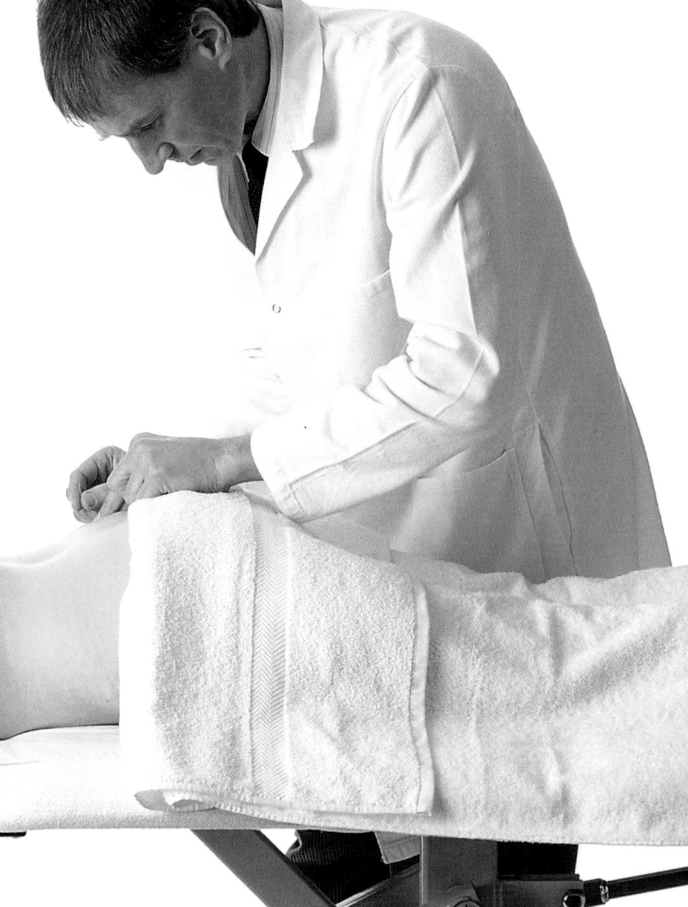

ADDITIONAL TREATMENTS

OTHER TECHNIQUES may be applied as part of the treatment during an acupuncture session.

ELECTROACUPUNCTURE

In certain conditions it may be appropriate to stimulate the flow of Qi by connecting a pair of needles to a small DC charge from a specially designed electroacupuncture stimulator. Several pairs can be connected at the same time, and the frequency and strength of the electric pulse can be varied in order to achieve the desired effect.

MOXABUSTION

It is quite common to combine acupuncture treatment with moxabustion. Direct or indirect moxabustion may be used, and loose moxa is often burned on the handle of a needle that is inserted in a particular point. *(See page 142 for further details on moxabustion.)*

CUPPING

Cupping may precede an acupuncture treatment in some conditions; in other specific situations a cup may be placed over a needle and retained there for some time. In some specialized treatments the cup may be placed over a point that has deliberately been bled, thus stimulating the flow of blood. *(See page 145 for further details on cupping.)*

AURICULAR ACUPUNCTURE

Ear points are sometimes needled during a more general acupuncture session. Press needles or ear seeds are put in position and kept there between sessions.

LEFT
There can be various mild sensations when the needles are put in place.

SIDE EFFECTS

SOME PATIENTS are anxious about whether there will be any side effects and what they are likely to feel after the needles are taken out. The vast majority of patients show absolutely no adverse reactions. However, a very small number of patients have quite dramatic reactions to needling, including lightheadedness, nausea, and vomiting, and in some cases they may even pass out during treatment.

Such extreme "needle shock" reactions are very rare and are easily reversed by laying the patient down in the recovery position and removing the needles. Finger acupressure on specific points can bring around a patient who has fainted. The less dramatic reaction of slight lightheadedness or nausea usually wears off after a few minutes.

Patients should bear in mind that it is not advisable to give acupuncture to anyone who has been drinking alcohol in the hour or so before a treatment, or to anyone who has been taking illegal drugs.

Women patients should always inform the practitioner if there is any chance they may be pregnant: there are certain acupuncture points that have to be avoided in pregnancy. It is naturally also the responsibility of the practitioner to check with any woman patient whether pregnancy may be a possibility.

LEFT
A response may be felt flowing along a meridian. Adverse reactions are extremely rare.

MOXABUSTION

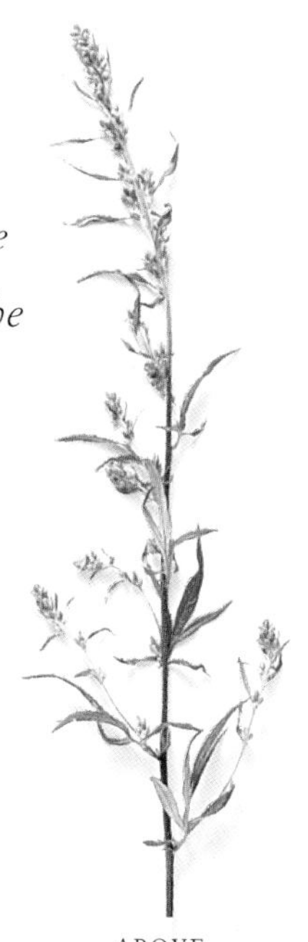

ABOVE
Mugwort, the wild plant used in moxabustion, is common in many parts of the world.

MOXABUSTION IS the process whereby moxa – a dried herb, usually the species mugwort (Artemisia vulgaris) *– is burned, either directly on the skin or indirectly above the skin, over specific acupuncture points. The mugwort is harvested in the early part of the summer, and the leaves are dried and allowed to age. It is then crushed and subjected to varying degrees of sifting. The highest-grade moxa almost exclusively consists of the fluffy underside of the leaf. This moxa is considered most appropriate for direct application to the skin. The less refined moxa contains a mixture of the fluffy underbelly of the leaf and parts of the leaf body. This lower-grade moxa tends to be used for indirect application.*

When lit, moxa burns slowly and provides a penetrating heat that can enter the channels to influence the Qi and Blood flow. Moxa burns with a characteristic musky odor and can give off a fairly copious amount of smoke, depending on the grade. Some patients may find the smell and the smoke difficult to tolerate, and the odor tends to be retained in the clothing and hair long after the treatment session. Smokeless moxa is available, but it can be very difficult to light and is not commonly used.

Moxa is also available in a loose form for making moxa cones or wrapping around an acupuncture needle. Alternatively, moxa comes packed and rolled in a long stick, about six to eight inches (15–20 cm) long and between one half and three quarter inch (1–2 cm) in diameter.

BELOW
Dried moxa is suitable for direct application to the skin.

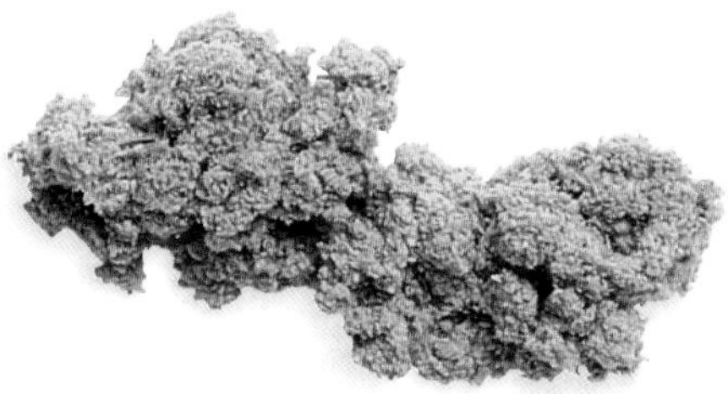

RIGHT
Loose moxa is prepared to be burned in a box.

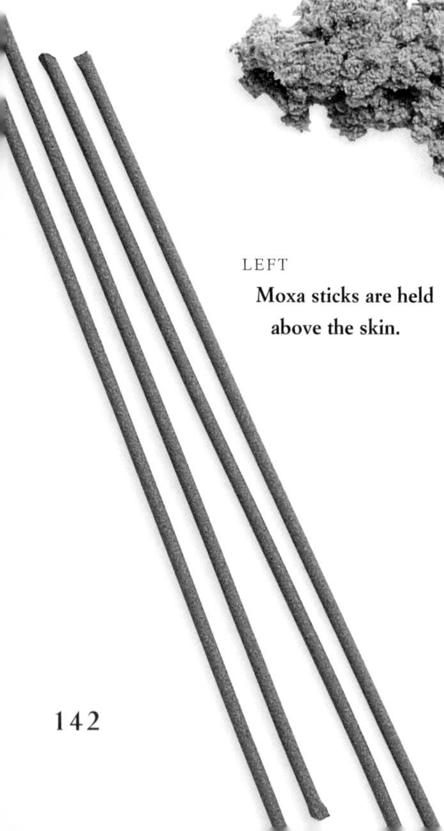

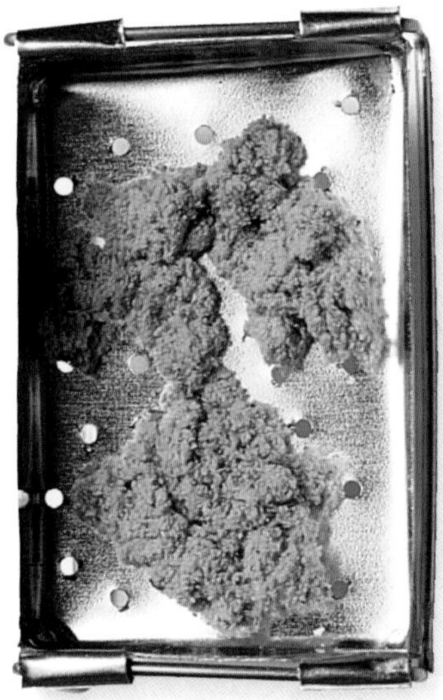

LEFT
Moxa sticks are held above the skin.

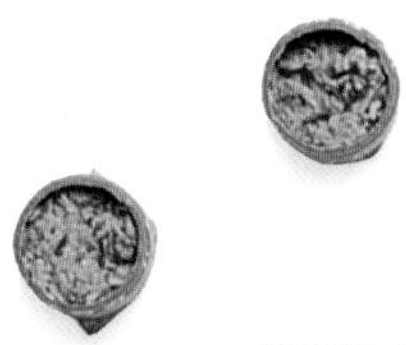

ABOVE AND BELOW
Moxa cones are placed on the body and then lit.

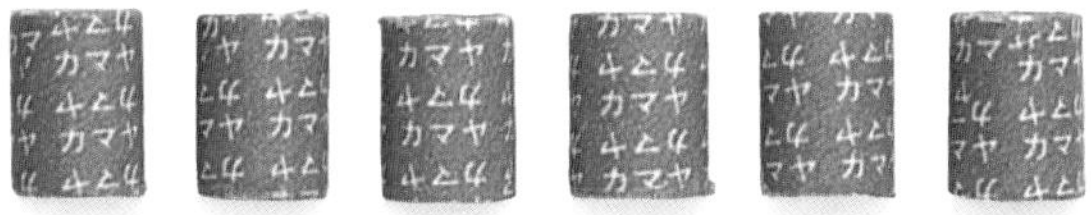

FEATURED MATERIALS BY COURTESY OF THE ACUMEDIC CENTRE, LONDON

DIRECT MOXABUSTION

MOXA IS formed into small cones that are placed on selected points on the body and then lit. The moxa cone is allowed to burn down until the skin turns red, and then the ash is removed and a new cone lit. The process is repeated until the treatment is concluded.

If the moxa burns right down to the skin, scarring will occur. Although scarring moxabustion is regularly referred to in Chinese texts, it is not regularly practiced in the West. In this technique, the cone burns the skin and a blister forms. The resultant scar can take a considerable time to heal, and the area must be cleaned and dressed regularly. Ancient wisdom has suggested that the formation of the blister is essential if healing is to be achieved, but modern Western practitioners find that moxa can be highly effective without resorting to scarring the patient.

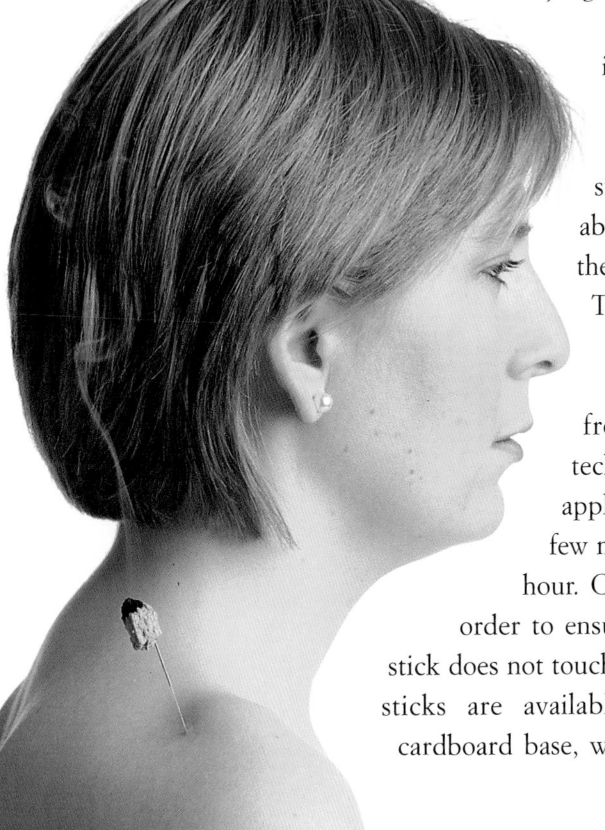

RIGHT
Moxa may be applied directly to the skin (where it is carefully watched so that it does not burn right down) or to the end of the acupuncture needle as shown. The warmth stimulates energy in the areas that are cold or painful because Qi is stuck or weak.

INDIRECT MOXABUSTION

MOXA IS burned indirectly, either above the skin or on another medium between the moxa and the skin. The substances most commonly used as a medium are

- salt – *often placed in the umbilicus (acupuncture point Ren 8); the moxa is then burned on the salt layer*
- garlic – *a slice of garlic, with perforations, is placed on the skin and the moxa is burned on this*
- ginger – *a slice of ginger is used in a similar fashion to garlic.*

The herb Fu Zi (aconite), which has very hot and acrid energetic properties, is also described in the literature as a moxa medium, but is unlikely to be used in Western practice: Fu Zi is toxic and its use is banned in many countries.

The choice of medium depends on the condition being treated and the clinical judgment of the practitioner.

A very common form of indirect moxabustion uses moxa sticks, a bit like large cigars or incense sticks. These are lit and held about an inch (2.5cm) above the point or area to be treated. They are usually turned in a rotational manner, or "pecked" toward and away from the skin. Using this technique, treatment can be applied for anything between a few minutes and a quarter of an hour. Care has to be exercised in order to ensure that the burning moxa stick does not touch the skin. Very small moxa sticks are available mounted on a small cardboard base, which itself has an adhesive

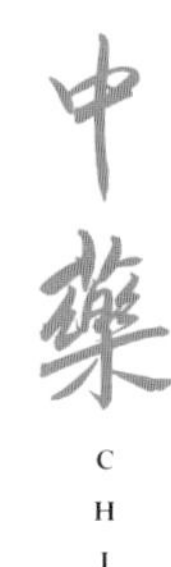

BELOW

The moxabustion process is carefully controlled by the practitioner.

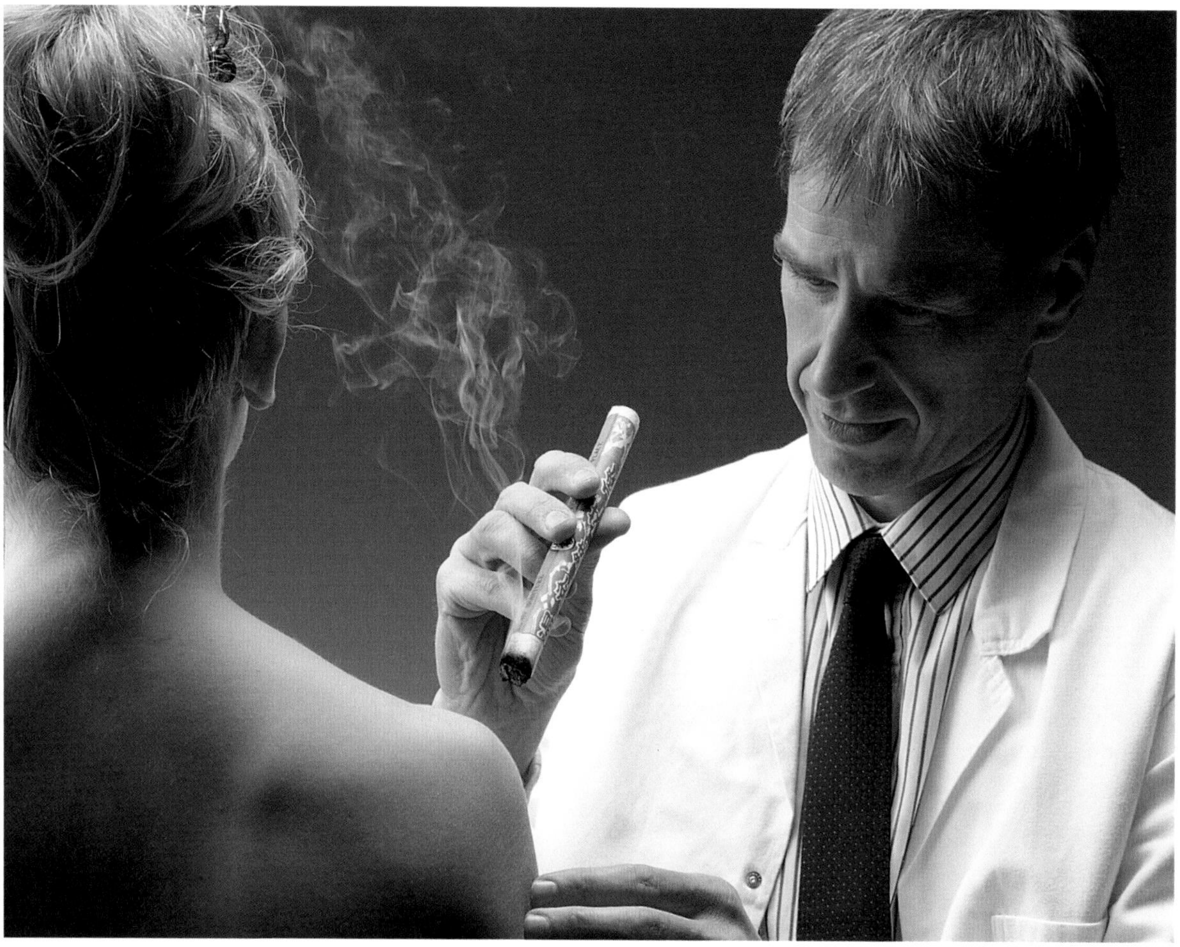

surface. When placed on the skin, these small sticks produce indirect moxabustion, but the cardboard base acts as a more neutral conductor than the mediums described above.

Moxa sticks can be cut into smaller lengths – between a half and one and a quarter inches (1–3 cm) – and burned on the handle of a stainless steel needle, which is then inserted into an acupuncture point. In this way, the heat not only warms the skin but is also drawn into the channel through the needle. Loose moxa can also be wrapped around the needle and burned in the same way.

The other common method of applying indirect moxabustion involves the use of a moxa box. These boxes come in various designs but work on the common principle of allowing the heat from the moxa – either stick or loose – to be distributed over a larger area. For example, when there is low back pain due to a deficiency of Kidney Yang, moxa is burned in a box that is placed over the lower back area. This allows the warming effect of the moxa to penetrate a wide area.

The choice of when and where to use moxabustion, either on its own or in conjunction with acupuncture, is a matter of clinical judgment for the practitioner, in consultation with the patient.

LEFT

A moxa box allows moxa to be burned over a wider area.

CUPPING

CUPPING IS a technique that is especially useful in the treatment of problems of local Qi, or Blood stagnation in the channels. It can also be very helpful in expelling the external pathogenic factor of Wind-Cold that can invade the Lungs. Cupping is an ancient technique that is still used by modern practitioners. This form of treatment is usually performed as an alternative to acupuncture: the cups are placed over acupuncture points but they treat a larger area of the body.

CUPS ARE either of robust, rounded glass construction or of bamboo. Other materials have been used, but practitioners in the West tend to use glass. (Caution: on no account should "do-it-yourself" cupping be undertaken with items such as jars and glasses. Cupping creates a strong vacuum, and an inappropriate vessel may shatter and cause injury.)

In this technique, a burning taper is held for a very short period of time inside the cup, before the cup is immediately placed down over the selected area. Because the taper flame exhausts all the oxygen in the cup, a vacuum is created; this anchors the cup to the skin and draws up the skin beneath the cup. The effect of this is to encourage the flow of Qi and Blood in the area beneath the cup. By this means, local stagnation begins to clear.

The strength of the vacuum depends on the amount of oxygen burned in the cup and on the skill of the practitioner in quickly placing the cup in the appropriate position. In some instances the cup is retained in the same position for a considerable time, while in others it is removed quickly and placed elsewhere on the body. For example, when cupping is used to expel Wind-Cold from the Lungs, several cups may be placed over the lung area on the back, and regularly removed and replaced until the whole area to be treated has been thoroughly covered.

In "moving cupping," an area of the body is lightly smeared with oil or soap and the applied cup is drawn around with the vacuum intact, thus encouraging a more generalized movement of Qi and Blood in the area.

Cupping draws blood to the external capillaries of the body, and as a result minor weals or bruises may be left after treatment. If cups are retained in one spot for any length of time, the marking may be quite considerable. If a practitioner is using cupping, this possible consequence of treatment should be explained to the patient.

ABOVE
Absorbent cotton soaked in surgical spirits is burned inside the cup.

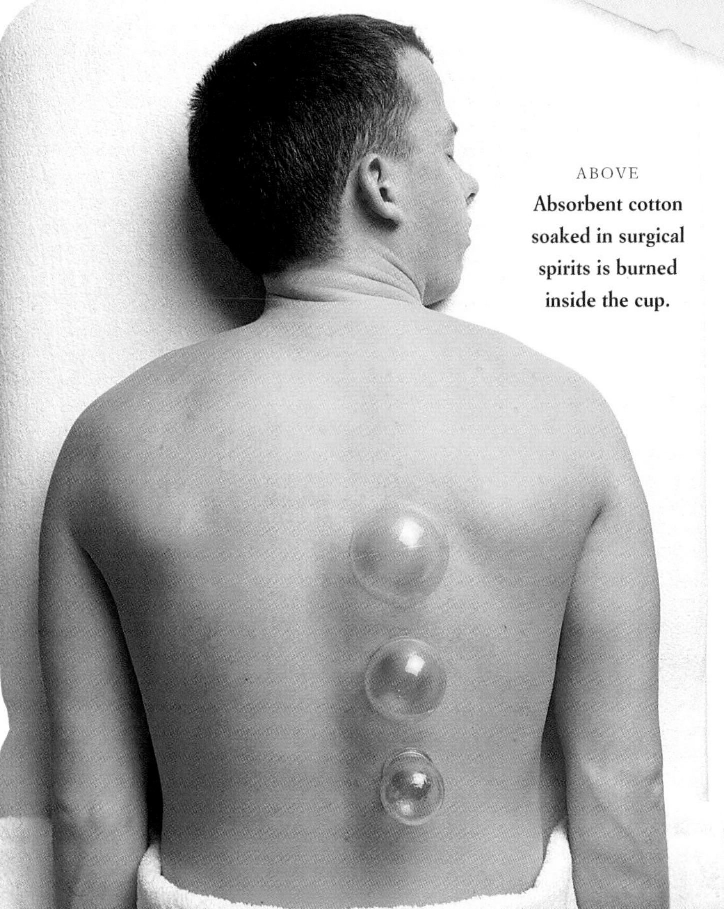

RIGHT
Here, cups are used to draw fresh Qi to muscles in spasm beside the spine and disperse the stagnant Qi resulting from the spasm.

HOW WILL I FEEL AFTER TREATMENT?

AFTER TREATMENT some patients will step off the couch and go about their daily life as if nothing had happened at all. Others may well experience a residual reaction.

By far the most common reaction is that patients feel very tired and washed out for several hours afterward. If treatment is given in the evening, this rarely causes a problem, but if it is given earlier in the day, patients need to be warned of this possibility. Less commonly, patients feel very energized after a treatment.

Another point to remember is that there may be an exacerbation of the symptoms after treatment. This does not usually last long and is followed by an improvement in the condition. Early on in a course of treatment, it may happen that after a visit to the acupuncturist, the patient has a period when things feel worse, then a period of no change at all.

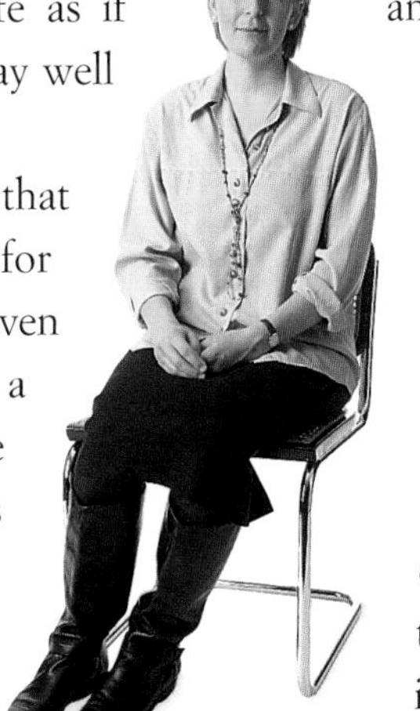

ABOVE
After treatment the patient often feels tired, though calm and relaxed.

All these possible reactions to acupuncture and related treatment should be fully explored by the practitioner with the patient as part of the contractual discussion before treatment begins.

In most cases the changes brought about by acupuncture treatment are gradual, although in some instances they can be both immediate and dramatic. The patient and the practitioner should discuss progress on a regular basis, with the practitioner revisiting the diagnostic interview information to check for specific changes. Together they map the progress of the treatment program.

Treatment sessions may be terminated at any appropriate point, but often patients are "weaned off" by decreasing the frequency of visits. No professional practitioner will continue to treat a patient with acupuncture for any longer than is necessary.

CHOOSING A PRACTITIONER

The situation regarding training, accreditation, and registration varies from country to country, and in the United States between individual states. However, some general points can be made.

✦ Registered orthodox medical practitioners who offer acupuncture are not necessarily trained in Chinese medicine. While they may be able to use acupuncture to treat minor problems such as local channel pain, they are not able to diagnose and treat in terms of the principles and theories of Chinese medicine.

✦ Fully registered practitioners of acupuncture have undertaken an agreed and recognized training in the practice of Chinese medicine. They have also reached curricular standards in Western anatomy, physiology, and pathology. Thus, they have an understanding of the patient from the perspective of orthodox medicine, although they do not offer treatment in that modality. Such practitioners are required to adhere to a professional code of conduct and are bound to comprehensive ethical standards. They also carry comprehensive professional indemnity insurance.

It is advisable to check the register of the professional body of the state or country concerned to ensure that the practitioner is currently registered.

A CASE HISTORY

DIANE IS 29 years old. She is complaining of what she calls depression. It started two years ago when she suddenly felt faint at work and had to be sent home. She had a complete nervous breakdown and hasn't been able to work since. She has been attending the psychiatric outpatients department at her local hospital and has been on various forms of medication. The drugs tend to relieve the symptoms for a short while, but they soon return.

Diane describes the problem as feeling anxious and agitated. She feels hot most of the time, and although she used to have a lot of energy she complains she is constantly tired. Her sleep pattern is poor – she gets off to sleep but invariably wakes between 1 and 3 a.m., after which she cannot get back to sleep. She has palpitations, both in bed at night and more recently during the day, for no apparent reason. She gets very hot at night and sweats profusely in bed, sometimes waking up with her body soaking wet. Her skin is very dry, her nails are ridged, and she complains that her hair is thinning. Constipation has started to be a problem, although she says her appetite is good and she has a balanced diet (except for drinking up to fifteen cups of coffee a day). Her urine is quite dark. She complains of "ringing" in her ears and sometimes gets a sudden sensation of deafness, which usually passes after a few minutes. Her periods are normal, but the blood flow is quite scant. She says that her once period-related back pain now tends to last all the time. Although unmarried, she has regular and varied sexual partners, but nothing seems to develop into a lasting relationship. She would like to have a child and is desperate to get pregnant – either within or outside a stable relationship. Her pulse is rapid and somewhat superficial, and her tongue is quite dry and red, with a very red tip.

WHAT CAN ACUPUNTURE TREAT?

Patients may seek out an acupuncturist for a variety of reasons. Very often, it is a last resort for a chronic condition. The acupuncturist takes a holistic approach and will often find that emotional factors and unexplained – and unremarked – symptoms are all linked to the "main" problem. A myriad of health and emotional problems is often solved during treatment.

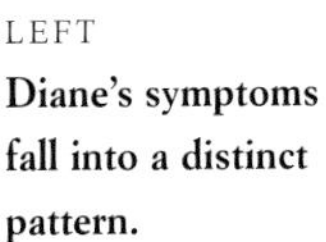

LEFT
Diane's symptoms fall into a distinct pattern.

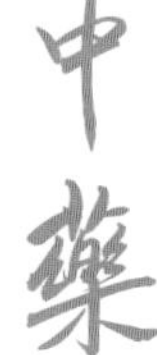

CHINESE MEDICINE

What is going on with Diane?

It is useful to consider her symptoms in terms of the Eight-Principle patterns. What is most obvious is the many Heat signs – feeling hot, sweats, rapid pulse, red tongue, dark urine.

Second, the Heat signs appear to be those of empty rather than full Heat. This tends to suggest that the Heat is caused by a deficiency of Yin. This is a chronic problem affecting the Zangfu system and is clearly an internal disharmony. Thus, in terms of the Eight-Principle patterns, there is evidence to suggest

✦ *Heat* ✦ *Deficiency* ✦ *Internal* ✦ *Yin.*

The next stage is to consider what Zangfu are involved. There is evidence that there are disharmonies affecting the Kidneys, the Liver, and the Heart.

- *Kidney Yin deficiency* – suggested by night sweats, lower back pain, rapid pulse, constipation, dark urine, tinnitus, deafness.
- *Liver Blood deficiency* – suggested by dry skin, ridged nails, poor energy, thinning hair, scanty menstrual flow, sleeplessness between 1 and 3 a.m. (Liver time in the daily cycle).
- *Heart Yin deficiency* – suggested by palpitations, poor sleep pattern, red tongue tip, and general Yin deficiency signs.

In terms of a diagnosis in Chinese medicine it would appear that Diane exhibits a combined pattern of Kidney and Heart Yin deficiency (usually referred to as "Kidney and Heart not Harmonized"), together with an associated Liver Blood deficiency.

How might these patterns have developed?

Diane has had a lot of emotional problems in her life, with associated anxiety and sadness, and this can deplete the Heart Yin. Excessive sexual activity can weaken the Kidney Yin. She also has obvious emotional problems concerning relationships and her desire for a child. It is probable that these factors are combining to weaken the Kidney Yin energy. The Kidney Yin fails to nourish the Liver Yin, which is closely related to Liver Blood, thus causing the Blood deficiency problems. The Kidney Yin also fails to nourish the Heart Yin, causing empty Heat to flare up in the Heart. This leads to palpitations and the Heart's failure to house the Shen – hence the sleep problems. The tinnitus and the deafness result from the Kidney Yin's failure to nourish the ears (the sensory organ related to the Kidneys).

What can acupuncture do to help?

The principle of treatment in Diane's case was to tonify the Kidney and Heart Yin, clear the empty Heat, calm the Shen, and tonify the Liver Blood. Diane required on-going acupuncture sessions and was advised to revise various lifestyle factors – in particular her gross overconsumption of coffee and her excessive sexual activity.

Acupuncture proved of considerable help to Diane. Six months after starting treatment she was back at work, feeling much more positive about life, and in a stable relationship that she also felt positive about. She was virtually symptom free, and although she experienced flareups from time to time, she felt more able to cope with them.

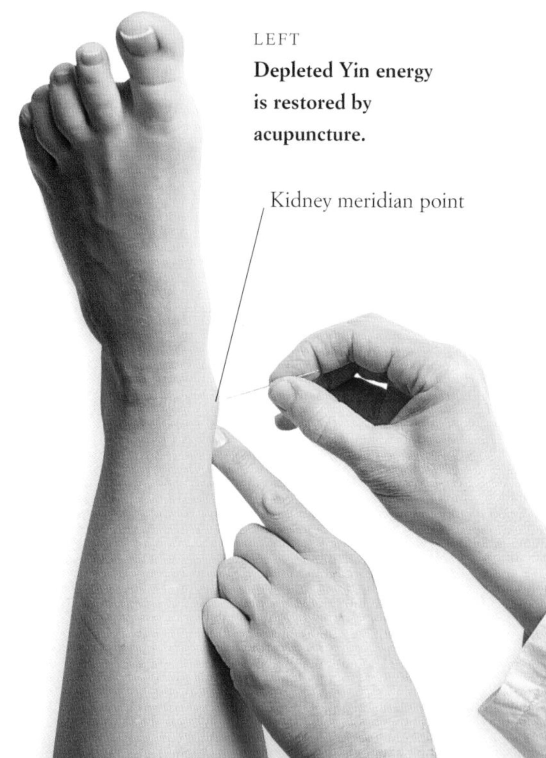

LEFT
Depleted Yin energy is restored by acupuncture.

ACUPRESSURE

MASSAGE IS widely used in Chinese medicine, and a whole range of techniques has been developed as part of the evolution of Chinese medicine in general. Acupressure massage can be used over general areas of the body to promote Qi and Blood flow through the meridian system. This form of treatment can be invaluable for minor channel disharmonies involving the local stagnation of Qi and Blood. It can be used on its own, or in conjunction with other treatment strategies. For example, acupressure massage is often used prior to acupuncture treatment.

A common question that is asked is "What is the difference between acupuncture and acupressure?" In terms of the underlying philosophy and principles there is no essential difference, but in terms of treatment approaches, acupressure obviously is noninvasive.

Cavity-press massage concentrates on applying pressure to specific acupuncture points in order to achieve specific systemic changes in the body. Different forms of pressure are applied depending on whether the aim is to tonify, to reduce, or to achieve a more neutral, calming effect. The choice of points is based on the same type of differential diagnosis that is used in acupuncture treatment.

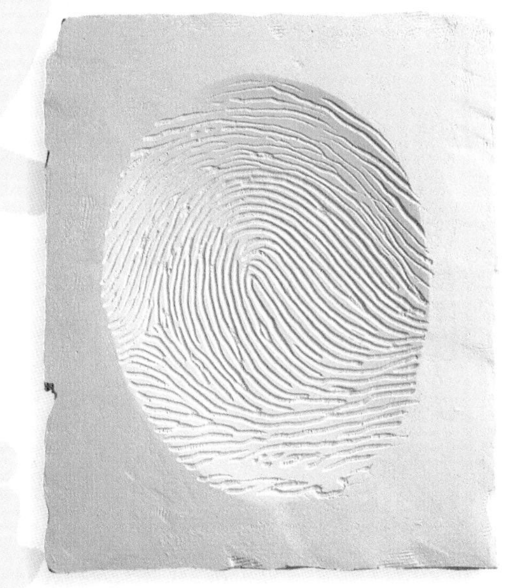

ABOVE
Acupressure is a specific form of therapeutic massage.

Specific forms of acupressure massage have developed as part of the overall development of Chinese medicine. Tui Na therapy uses pressure, manipulation, and a variety of other approaches to promote Qi and Blood flow, which in turn helps to address a whole range of presenting disharmonies. The Japanese development of acupressure massage is most clearly articulated in the practice of Shiatsu, and numerous practitioners now train and practice in this field. In more recent times, the more specialized approach of Zero Balancing (developed by Fritz Smith) encourages energetic harmony in the body through a sequence of well-defined protocols.

Anyone seeking professional help in the field of acupressure massage should look for a registered practitioner who is fully qualified in either Chinese medicine or one of the more specialized therapies such as Shiatsu and Zero Balancing (both of which operate a register). Details of register contacts can be found on pages 246–247.

SELF-HELP ACUPRESSURE

ALTHOUGH PROFESSIONAL help should be sought where possible, it is fairly easy to learn some very simple and straightforward acupressure techniques that can be used as "first-aid" measures. The following techniques can be used on friends and relatives, and some of the more simple ones can be self-applied. Fingers, thumbs, or the whole hands may be used, as shown in the following examples. Conditions that often respond well to do-it-yourself acupressure are tension headache and travel sickness. Acupressure is safe, as long as the following precautions are observed.

PRECAUTIONS

WHILE THE techniques described here are generally very safe and straightforward, several cautionary points need to be made.

- Never use acupressure massage on someone who is suffering from an acute infectious disease.
- Always avoid massage or pressure on areas where there is a lump or tumor, and in the area immediately surrounding it.
- Do not use massage or acupressure on areas where there are skin lesions or sores.
- Avoid massage on areas where the skin has been broken as a result of injury or illness.
- Do not use massage on areas that have been burned or scalded.
- Do not use massage on patients with severe cardiovascular or Liver disease.
- Avoid massage on patients who exhibit psychotic disorders or other evidence of severe mental illness.
- Take extreme care with acupressure and massage if the patient is pregnant. Certain acupoints can trigger miscarriage if over-stimulated. (In the following techniques, a caution will indicate any points that are clearly contraindicated in pregnancy.)
- Take care when massaging patients during menstruation.
- Take care when using massage or acupressure on elderly and infirm patients, especially if they are seriously ill.

ACUPRESSURE TECHNIQUES FOR SELF-HELP TREATMENT

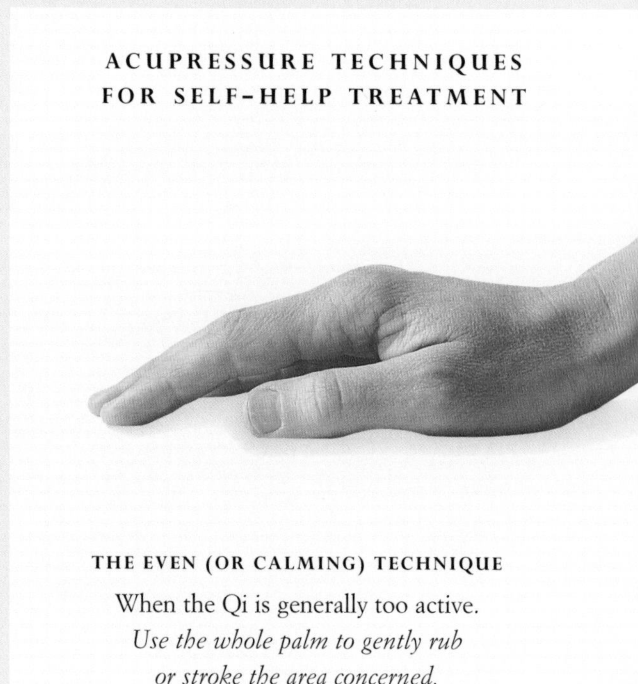

THE EVEN (OR CALMING) TECHNIQUE

When the Qi is generally too active. *Use the whole palm to gently rub or stroke the area concerned.*

GENERAL PRINCIPLES

WHEN MASSAGING yourself or someone else, remember that as a general rule, whichever massage technique is being used, you should apply the pressure for between two and three minutes on each point. With bilateral acupuncture points (situated on both sides of the body), apply the pressure first on one side, then on the other, for the same length of time on each side. You may wish to vary this slightly in the light of your own experience as you develop your own technique.

Finally, it is important to remember that your conscious intent is crucial when carrying out acupressure massage. When reinforcing, your intent should be focused on "reinforce," and so on. If you try these techniques with your hands while your mind is elsewhere, the effectiveness of your treatment will be seriously impaired, and in some instances may be positively harmful.

THE ENERGETIC CIRCUIT

At all times it should be remembered that as soon as you touch another person an energetic Qi circuit is set up between you. As Qi follows mind intent, your frame of mind when using these techniques is absolutely vital. Inappropriate emotions or thoughts always impair the relationship, and hence the treatment. Make sure you are calm and that your mind is focused on what you are trying to do. If necessary, take five minutes to meditate or do breathing exercises before you start.

Whenever possible make sure that both your hands are on the recipient at all times, even if only one hand is actively working. The use of both hands ensures that the energetic circuit is complete, even if one hand is only taking a holding or supporting role.

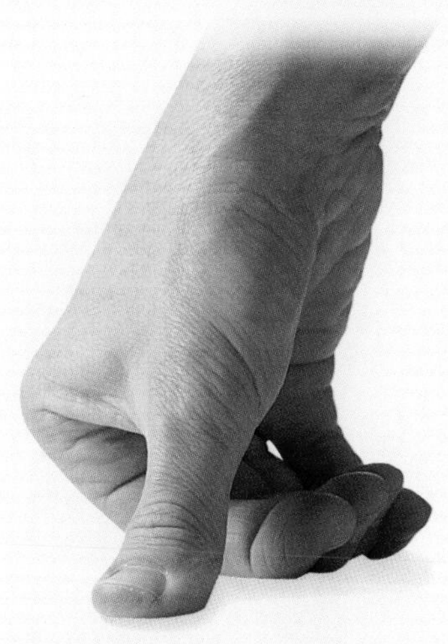

THE REINFORCING TECHNIQUE

Used when there is deficient Qi.

Apply firm and stationary pressure, with the thumb or middle finger, to the chosen point.

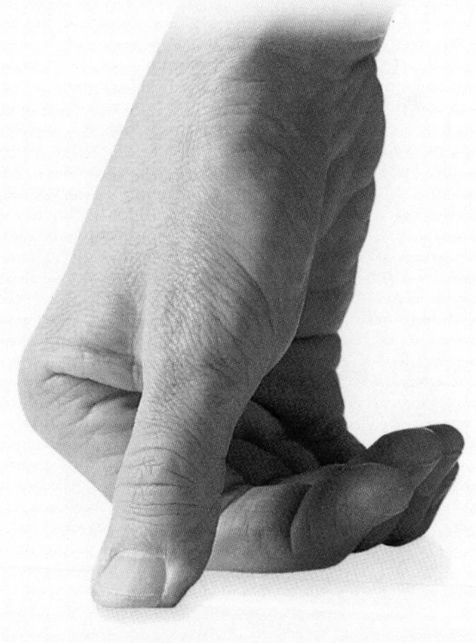

THE REDUCING (OR DISPERSING) TECHNIQUE

Used for an excess of blocked or stagnant Qi.

Apply firm pressure, but then move the pressure by making a small rotation of the thumb or finger around the point (varying between clockwise and anticlockwise directions) or pressing/pumping in and out on the point.

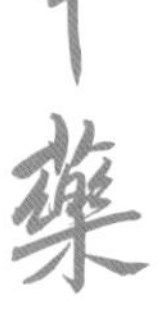

TECHNIQUES

ACUPRESSURE MASSAGE is given along the meridians, and special attention is paid to the acupuncture points, which the person giving the massage may sometimes feel as nodules under the skin and the person being massaged will usually feel as trigger points. The pressure on these points may cause something close to pain, but it feels like therapeutic pain that is helping to heal. Do not massage if pain is felt in any other way.

Note: In the following protocols for specific problems, it is important to remember that they are offered only as a first-aid approach. If the problem continues or worsens, it is important that the acupressure massage be terminated and professional help sought, either from a Chinese medical practitioner or from an orthodox doctor.

GENERAL MASSAGE

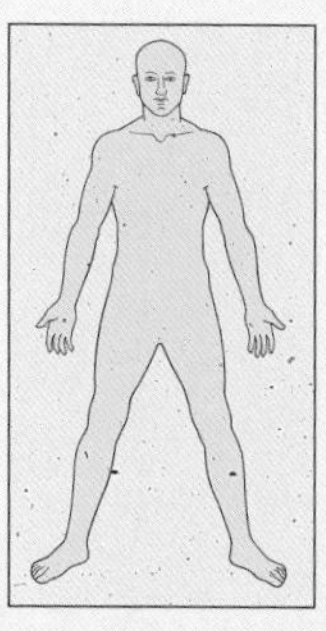

GENERAL MASSAGE treats the Back Shu points of the Bladder channel, which runs from the head, down the back of the body to the legs, and terminates at the end of the little toes. The Back Shu acupuncture points are situated about an inch to an inch and a half (2.5–3.5cm) on either side of the spine. Running down the back from top to bottom, these points link in with the Zangfu organ system. For example, Bladder 10 (Tianzhu) is connected to the functions of the Lungs, and Bladder 23 (Shenshu) is connected to the functions of the Kidneys. In the Bladder channel, the Qi flows down the body; gentle massage of the Back Shu points from top to bottom thus encourages the smooth flow of Qi and stimulates the general functioning of the whole of the internal Zangfu system.

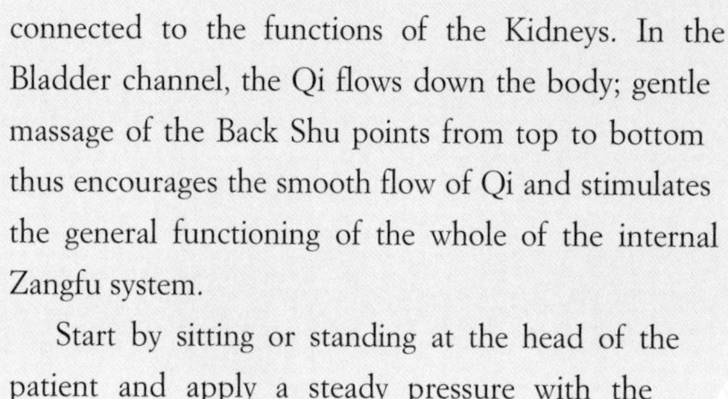

Start by sitting or standing at the head of the patient and apply a steady pressure with the thumbs or the whole hand, down and along the Bladder channel. Use small amounts of massage oil to smooth the flow. This can be continued for between three and five minutes; not only is it very relaxing but it also gives a general stimulus to the whole system.

RIGHT
A massage of the Bladder channel has a generally relaxing and stimulating effect.

HEADACHES

MINOR HEADACHES are an irritation that we all experience at some time. The following simple techniques may help.

REDUCTION OF LI 4 (HEGU)

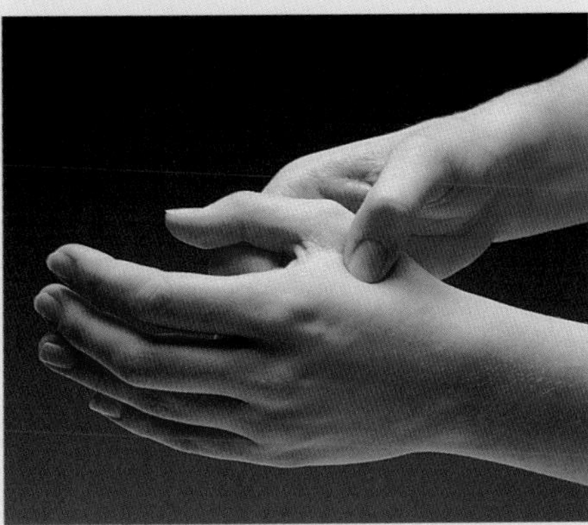

This point is found on the web between the thumb and forefinger. Apply a firm reducing pressure on Hegu for about two minutes, then repeat on the other hand.

REDUCTION OF YINTANG

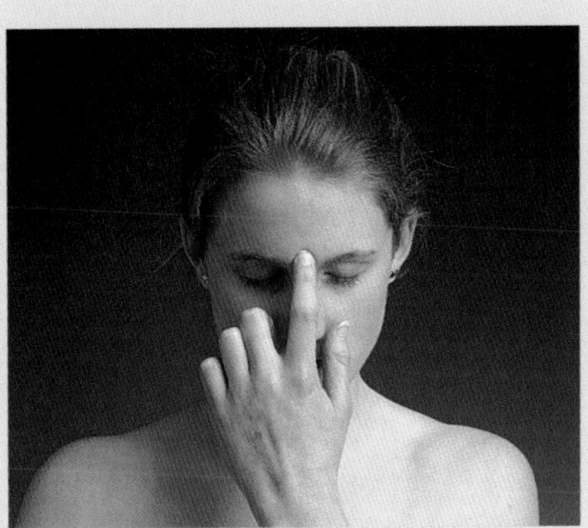

The Yintang point is located between the eyebrows in the middle of the forehead. Gently reduce this point with fingertip pressure. This can help clear the mind as well as lift the headache. Continue the pressure for between two and three minutes.

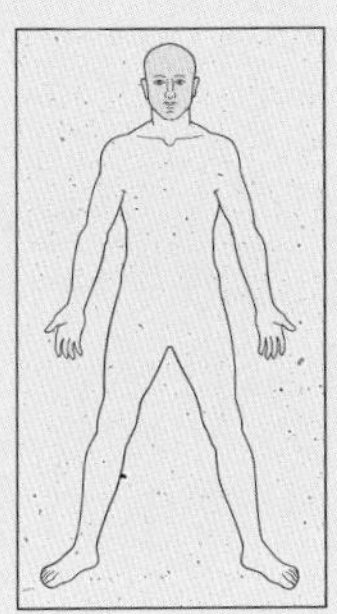

CAUTION

Do not massage the Hegu point on anyone who is pregnant.

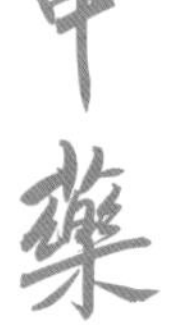

NAUSEA / SICKNESS

THESE TWO protocols can ease the symptoms of nausea or vomiting – especially when caused by indigestion or travel sickness.

GENTLE REDUCTION OF REN 12 (ZHONGWAN) AND LIV 13

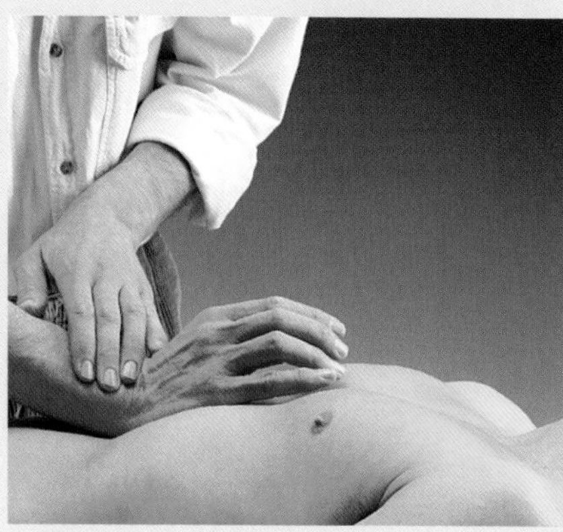

Overeating or eating too quickly can cause digestive problems and stagnation of Qi in the Spleen and Stomach. This can lead to feelings of nausea; actual vomiting may occur if the stagnant Qi "rebels" upward against the natural flow.

This protocol is best performed with the patient lying flat on the back. However, if vomiting is a possibility, the patient must not lie down. The protocol can be done with the patient in a sitting position, although it may be more difficult.

With the heel of the hand, gently reduce over the area of Zhongwan (on the body midline, midway between the bottom of the breast bone (sternum) and the umbilicus), and the area around Zangmen (below the eleventh rib at the side of the rib cage, on both sides of the body). Continue for several minutes until the sensation of nausea passes.

STRONG REDUCTION OF P6 (NEIGUAN)

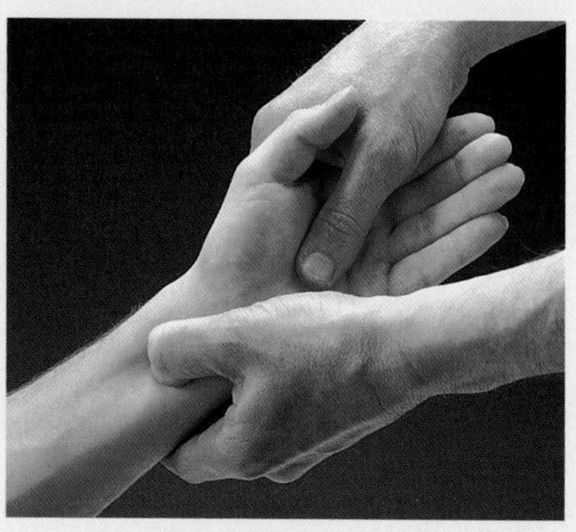

This point is especially useful for nausea, particularly when it is associated with movement (travel sickness, for example). Commercially available bands, worn around the wrist, work on the principle of stimulating Neiguan.

Pressure can be self-applied on this point. With the thumb or middle finger, apply strong reduction on Neiguan (on the forearm, about two inches (5cm) up from the wrist crease and between the two tendons that can be felt there).

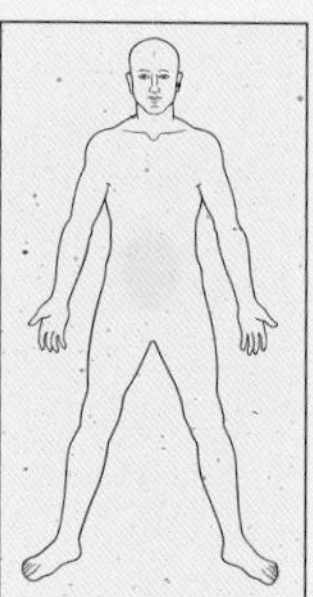

ACHES AND PAINS

JOINT AND muscle problems are common – especially in older people, or after an accident – and produce local aches and pains, which can be very severe. With a local trauma, before using any acupressure massage it is important to allow any initial swelling to go down. It is also essential to ensure that there is no serious underlying trauma or problem, such as a fracture.

WRIST/HAND

Apply gentle reduction on any of the following points, depending on where the pain is.

REDUCTION OF LI 4 (HEGU)

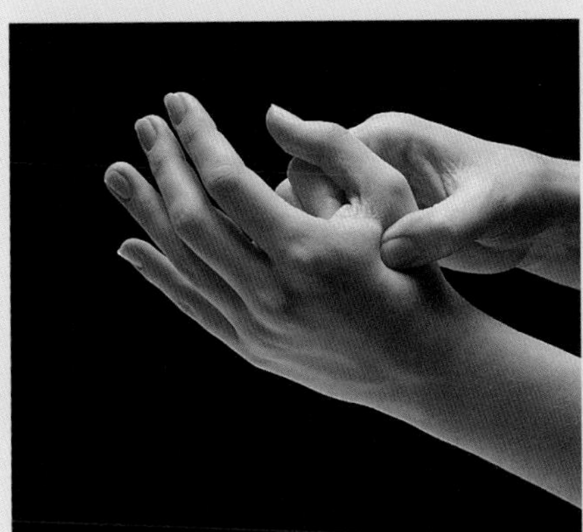

Apply pressure on the web between the thumb and forefinger. Caution: do not use on pregnant patients.

REDUCTION OF SI 3 (HOUXI)

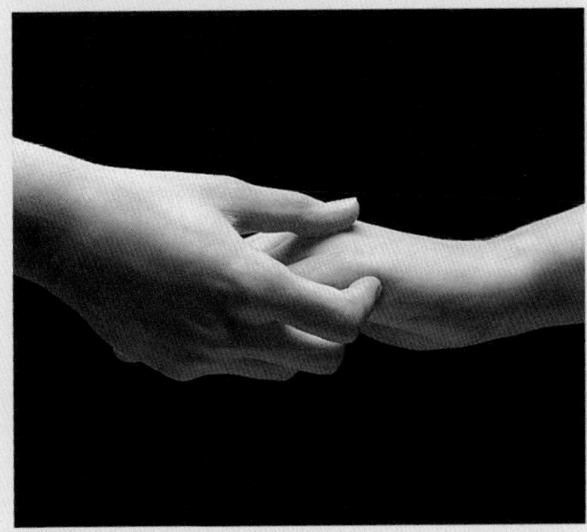

Apply pressure on the side of the hand, in the hollow below the joint of the little finger.

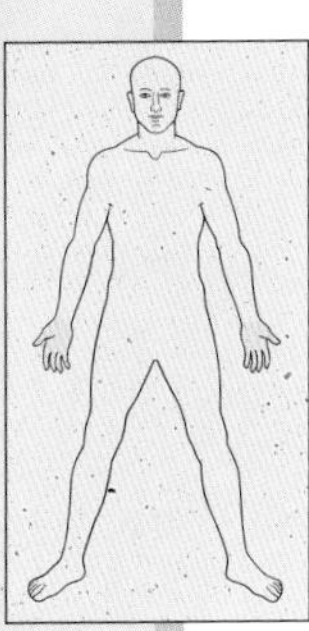

REDUCTION OF LI 15 (YANGXI)

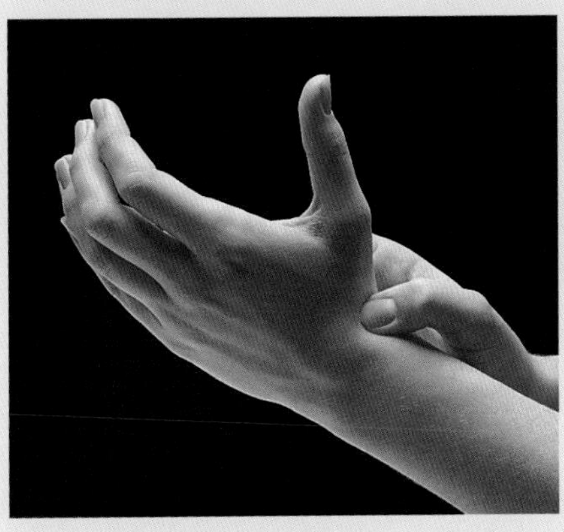

Apply pressure in the hollow below the tendon when the thumb is bent back.

REDUCTION OF SI 5 (YANG GU)

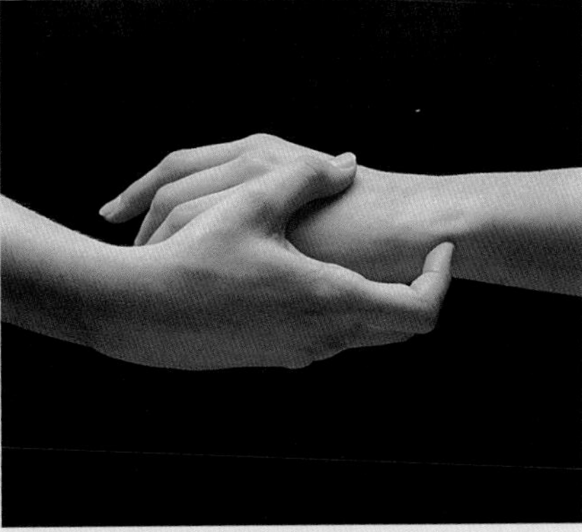

Apply pressure on the outside of the hand in the hollow before the wrist joint.

REDUCTION OF SJ 4 (YANG QI)

Apply pressure on the middle of the wrist crease on the back of the hand.

ELBOW

Apply gentle or firm reduction, depending on the level of pain, on the following points:

REDUCTION OF LI 11 (QUCHI)

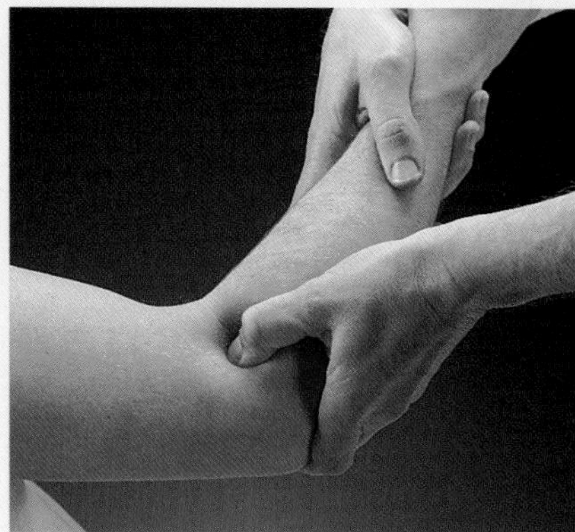

Apply pressure on the outside back of the arm at the elbow. Locate the point by bending the arm and following the crease formed at the elbow to the end.

REDUCTION OF SJ 5 (WAIGUAN)

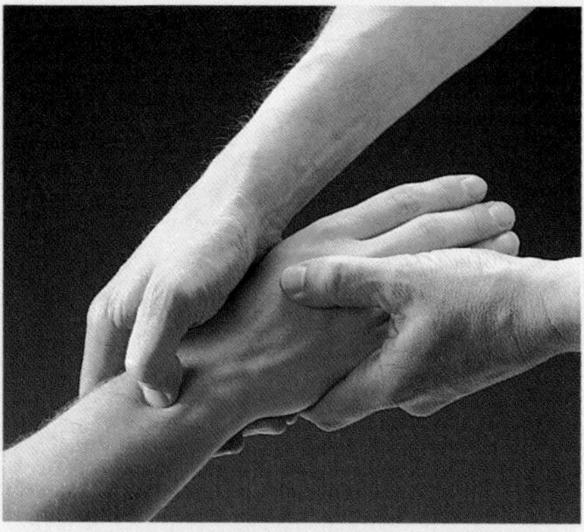

Apply pressure on the back of the forearm between the tendons, about one and a half inches (3.5cm) above the wrist crease.

SHOULDER

Apply gentle or firm reduction, depending on the level of pain, on the following points:

REDUCTION OF SJ 14 (JIANLIAO)

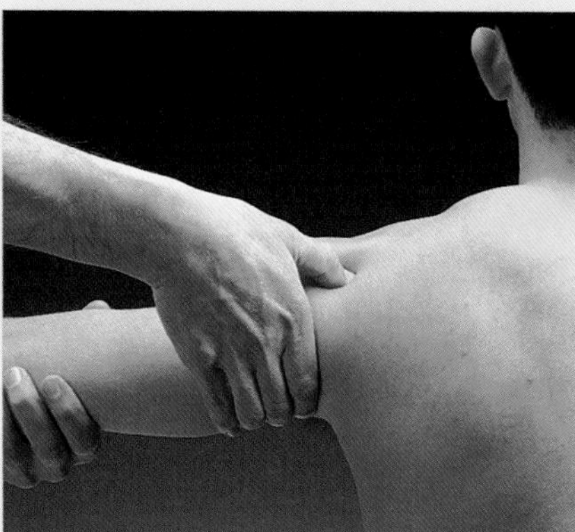

Apply pressure in the "eye" below the shoulder joint at the back.

REDUCTION OF LI 15 (JIANYU)

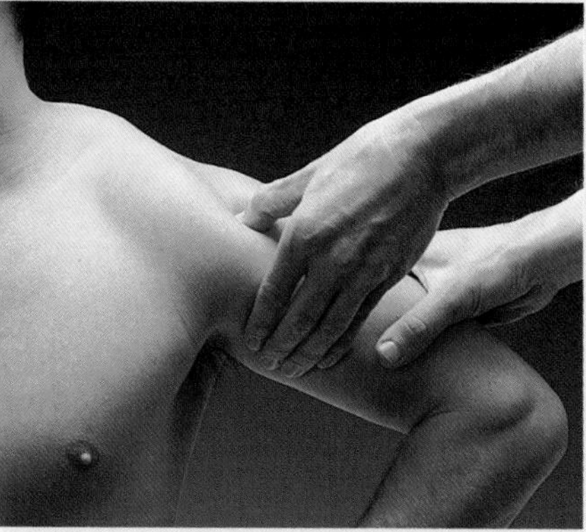

Apply pressure in the "eye" below the shoulder joint at the front.

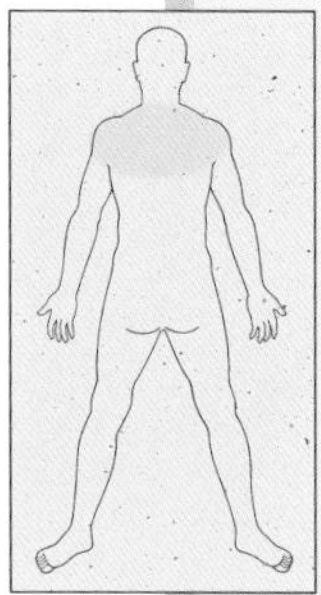

REDUCTION OF SI 12 (BINGFENG)

Apply pressure in the muscle area, about half an inch (12mm) from the spine at the shoulder blade.

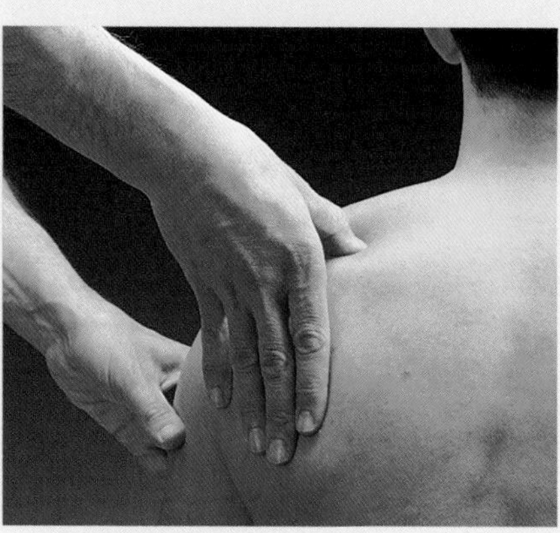

NECK

Apply gentle or firm reduction, on one or more of the following points:

REDUCTION OF SI 12 (BINGFENG)

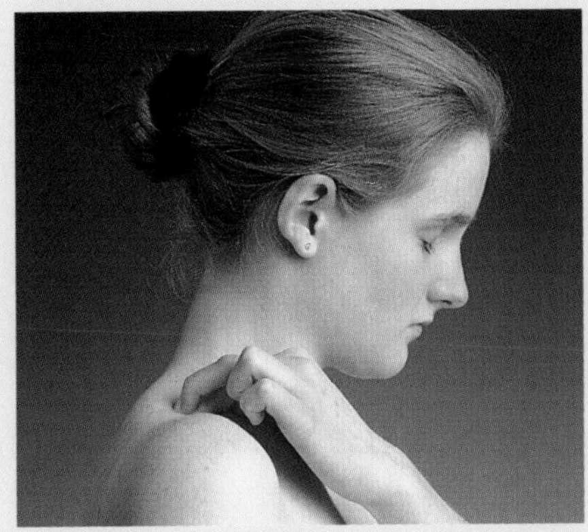

Apply pressure in the muscle area, about half an inch (12mm) from the spine at the shoulder blade.

REDUCTION OF GB 20 (FENG CHI)

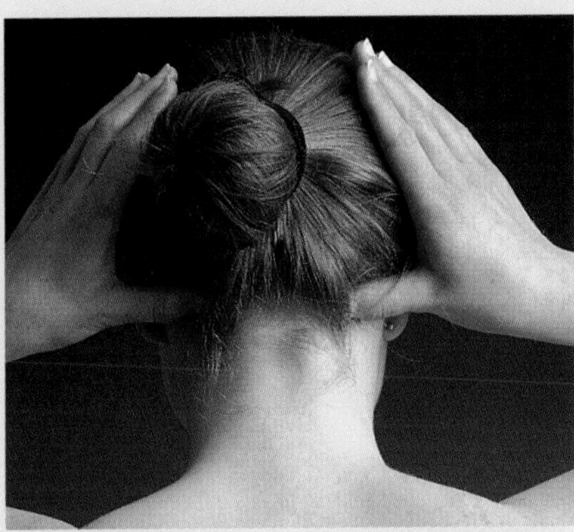

Apply pressure in the depressions below the skull bone, slightly to the side of the midline at the back.

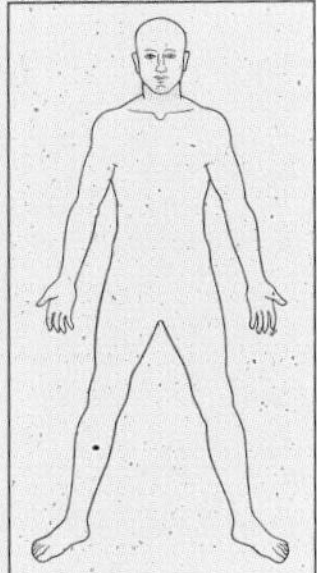

REDUCTION OF GB 21 (JIANJING)

Apply pressure on the muscle at the top of the shoulder, midway between the shoulder and the neck.

CAUTION

Do not massage the Jianjing point on anyone who is pregnant.

LOWER BACK/LUMBER SPINE

Apply firm reduction on the following points:

REDUCTION OF BL 23 (SHEN SHU)

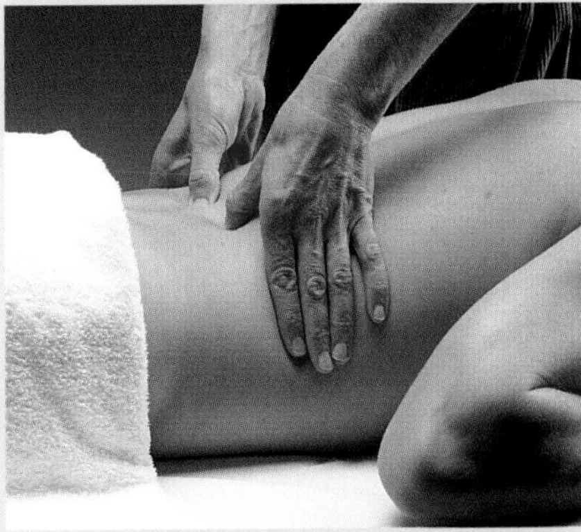

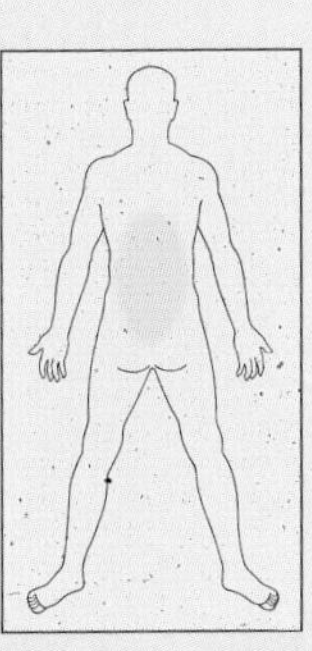

Apply pressure about one and a half inches (3.5cm) either side of the spine, in the small of the back.

KNEES

Apply firm or gentle reduction on the following points:

REDUCTION OF ST 35 (DUBI)

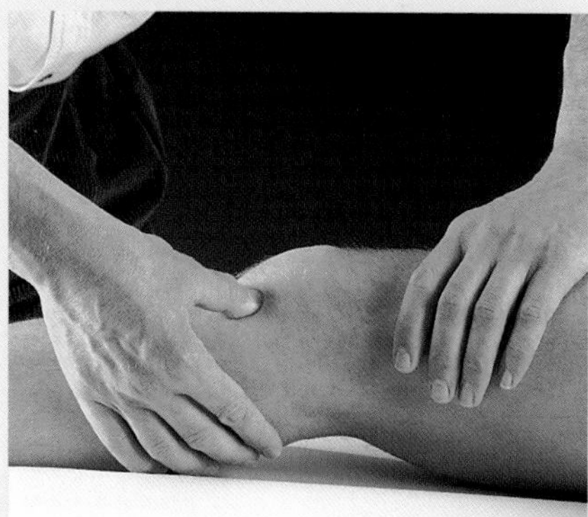

Apply pressure in the eye of the knee below the knee cap, on the outer side.

REDUCTION OF XIXAN

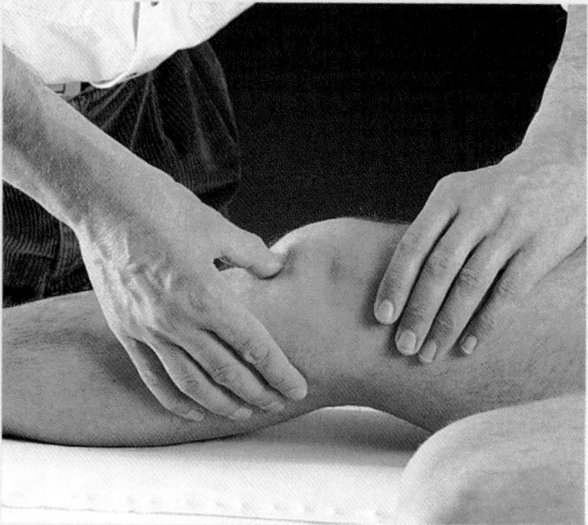

Apply pressure in the eye of the knee below the knee cap, on the inner side.

REDUCTION OF BL 40 (WEI ZHONG)

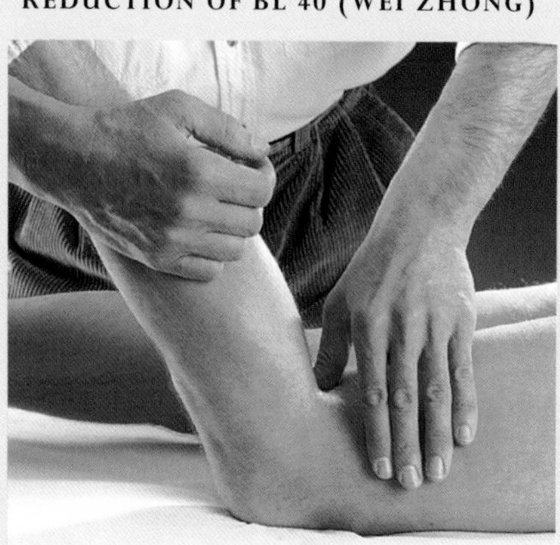

Appy pressure in the middle of the knee, between the tendons at the back.

REDUCTION OF SP 9 (YIN LING QUAN)

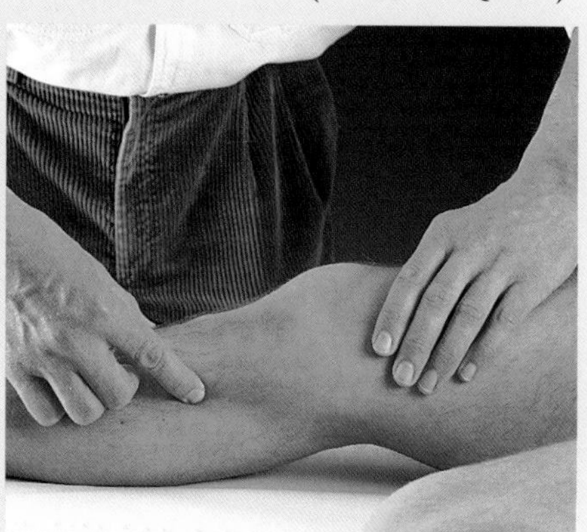

Apply pressure in the depression at the top of the tibia, just below the knee, on the inner side.

LEFT
Problems in hips, legs, knees, and ankles can all be treated with acupressure.

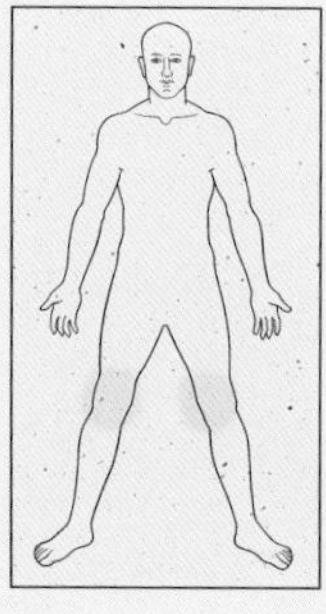

治療
ACUPUNCTURE

SCIATICA

Apply firm reduction on the following points:

REDUCTION OF BL 23 (SHEN SHU)

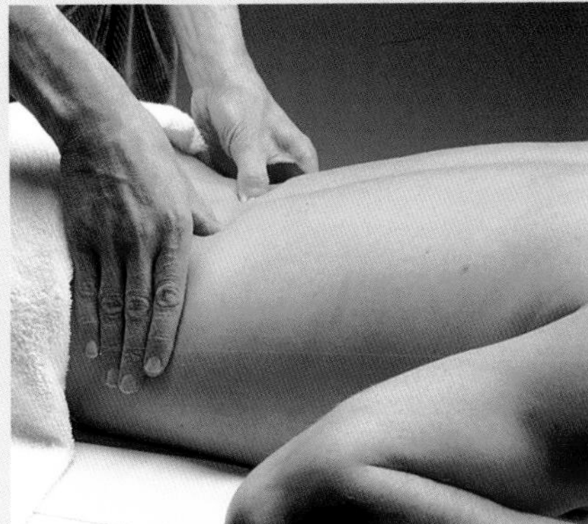

Apply pressure about one and a half inches (3.5cm) either side of the spine, in the small of the back.

REDUCTION OF GB 30 (HUAN TIAO)

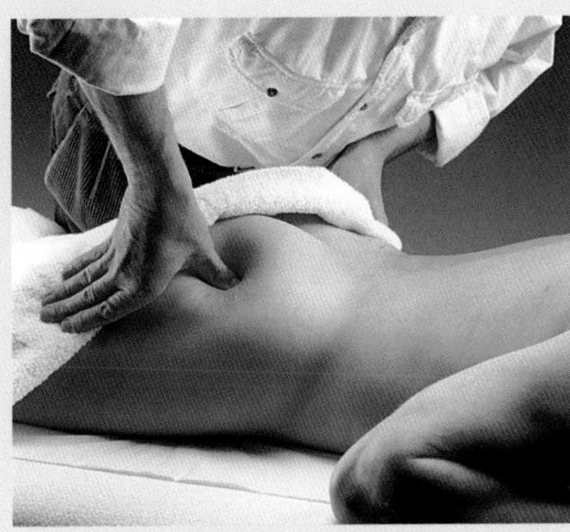

Apply pressure in the buttocks, one third of the way along a line joining the top of the femur and the bottom of the spine.

ANKLE

Apply gentle or firm reduction, on one of the following points:

REDUCTION OF KID 3 (TAIXI)

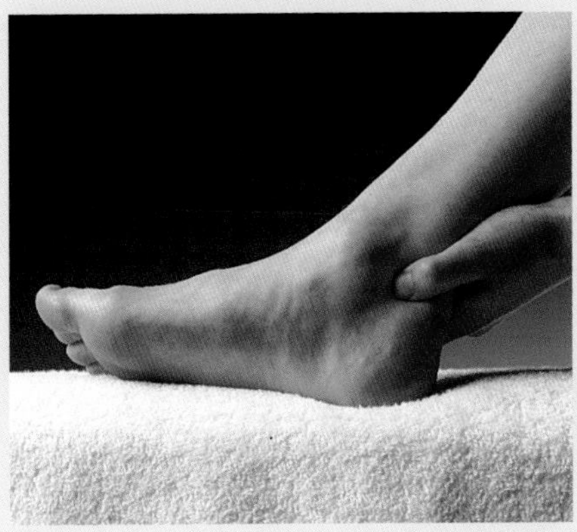

Apply pressure in the depression between the ankle bone and the Achilles tendon, on the inside of the ankle.

REDUCTION OF BL 60 (KUNLUN)

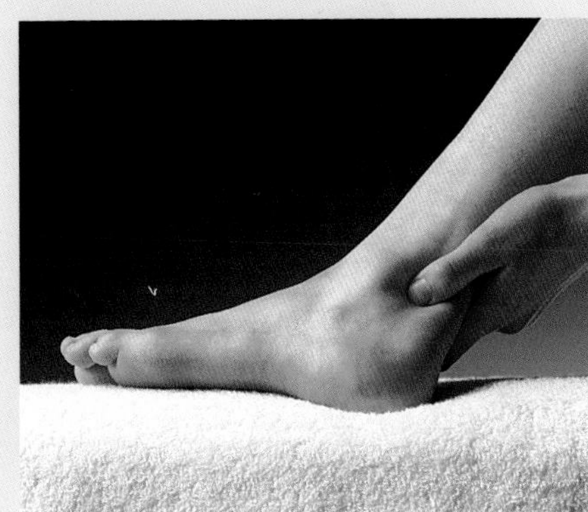

Apply pressure in the depression between the ankle bone and the Achilles tendon, on the outside of the ankle.

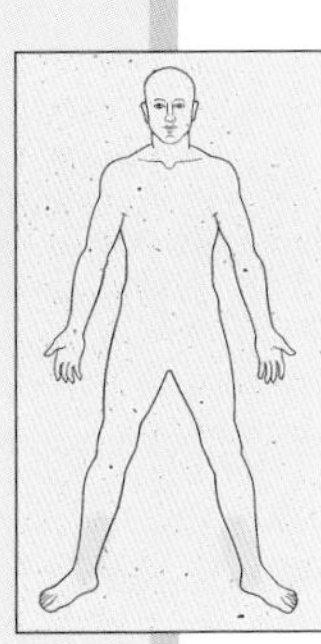

CAUTION

Do not massage the Kunlun point on anyone who is pregnant.

REDUCTION OF ST 41 (JIEXI)

Apply on the top of the foot, in line with the ankle bones, between the tendons.

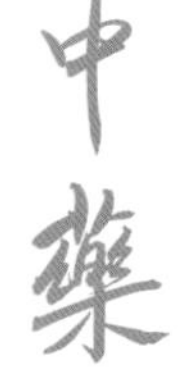

CHINESE MEDICINE

SHEN DAO NECK RELEASE PROTOCOL

THIS PROTOCOL is one involving a professional practitioner and belongs to a more subtle form of acupressure in which emphasis is placed on the energetics of the Qi flow between patient and practitioner rather than on physical pressure. It involves the very light touching of a series of acupuncture points, in a predetermined sequence, and requires the practitioner's energy to be at its peak. It is extremely helpful for relieving the general physical and emotional tension that builds up throughout the day and can bring tremendous relaxation to those who receive it.

OPENING

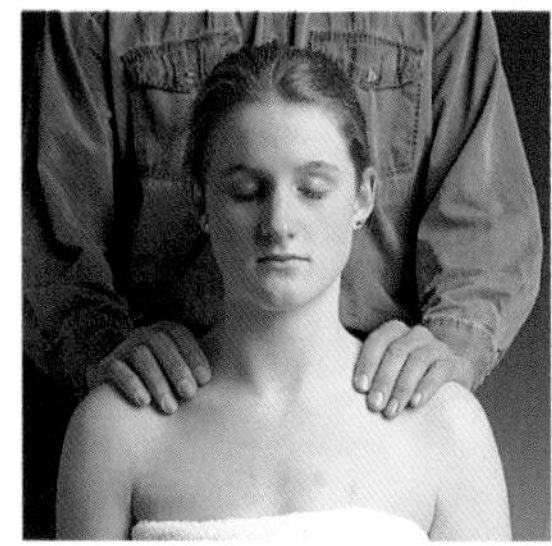

The practitioner stands behind the patient, who sits upright on a straight chair. With the palms resting lightly on the patient's shoulders, the practitioner should take several minutes to become focused – the use of simple Qigong stances is usually recommended (see pages 194–195). *Once both practitioner and patient feel calm and settled the sequence can begin. Each point is usually held for about one minute.*

POSITION 1

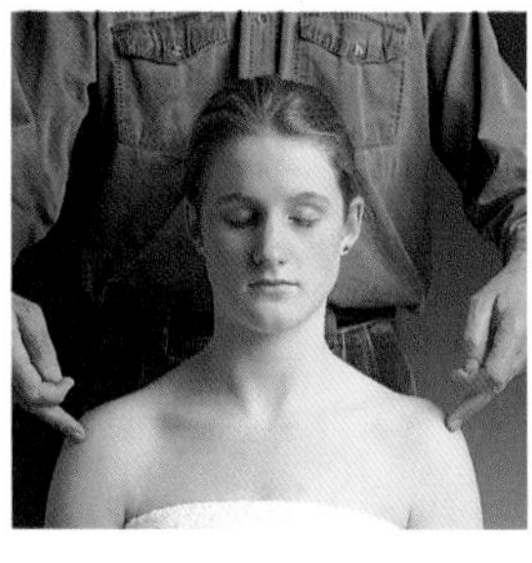

The practitioner gently places the tip of the middle finger of both hands – the acupuncture point P 9 (Zhong Chong) – on the points LI 15 (Jianyu) at the patient's shoulder.

POSITION 2

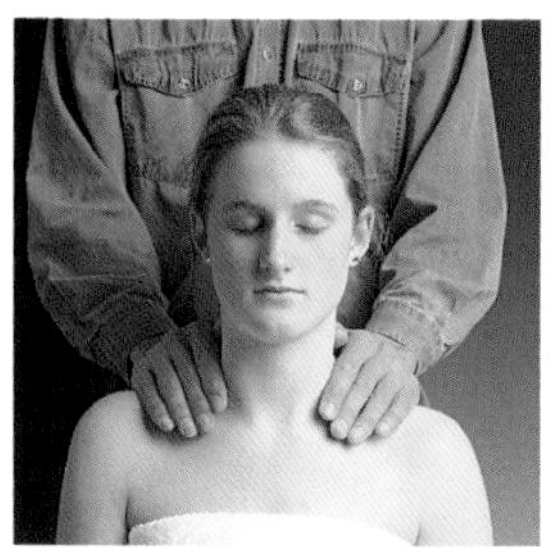

The practitioner gently places the palm along the patient's shoulder, aligning the point in the palm – P 8 (Laogong) – with the point on the shoulder – GB 21 (Jianjing).

POSITION 3

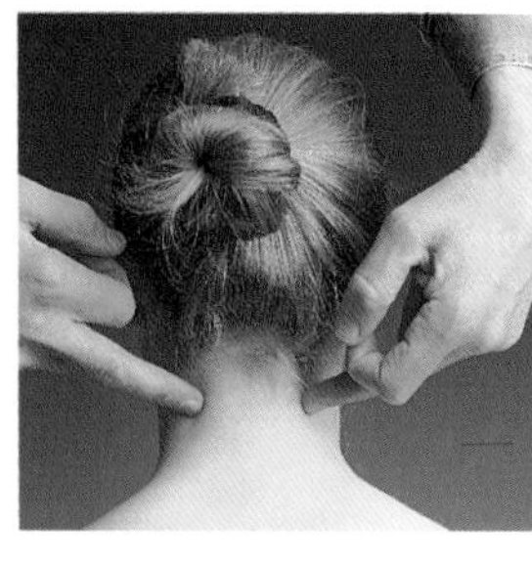

The practitioner gently places the tips of the middle fingers along the line of the Bladder channel at each side of the patient's neck.

POSITION 4

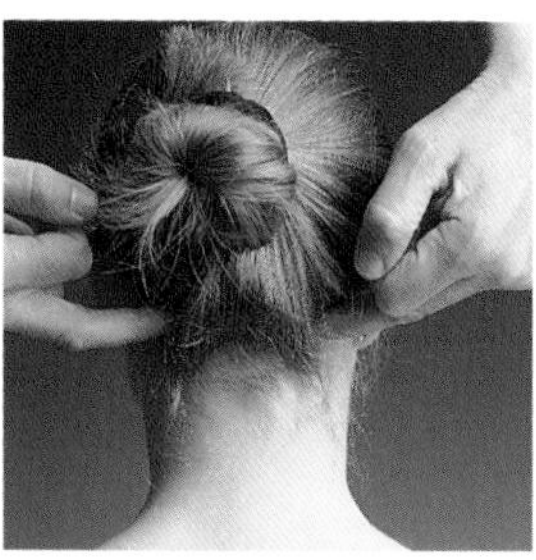

The practitioner gently places Zhong Chong on the patient at the point GB 20 (Feng Chi).

POSITION 5

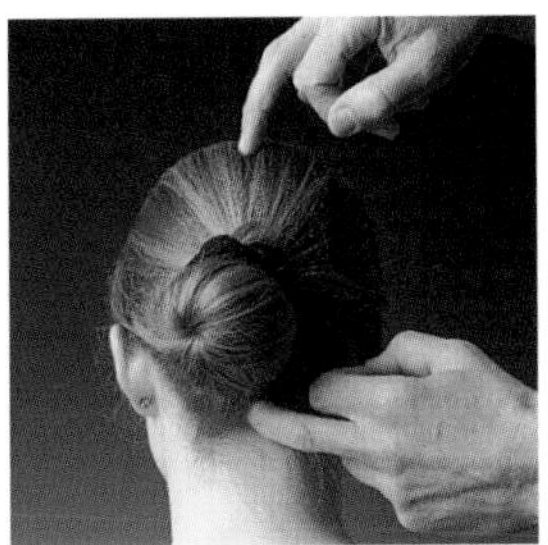

The practitioner gently places the Zhong Chong point of the left hand at point Du 16 (Feng Fu) on the patient, and the Zhong Chong point of the right hand at point Du 20 (Baihui).

POSITION 6

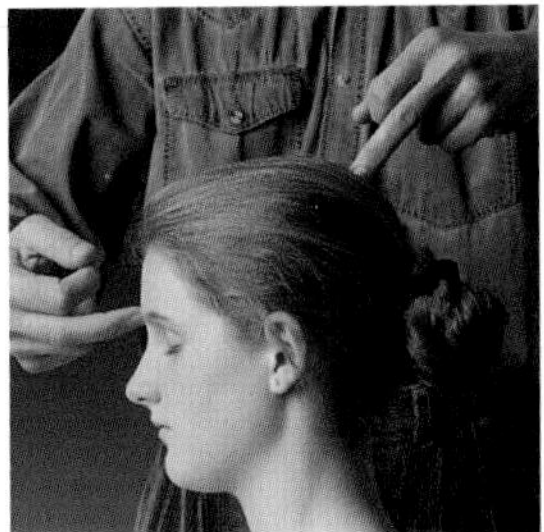

The practitioner gently places the Zhong Chong point of the left hand on Baihui and the Zhong Chong point of the right hand on Yintang.

POSITION 7

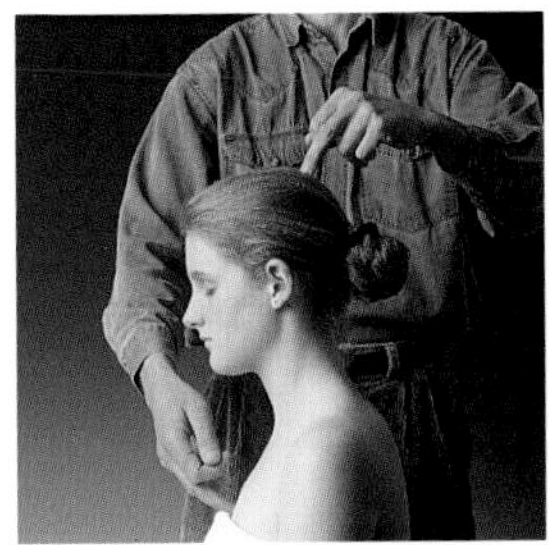

The practitioner keeps the left hand at Baihui and places the Zhong Chong point of the right hand on the patient's point Ren 17 (Tan Zhong).

POSITION 8

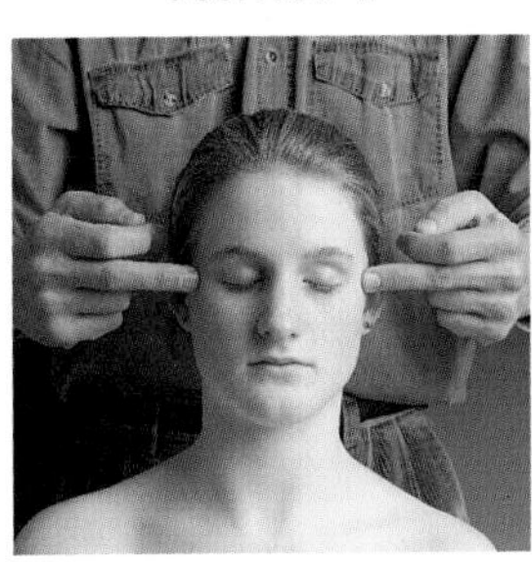

The practitioner places the Zhong Chong points on both hands on the patient's Taiyang points.

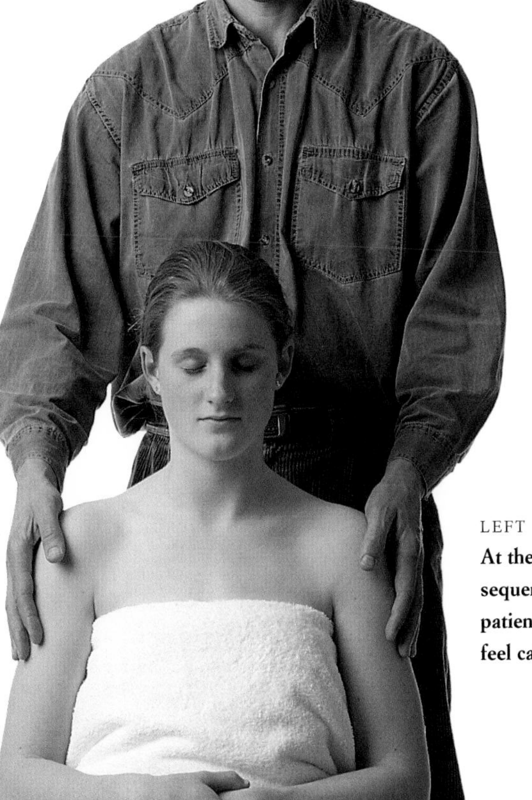

POSITION 9

The practitioner closes by resting the full palm on the patient's shoulder, as shown.

LEFT

At the end of the sequence, both patient and therapist feel calm and still.

POINT POSITIONS

P 9 (Zhong Chong)
at the tip of the middle finger.
P 8 (Laogong)
in the middle of the palm of the hand.
Du 16 (Feng Fu)
on the midline at the back of the neck, immediately below the skull bone.
Du 20 (Baihui)
on the midline at the top of the skull, on a line joining the tips of the ears.
Ren 17 (Tan Zhong)
in the middle of the breastbone on the midline, below the fourth rib in line with the nipples.

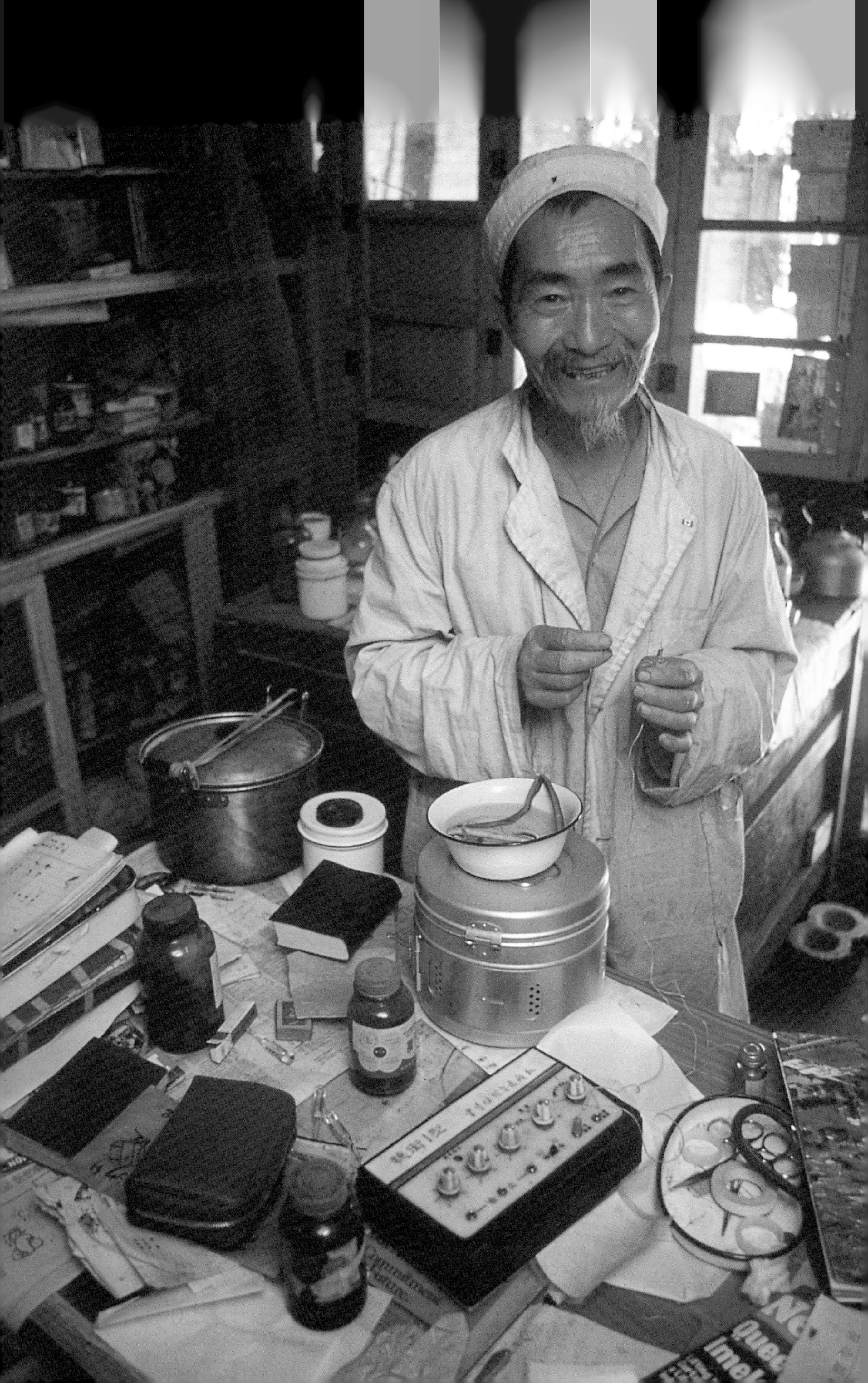

CHINESE HERBALISM

*A*LONGSIDE ACUPUNCTURE, *herbal medicine is the other major pillar of Chinese medicine. Herbal preparations have long been used in China, and there is evidence from as far back as 2000* B.C. *of a shamanic culture that used plant, mineral, and animal substances to treat ailments. Over the succeeding centuries the use of such substances was refined and developed: by about* A.D. *659 a comprehensive "materia medica," which listed the herbal components and described their actions and properties, was beginning to emerge.*

Acupuncture and herbal medicine share the same underlying theories and principles, but the descriptions of how herbs work comprise a subtle component of the theoretical blueprint. Herbs tend to be highly specific in their actions, and herbal formulae contain a range of herbs that not only possess different qualities and properties but also target different aspects of the patient's disharmony. In addition, certain individual herbs address several different functions at the same time. Overall, the herbal practitioner has to weigh up many factors when preparing a formula, but the benefits for patients can be substantial.

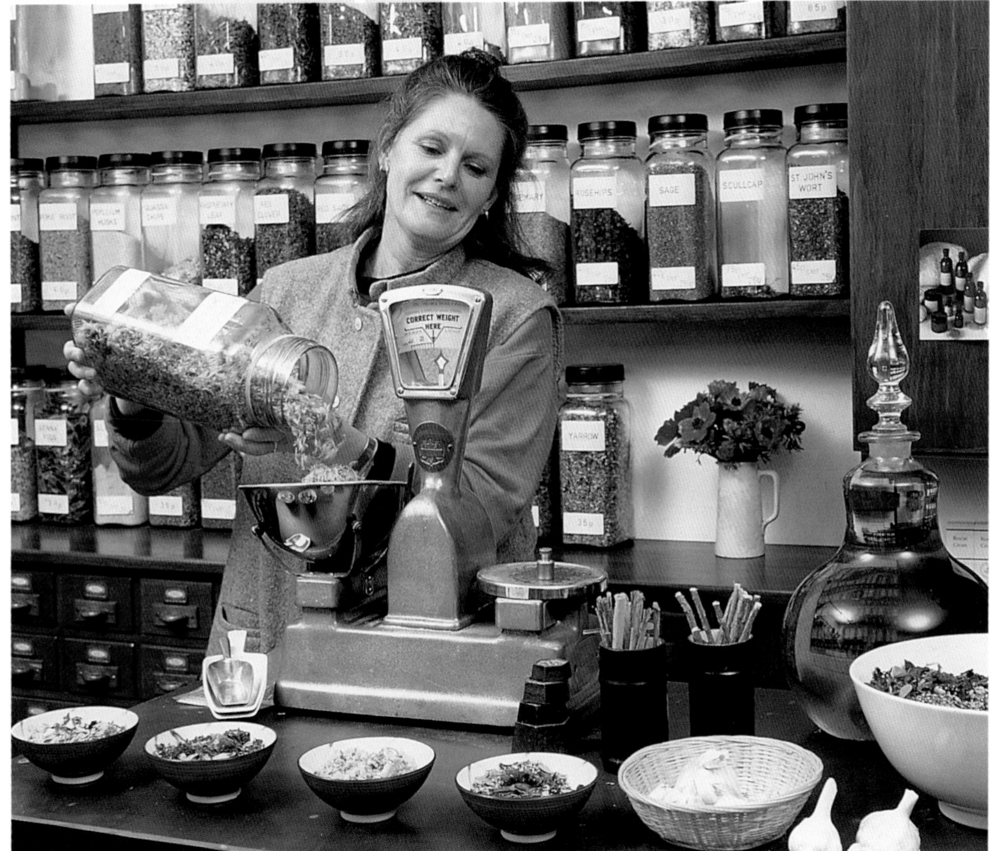

RIGHT AND ABOVE
Chinese herbalists once prepared their own remedies. Now herbs and other ingredients are usually obtained from specialist suppliers.

LEFT
A traditional Chinese herbalist with his ingredients and remedies.

HERBS THROUGHTOUT THIS CHAPTER SUPPLIED BY COURTESY OF MAYWAY, LONDON.

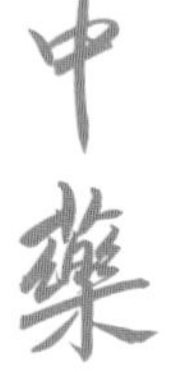

CHINESE MEDICINE

PROPERTIES OF HERBS

CHINESE HERBS can be considered in terms of the following classifications:

THE FOUR ENERGIES

The four essential energetic qualities of herbs, and their corresponding actions, relate to their perceived temperatures:

Cool or cold herbs relieve conditions where there is Heat in the body, while warm or hot herbs relieve Cold symptoms. Some herbs are neither hot nor cold, and in essence they describe a fifth energy, that of neutral herbs. For example: ✦ Sheng Di Huang (fresh rehmannia root) – cool/cold – relieves Heat. ✦ Rou Gui (cinnamon bark) – warm/hot – relieves Cold symptoms. ✦ Fu Ling (poria) – neutral.

FU LING

SHENG DI HUANG

THE FIVE TASTES

The five taste qualities of herbs relate to their action on the Qi of the body:

These tastes describe the therapeutic effect of herbs. Pungent/acrid herbs disperse and promote the movement of Qi in the body and invigorate the Blood; sweet herbs tonify and strengthen the Qi and nourish the Blood; sour/astringent herbs absorb body substances and control the functions of the Zangfu; bitter herbs reduce excess Qi and dry excess moisture; salty herbs soften lumps. Some herbs, described as "bland," are relatively neutral in terms of taste. For example: ✦ Hong Hua (safflower) – pungent/acrid – invigorates the Blood. ✦ Ren Shen (ginseng root) – sweet – tonifies the Qi. ✦ Wu Wei Zi (schisandra fruit) – sour – relieves spontaneous sweating. ✦ Huo Po (magnolia bark) – bitter – dries and transforms dampness. ✦ Mang Xiao (Glauber's salt) – salty – clears constipation.

RIGHT
Through their differing properties, herbs treat Heat or Cold and influence different parts of the energetic system. The way they are prepared affects their action.

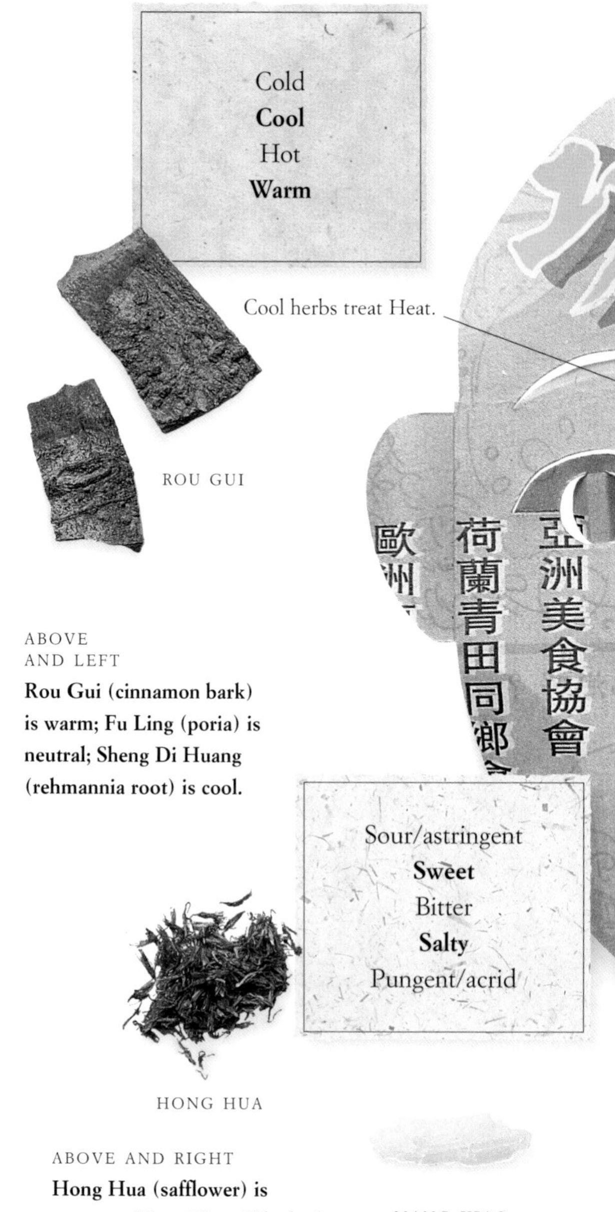

ABOVE AND LEFT
Rou Gui (cinnamon bark) is warm; Fu Ling (poria) is neutral; Sheng Di Huang (rehmannia root) is cool.

MANG XIAO

ABOVE AND RIGHT
Hong Hua (safflower) is pungent; Mang Xiao (Glauber's salt) is salty; Wu Wei Zi (schisandra fruit) is sour.

The classification of the herbal qualities into energies and tastes shows what each herb can do. However, these qualities are not absolute; they all exist on a continuum. It is thus possible to differentiate herbs in terms of their position on these energetic continua. A herb may be slightly warm, warm, very warm, hot, and so on, together with the other qualities of energy and taste.

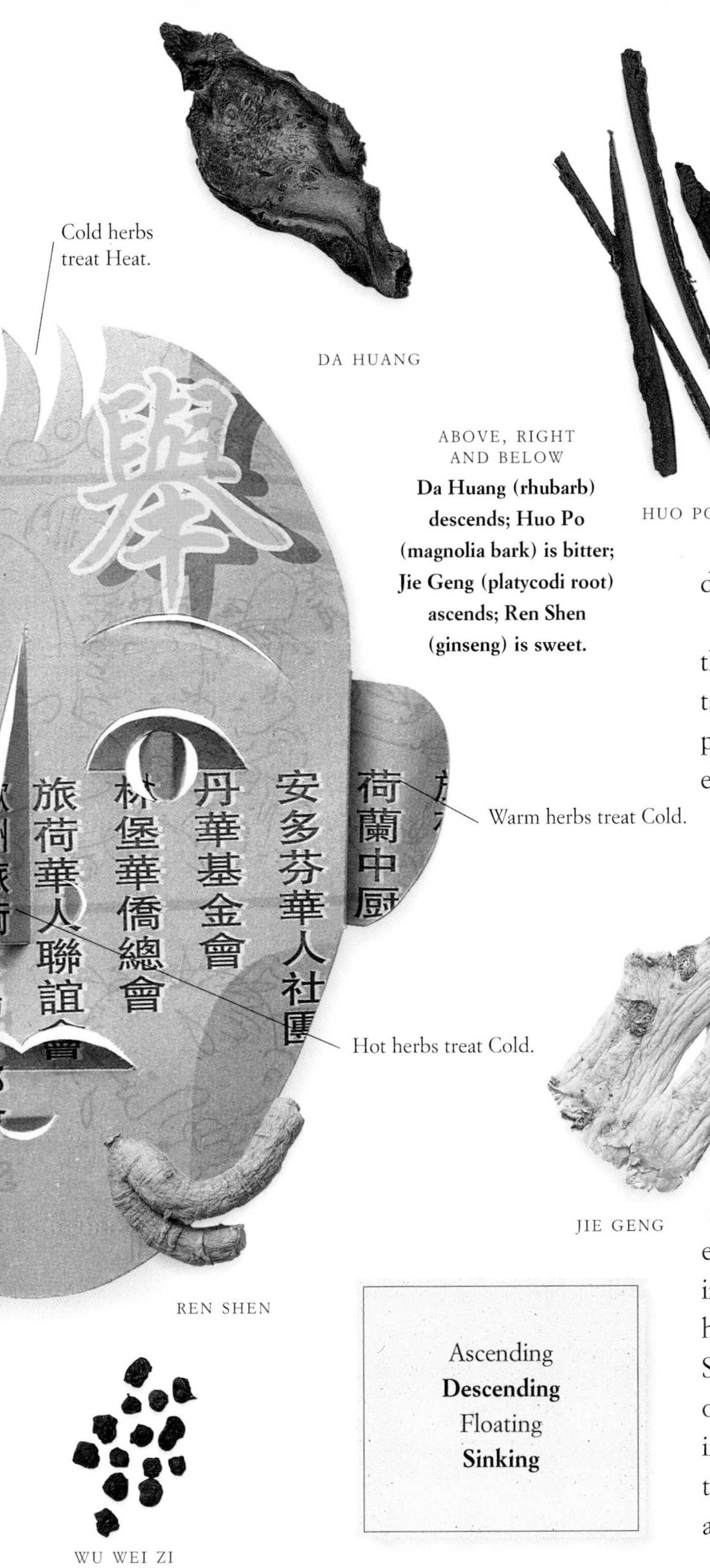

DA HUANG

HUO PO

JIE GENG

REN SHEN

WU WEI ZI

ABOVE, RIGHT AND BELOW **Da Huang (rhubarb) descends; Huo Po (magnolia bark) is bitter; Jie Geng (platycodi root) ascends; Ren Shen (ginseng) is sweet.**

Ascending
Descending
Floating
Sinking

The "movement" of herbs

Since herbs are said to move through the energetic system of the body, specific herbs can be used to target specific parts of the body, or to facilitate the movement of other active herbal ingredients. The four basic "movements" are as follows:

Herbs that ascend and float tend to move upward and outward, influencing the top part of the body and the extremities. Herbs that descend and sink, on the other hand, move both downward and inward, influencing the lower part of the body and the interior. For example: ✦ Jie Geng (the platycodi root or "balloon flower") – ascending – opens and dispels Lung Qi. ✦ Da Huang (rhubarb) – descending – relieves constipation.

In reality these functional tendencies involve the complex interaction of the basic energies and tastes. In addition, the manner in which herbs are processed also influences their function. For example, frying a herb encourages it :while preparing a herb with salt promotes a descending action.

Entering the channels

In Chinese herbal medicine, individual herbs are thought to "enter" specific channels or meridians and are therefore targeted toward the Zangfu system associated with that channel. It is probably more accurate to state that specific herbs energetically influence particular Zangfu systems in the body. For example, when it is said that the herb Da Zao (Chinese date) enters the Spleen and Stomach channels, it is suggested that the function of the herb relates to the function of these organs in terms of the theory of the Zangfu. Da Zao is therefore used by herbalists to tonify the Spleen and augment the Qi.

The practitioner of Chinese herbal medicine has to consider how the energetic qualities of a herb, in terms of the Four Energies and the Five Tastes, interact to describe its function and action. At the same time, the practitioner must be aware of which Zangfu system is being influenced. A Chinese herbal formula is a complex cocktail of energetic qualities, functions, directions, and foci, and it takes skill to pitch ingredients and dosage at the correct level in order to address the symptoms of a patient's disharmony.

Not all herbs are plants

Patients are often surprised to learn that not every substance in the "materia medica" comes from a vegetable or plant source. In the West, the tendency to equate the term "herb" with something that grows in the garden leads to quite serious misconceptions when considering Chinese "herbs." Certainly, the majority of herbal remedies are made from parts of plants – roots, stalks, bark, leaves, fruit, seeds, and so on. However, some substances are animal or mineral in origin. Shi Gao (gypsum), for example, is a very cooling mineral herb, commonly used to treat conditions where there is a lot of Heat.

The use of animal parts in herbal medicine is a somewhat controversial issue. Culturally, the Chinese view the use of animals in a far more pragmatic way than is generally the case in the West. They have never avoided using animal products and have found many to be very effective. However, certain animal parts have been the focus of much controversy and outrage, and in real terms these products are rarely used, if ever, today. That said, several "animal" herbs are still a very important constituent of many common and important formulae. For example, Chan Tui (cicada husks) are used regularly to treat skin conditions since they are very effective in relieving the itch associated with these complaints.

There are no absolutes here: some patients feel very unhappy about using animal products, others do not mind. If you have a problem in this area, it is important to discuss it with your herbal practitioner before a prescription is made up. In most instances, alternatives can be used.

MU LI

LEFT
Mu Li (oyster shells) may be used for hypertension, dizziness, headache, and other problems.

Toxicity

A perfectly natural question with respect to Chinese herbs is the extent to which they may be toxic or in any way dangerous to take. The reality is that taking herbs is no different from taking any other substance into the body. Too much can be harmful, and in some instances doses need to be monitored very carefully to ensure that there are no unwelcome toxic side effects.

The vast majority of herbs are quite safe and pose no threat if taken in the specified dose. With most herbs, the practitioner has a wide dosage range within which to work; but with some herbs the range is much narrower, and their use may need to be limited in order to avoid side effects. A few herbs that are regularly used in China are not generally prescribed in the West. The most notable example is Fu Zi (aconite), which has very hot qualities. Appropriate substitutes are generally available.

To avoid any problems, the best advice, as always, is to make sure that you consult an appropriately trained and experienced practitioner of Chinese herbal medicine.

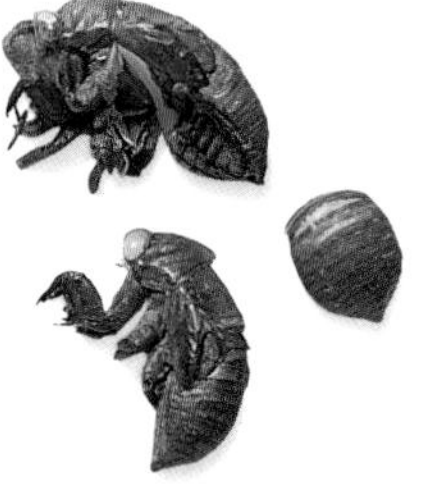

CHAN TUI

LEFT
Chan Tui (cicada husks) are helpful for skin conditions.

BELOW
Shi Gao (gypsum) is used for thirst, heat rash and other conditions caused by Heat excess.

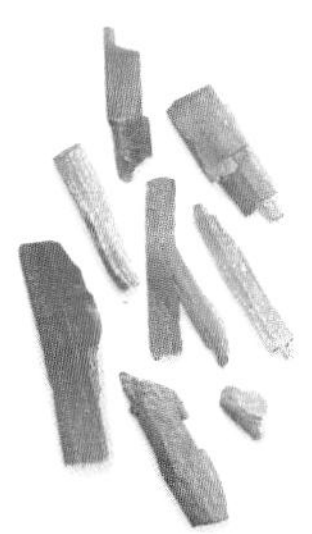

SHI GAO

BELOW

Many powerful ingredients are used in Chinese herbalism. Dangerous ones, such as arsenic, can be sold only to those with a doctor's prescription.

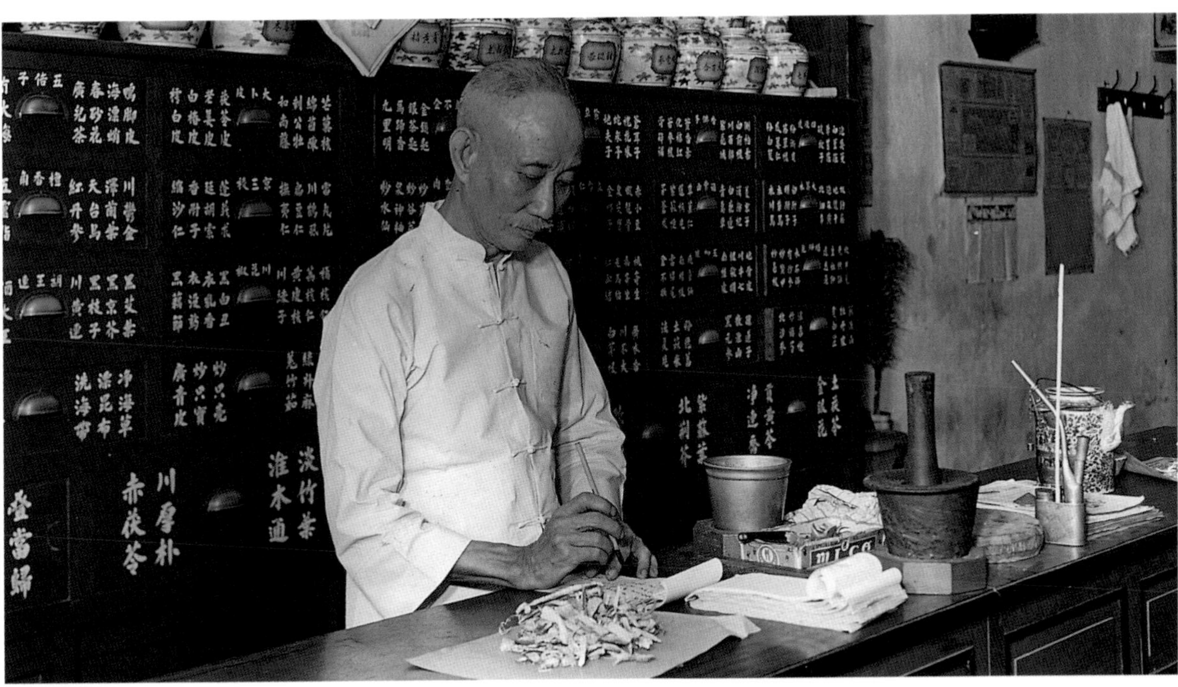

WHO CAN BE HELPED BY CHINESE HERBALISM?

IN TERMS of fundamental principles, the approach taken to the use of Chinese herbs is essentially the same as that taken when considering acupuncture. The essence of Chinese herbal medicine lies in the skill of the practitioner in modifying and fine-tuning the herbal formulae in order to match the characteristics and variations in a patient's disharmony – in the same way that an acupuncturist selects an appropriate set of points on the body.

The answer to this question, therefore, is the same as for acupuncture – there are few problems that cannot be helped by Chinese herbalism, although there are some contraindications. With herbal medicine, though, more attention needs to be paid to situations where caution must be exercised and/or contraindications noted.

Unlike acupuncture, where (with one or two exceptions) the wrong choice of point to be needled is unlikely to be significantly detrimental, herbs can have very specific actions, and problems may arise if the choice of herb or the dosage is inappropriate. The experienced herbal practitioner has to bear in mind the following points:

- Certain herbs are contraindicated in pregnancy.
- Certain herbs are toxic.
- Herbs may be totally contraindicated in patients who have a Liver function problem (Liver function tests are sometimes performed as a matter of course before prescribing.)
- The herb chosen must always be sensitive to features of the patient's disharmony; for example, very hot and drying herbs should not be used where there is evidence of a Yin deficiency.
- Some patients will not use herbs of animal origin, and this must be ascertained before prescribing.

In the West, most practitioners of Chinese herbal medicine are also trained in acupuncture, although the reverse is not the case. In China, herbs and acupuncture are complementary aspects of Chinese medicine and would never be considered separately. It is only in order to clarify certain distinctions that the two modalities are distinguished in this book.

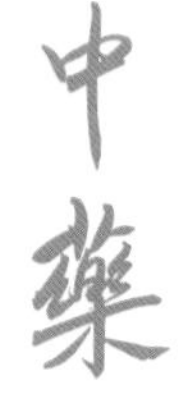

TOOLS AND TECHNIQUES

MATCHING ENERGETIC QUALITIES AND DIAGNOSIS

The practitioner of Chinese herbal medicine must match the qualities of individual herbs with the nature of the patient's energetic disharmony, which is defined in terms of the Eight-Principle patterns. By using the same diagnostic principles described for acupuncture *(see pages 138–140)*, the practitioner arrives at a detailed understanding of the patient's energetic disharmonies, and this suggests the types of herbs that are required. The diagnostic approach is summarized below.

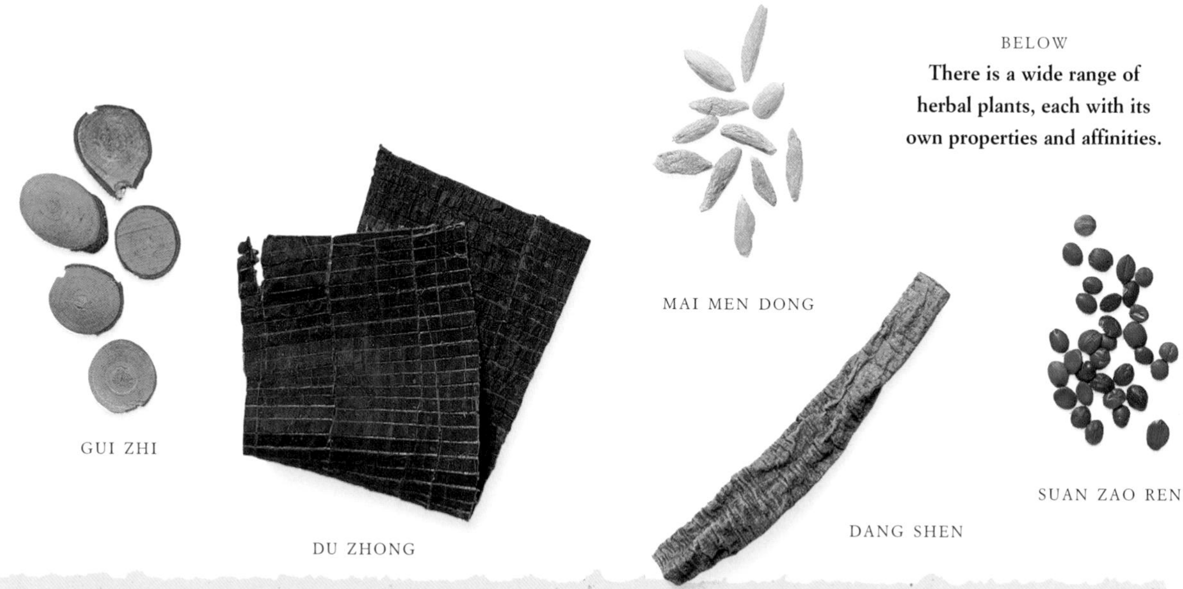

BELOW
There is a wide range of herbal plants, each with its own properties and affinities.

DISHARMONIES AND HERBS TO REMEDY THEM

NATURE OF DISHARMONY	HERB	ACTION
Qi deficiency	Dang Shen (*Codonopsis* root)	*Qi tonic*
Blood deficiency	He Shou Wu (*Polygonum* root)	*Blood tonic*
Yang deficiency	Du Zhong (*Eucommia* bark)	*Yang tonic*
Yin deficiency	Mai Men Dong (*Liriope* root tuber)	*Yin tonic*
Stagnant Qi	Chen Pi (*Citrus* rind)	*regulates Qi*
Stagnant Blood	Chuan Xiong (*Ligusticum* root)	*invigorates Blood*
Interior Cold	Rou Gui (*Cinnamomum* bark)	*warms and expels Cold*
Interior Heat/toxicity	Tu Fu Ling (*Smilacis* rhizome)	*clears Heat and toxins*
Exterior invasion (Cold)	Gui Zhi (*Cinnamomum* stems)	*expels/disperses Cold*
Exterior invasion (Heat)	Chai Hu (*Bupleurum* root)	*expels/disperses Heat*
Extreme interior Heat	Shi Gao (*Gypsum*)	*drains Fire/Heat*
Interior Damp	Cang Zhu (*Atractylodes* root)	*transforms Damp*
Disturbed Shen (spirit)	Suan Zao Ren (*Ziziphus* seeds)	*calms Shen*

This shows how herbs are matched with symptoms, but it does not suggest how the herbs may be combined, since this decision can be taken only by the practitioner.

HERBAL FORMULAE

THE DEVELOPMENT of herbal formulae has followed the same historical pattern as that of acupuncture points. Essentially it has been an empirical process in which the properties of herbs – and the effects of combining them – have been observed and recorded over many centuries. The resulting classic formulae comprise the basis of treatment in Chinese herbal medicine. The process is one of gradual evolution.

For example, over the years, once a formula is found to be effective in treating a particular type of disharmony, slight variations to this formula develop, although they usually retain the original name. When a practitioner first uses this formula, it may be necessary to alter it slightly in order to match the patient's disharmony. As the treatment process continues and the pattern of the disharmony shifts, the original formula may be adapted and changed several times. Indeed, it is quite possible that the patient's final formula, although still bearing the name of the classic original, has been significantly changed – and in some instances it may be almost unrecognizable as the original.

Thus, the art of prescribing Chinese herbs lies not so much in identifying which basic formula to use but in knowing how and when to adapt that basic formula to meet the changing therapeutic needs of the patient.

> **CAUTION**
>
> Do not prepare your own remedies except under the instructions of a qualified herbalist.

Many of the classic formulae are so consistently used that they are prepared as patent remedies available in health stores.

How is a herbal formula made up?

Du Huo Ji Sheng Tang *(Angelica pubescens* and Sang Ji Sheng Decoction), a commonly used and fairly complex herbal formula, provides a good example of how a formula is put together.

The name

Herbal formulae are often defined by the names of the main herbs they contain. In this instance, the name is built up from the two main herbs – Du Huo *(Angelica)* and Sang Ji Sheng *(Ramulus)*. The end of the name very often describes how the formula is prepared. Thus, Tang means "soup" or "decoction." The formulae may also be prepared as a powder ("San"), a pill ("Wan"), or a tincture in alcohol ("Jiu").

BELOW
Formulae have developed over centuries of use and observation.

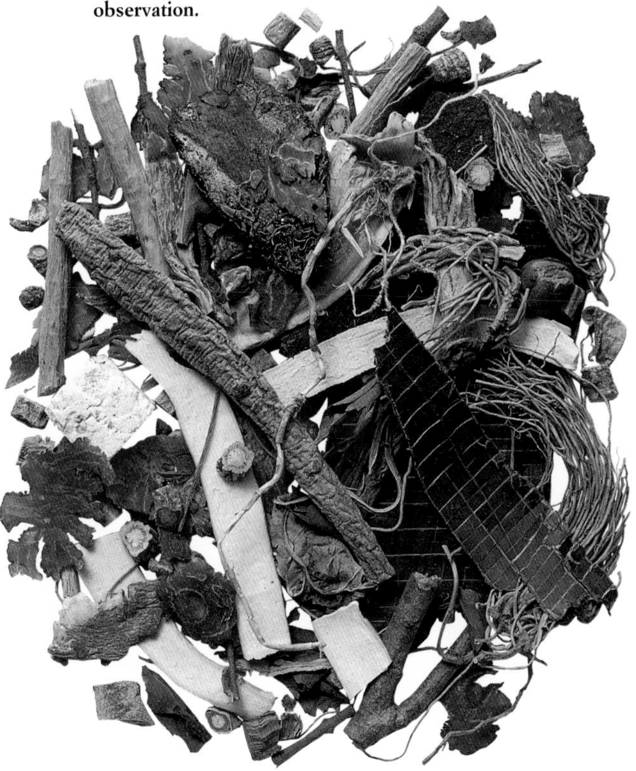

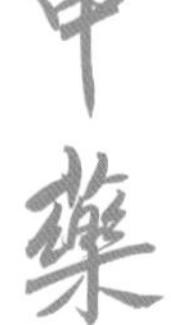

What is in the formula and what does it do?

To see how the Du Huo Ji Sheng Tang formula is made up, it is necessary to consider its ingredients and their action.

This particularly complex formula is prescribed for patients suffering from painful arthritic joints, stiffness, tiredness, and lethargy. In Chinese medicine, such a condition is seen as an external invasion of the channels by Wind, Damp, and Cold. The invading factors tend to lodge in the channels at the joints, producing the pain and swelling so characteristic of arthritis.

As can be seen, several herbs used in this formula warm the channels, expel Wind, Cold, and Damp and relieve pain. This is the main focus of the formula. In addition, other herbs move and nourish the Blood, encouraging the flow and lubricating and nourishing the joints, bones, and sinews. The formula also contains Qi tonic herbs to help strengthen the Spleen, promote the production of Qi, and build up the body's immunity, or Wei Qi (protective Qi).

In a complex formula containing a large number of different herbs with their own energies and tastes, it is important that they all work well together. Zhi Gan Cao (licorice) is included here, since it is a herb that harmonizes. The "Zhi" in front of its name indicates that it is fried (usually in honey) before being used.

A practitioner may well start treatment with the Du Huo Ji Sheng Tang formula as given, but, as the treatment process continues, the ingredients and doses may change in response to how the patient reacts.

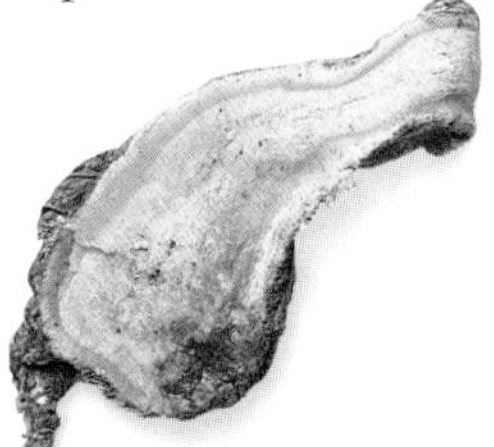

DU HUO

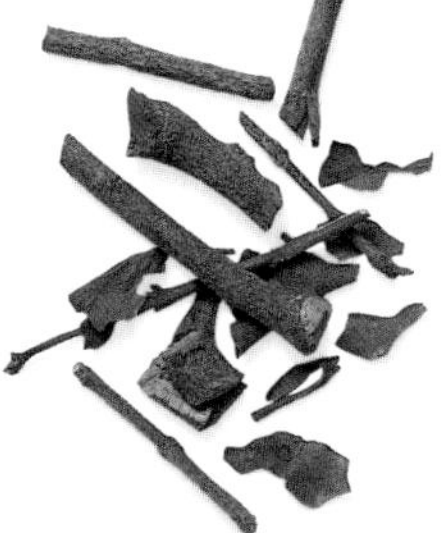

SANG JI SHENG

LEFT
Herbs with specific actions (see the table below) are used in combination.

HERBS IN DU HUO JI SHENG TANG AND THEIR ACTIONS

HERB	ACTION
Du Huo	*expels Wind, Damp, and Cold from the lower part of the body, and from bones and sinews*
Sang Ji Sheng	*expels Wind and Damp, tonifies the Liver and Kidneys*
Xi Xin	*clears Wind and Damp from bones, scatters Cold in the channels, stops pain*
Fang Feng	*expels Wind and clears Damp*
Qin Jiao	*expels Wind and Damp, relaxes the sinews*
Du Zhong	*expels Wind and Damp, tonifies the Liver and Kidneys*
Nui Xi	*expels Wind and Damp, tonifies the Liver and Kidneys*
Rou Gui	*expels Wind and Damp, warms the channels, strengthens the Yang*
Chuan Xiong	*nourishes and invigorates the Blood*
Sheng Di Huang	*nourishes and invigorates the Blood*
Bai Shao	*nourishes and invigorates the Blood*
Dang Shen	*tonifies the Qi, strengthens the Spleen*
Fu Ling	*drains Dampness, tonifies the Spleen*
Zhi Gan Cao	*tonifies the Qi, harmonizes the action of the other herbs*

HOW ARE HERBS PREPARED?

HERBS ARE prescribed in a variety of ways – raw, powdered, as a tincture, or as prepared pills.

RAW HERBS

The classic, and probably the best, way to take Chinese herbs is in their raw, dried form – although this is not always the most convenient way. The patient may well be given bags full of what appear to be twigs, roots, leaves, seeds, powders, hard bits, soft bits, light bits, heavy bits, and bits that are difficult to describe at all. The herbs are then usually cooked in a soup, following quite rigorous instructions. After cooking, the "water" or "decoction" is drained off for drinking, and the remnants discarded. All the herbs may be cooked together, or in some cases certain herbs may be added toward the end of the cooking in order to retain their properties. The decoction is drunk warm (not boiling), and the product of one brew is divided up into doses according to the prescription. Any decoction not taken immediately is usually stored in a glass jar in the refrigerator, and reheated as required. Glass or earthenware pots should be used to cook herbs. Metal pots are best avoided, although stainless steel is considered acceptable.

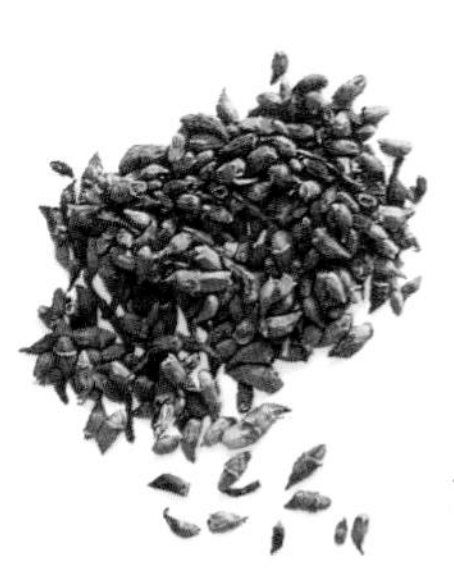

ABOVE
Dried, raw herbs are often made into preparations.

Herbs should never be cooked in a microwave: this can seriously impair their energetic qualities.

Decocted herbal preparations are rarely a gastronomic feast, and patients may find them difficult to take. This can be helped by taking a mouthful of dried fruit immediately before and after the decoction.

Without a doubt, decoctions are the best way to access the energetic qualities of herbs and bring about the most potent therapeutic effects. The disadvantage is in the preparation and actual consumption of the herbs. It can take up to an hour to prepare a herbal decoction, and the process can be messy and awkward.

Some raw herbal formulae can be taken by crushing the ingredients and forming them into "pills" with honey. Again, this can be an awkward and messy procedure, and one that is not always an appropriate form of treatment.

POWDERED HERBS

Dried, powdered herbs provide an alternative to raw herbs – and are much easier to prepare and slightly more pleasant to take. Raw herbs are dried and powdered and, since the resultant powder is up to six times more concentrated than the raw herb, doses are adjusted accordingly. The formula is made by mixing the selected ingredients together in the correct proportions. The stated dose is then normally mixed with boiling water to form a paste. More boiling water is added to make approximately half a mugful, but this quantity can be varied according to the taste preferences of the patient. This mixture is then stirred and allowed to cool for 15 minutes, stirring occasionally. It is best drunk in one go, but can be sipped if preferred.

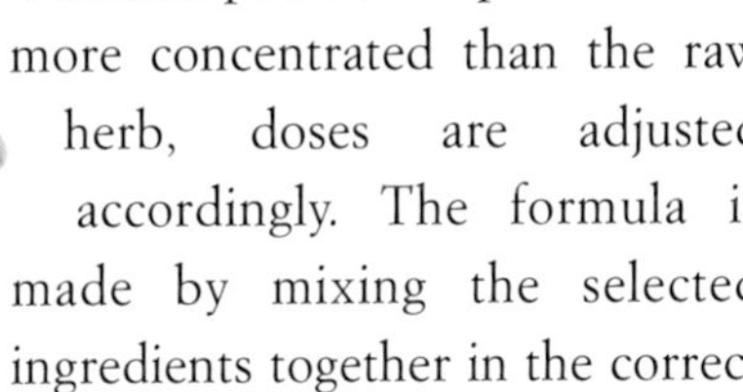

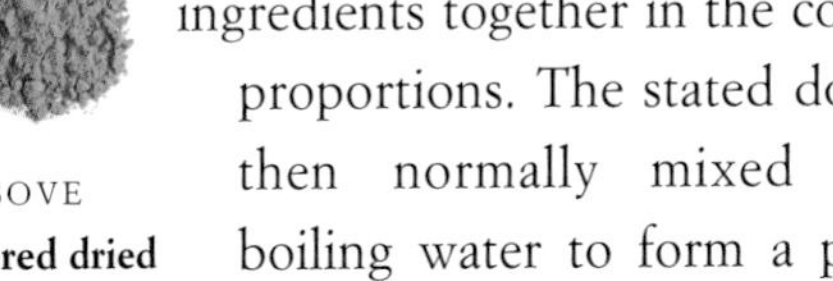

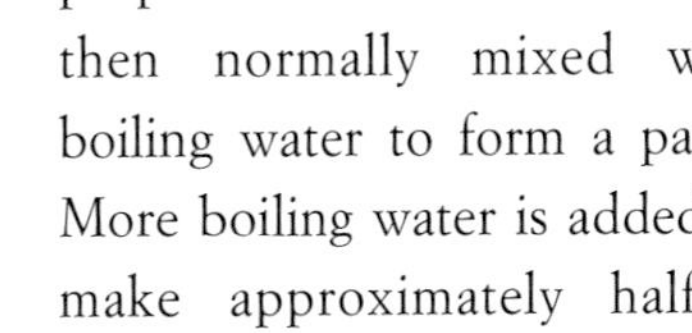

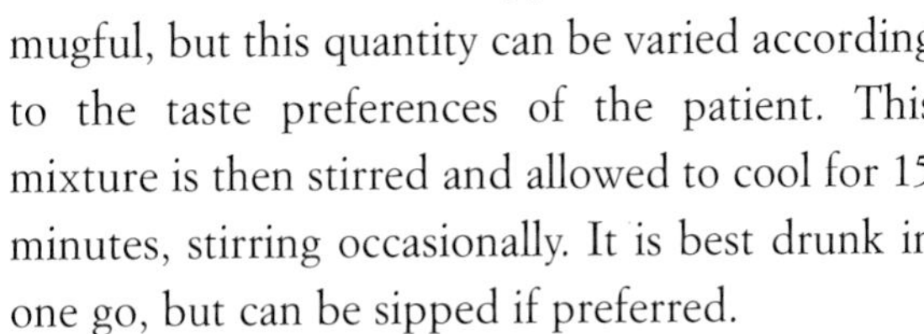

ABOVE
Powdered dried herbs are more concentrated.

The major advantage of powdered herbs is that they are easy to prepare and quite easy to take. They can also be supplied in capsule or other forms. On the other hand, they are generally considered less potent than raw herbs.

Many practitioners prefer to use powdered herbs because they have a higher patient compliance than raw herbs – in other words, there is no point in prescribing herbs in their most potent form (raw) if there is little likelihood that they will be taken.

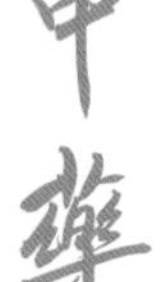

Herbal tinctures

Another method of preparation is to dry and suspend the herbs in a precise mixture of water and alcohol in order to extract their constituents. Most tinctures are prepared in a suspension of 25 percent alcohol, although in some instances this can be as high as 60 percent.

ABOVE
Herbs may be steeped in alcohol solution.

Each herbal tincture is mixed in the appropriate dosage ratio to make up the final formula tincture. This is then drunk in the prescribed dose.

Prepared patent herbs

Many of the classic formulae that have been developed over the centuries are considered so useful that they are manufactured in readily available patent forms. The herbs are usually available as pills, but some patents are offered as tinctures – or as rubs, creams, sprays, and poultices for external use. But the pill or capsule is by far the most important and common form of patent formulae available.

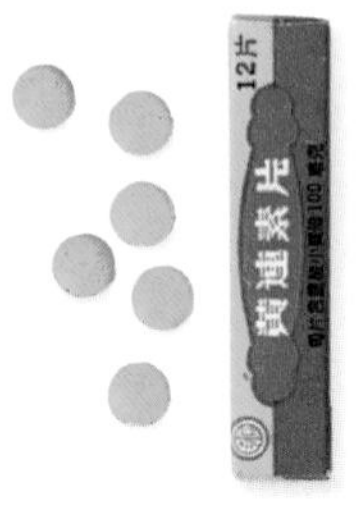

ABOVE
Patent preparations are available.

Many of the patents from the classic formulae are manufactured in China and exported to the West, although a growing number of manufacturers in both the United States and Europe are now offering their own variations on classic Chinese formulae in capsule or tincture form. This promises to be an interesting area of development for Chinese medicine.

Patents offer an easy way to take Chinese herbs, and they are readily available in Chinese supermarkets or from specialist Chinese herbal suppliers. There are advantages and disadvantages in taking patent remedies.

Advantages

Patent formulae offer a quick and easy way to take Chinese herbs, especially over a long period. Many can be remarkably effective, particularly with some acute conditions; and in problems of chronic Qi or Blood deficiency they can be taken safely over an extended period of time. Patents are probably most valuable as an adjunct to acupuncture and massage.

Disadvantages

Just as it would be considered inappropriate to take over-the-counter medicines for an extended period of time, or to exceed the recommended dose, so it is with patent herbal preparations. The following points must be emphasized:

- The majority of Chinese patent formulae should be taken only for as long as the energetic imbalance persists. As with prescribed formulae, it may be necessary to revise a formula, and this cannot be done readily with a patent. (The main exceptions to this rule are certain patent Qi and Blood tonic formulae – Ba Zhen Wan (Women's Precious Pills), for example – which can be taken safely over an extended period.)
- Many patent remedies produced in China have minimal or no translation of the Chinese on their packaging. Unless it is absolutely certain what a package contains, it should be avoided.
- As with all Chinese herbal formulae, there may be ingredients in a patent that are contraindicated in certain situations – during pregnancy, for example. Before taking a patent formula, it is essential to consult a Chinese herbal practitioner.

Patent formulae can be very helpful, but they should not be taken without seeking advice from a qualified practitioner of Chinese herbal medicine – the fact that a herbal product is available over the counter does not mean that it is either appropriate or safe.

COMMONLY USED PATENT REMEDIES

THE FOLLOWING patents may be prescribed on their own or as an adjunct to other forms of treatment. Under the advice and through the guidance of an experienced Chinese herbal practitioner they can be of tremendous value in overcoming certain disharmony problems, resulting in coughs, fatigue, menstrual disorders, nausea and insomnia.

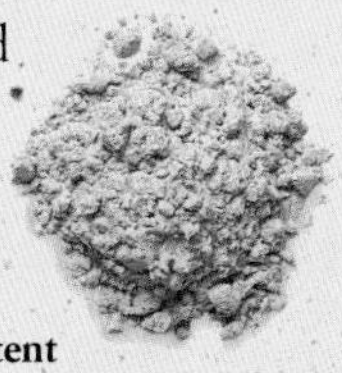

RIGHT
Loquat cough mixture patent remedy in powder form.

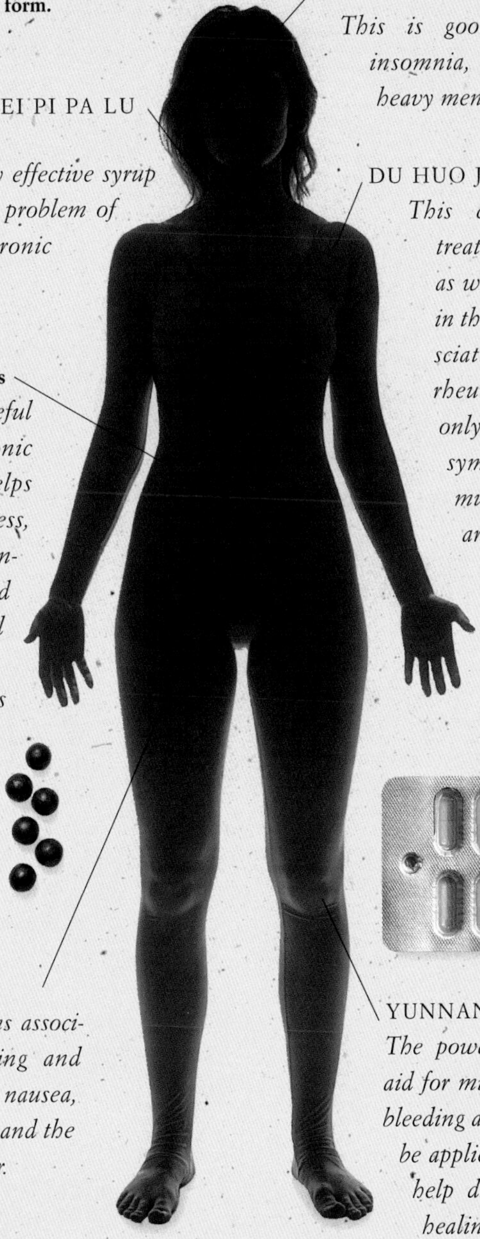

GUI PI WAN
This is good for restlessness, insomnia, and abnormal or heavy menstrual bleeding.

ZHI KE CHUAN BEI PI PA LU
Loquat cough mixture
This is an extremely effective syrup that can relieve the problem of an acute or chronic cough.

DU HUO JI SHENG WAN
This can be useful in treating conditions such as weakness and stiffness in the lower back, chronic sciatica, arthritis, and rheumatism. It should only be taken while the symptoms persist and must be avoided if there are signs of Heat such as hot, swollen joints.

BA ZHEN WAN
Women's Precious Pills
This is especially useful as a general tonic for women. It helps with fatigue, dizziness, palpitations, and menstrual disorders, and can be beneficial while recovering from more serious illnesses.

BELOW
Yunnan Pai Yao capsules in a bubble package.

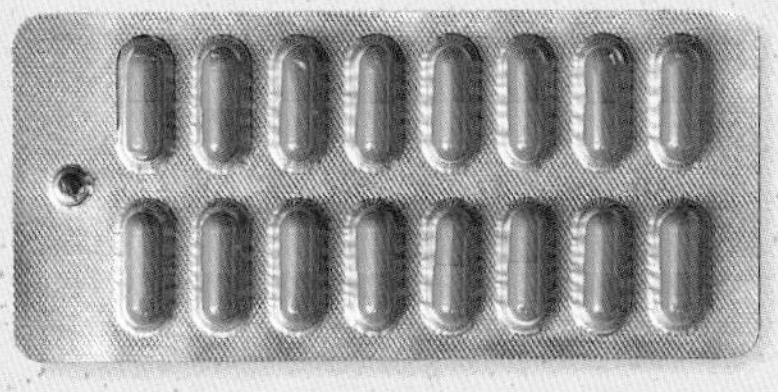

RIGHT
Er Chen Wan remedy available as pills.

ER CHEN WAN
Helps with problems associated with overeating and drinking. It relieves nausea, abdominal fullness, and the effects of a hangover.

YUNNAN PAI YAO
The powder is an invaluable aid for minor traumas, such as bleeding and insect bites. It can be applied externally and can help dramatically with the healing of such lesions.

ABOVE
Patent remedies take many forms. Although they can be useful, it is always best to consult a qualified herbalist before taking them.

FEATURED MATERIALS BY COURTESY OF THE ACUMEDIC CENTRE, LONDON.

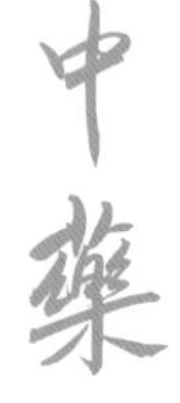

MAKING A DECOCTION

WHEN A patient leaves the practice of a Chinese herbalist, he or she will usually be armed with a week's supply of herbs, mixed by the herbalist to match the case. Often they will be separated into the appropriate quantities for daily treatment, with each day's remedies packed in a separate brown paper bag. The herbs are classified as Yin or Yang and are selected to balance the Yin or Yang of the patient's illness. The qualities of the four energies in the herbs – hot, warm, cold, and cool – are also used to balance the qualities shown in the illness.

Additionally, the herbs are chosen for their appropriate flavors, with the five flavors – hot, sweet, sour, bitter, and salty – matching the five elements – metal, earth, wood, fire, and water – and treating the related organ. The special affinity of a herb and its drying or moistening nature also affect the selection.

The practitioner will make sure that the patient has clear instructions on how to use the herbs. The simplest way of using them is to make a decoction or broth. This is done by boiling the herbs in a given amount of water to extract their substance.

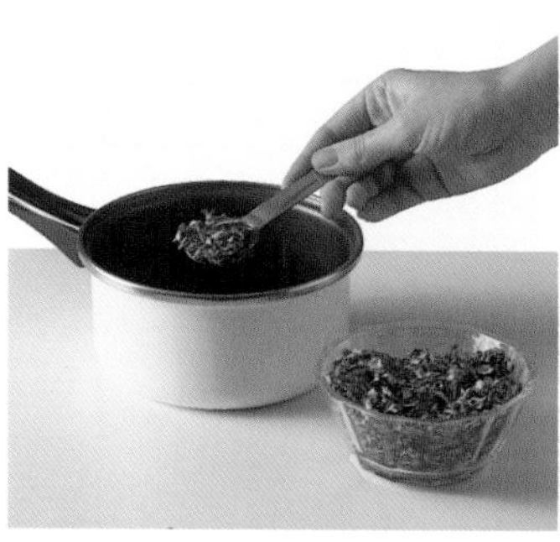

STEP 1 *Place the herbs in a clean pan and cover with the prescribed amount of water.*

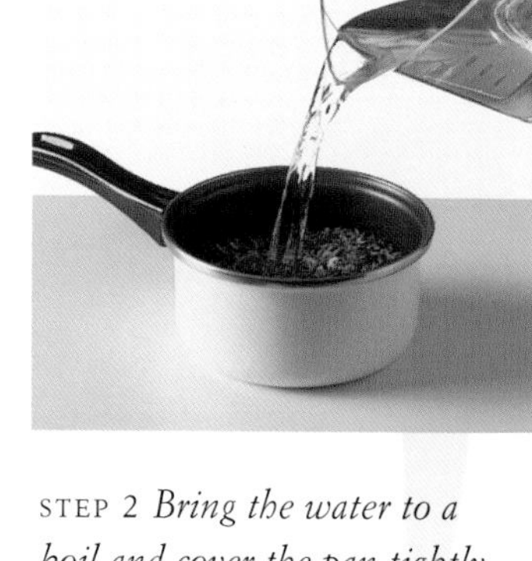

STEP 2 *Bring the water to a boil and cover the pan tightly.*

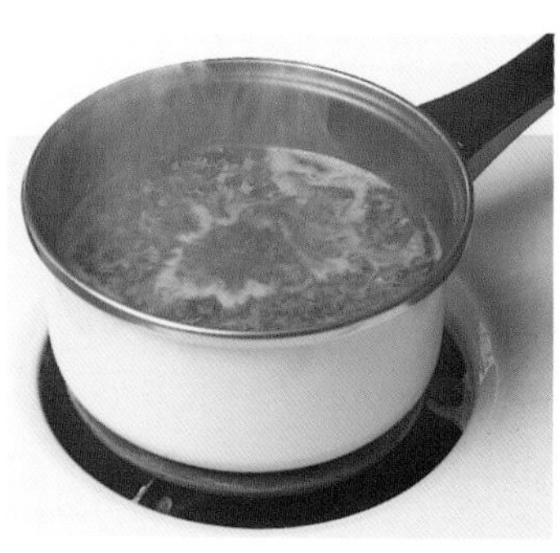

STEP 3 *Boil the ingredients for the time specified by the herbalist. Some mixtures require a shorter boiling time and a lower heat than others.*

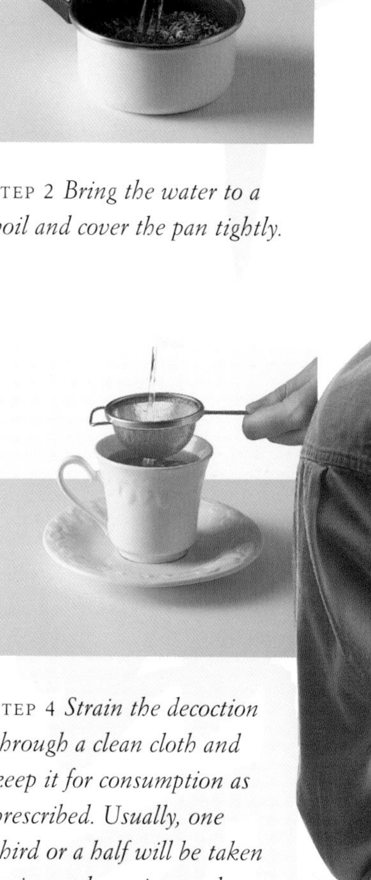

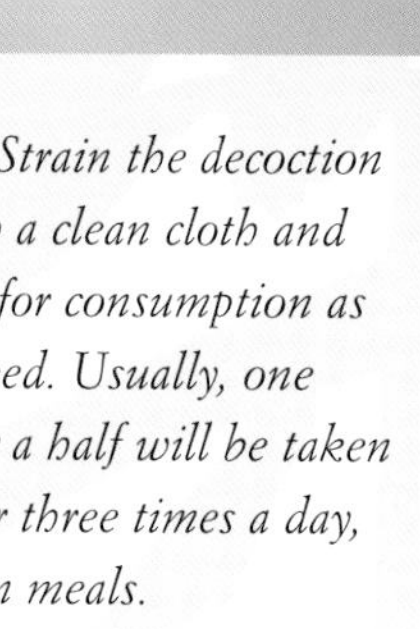

STEP 4 *Strain the decoction through a clean cloth and keep it for consumption as prescribed. Usually, one third or a half will be taken twice or three times a day, between meals.*

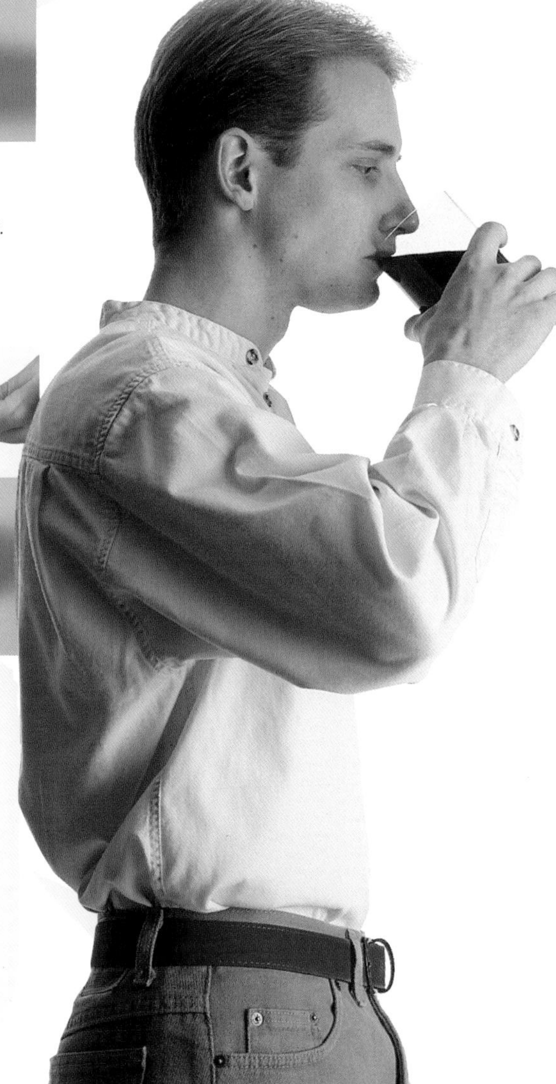

BELOW

A decoction is normally taken in two or three drafts a day.

MAKING A TINCTURE

A PRACTITIONER would prepare a tincture by steeping herbs in alcohol for six months, so that their essence is absorbed. The mixture is then filtered and stored in glass or pottery containers. It is sometimes known as 'medicine-wine'. A tincture is long-lasting, and fast in action.

Tincture formulae are manufactured under strict conditions and practices, and they are easy and not too unpleasant to take. Also, the alcohol ensures that they have a very long shelf life. Tinctures, too, are considered to be less potent than raw herbs. As with powdered herbs, some practitioners prefer them because of simplicity of preparation and higher patient compliance. Tinctures, however, tend to be markedly more expensive than other herbal preparations.

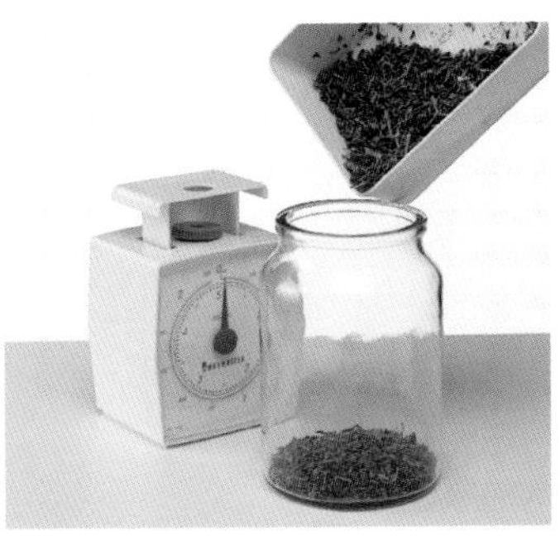

STEP 1 *To make a tincture put 4oz (120g) of chopped herbs in a glass or pottery container.*

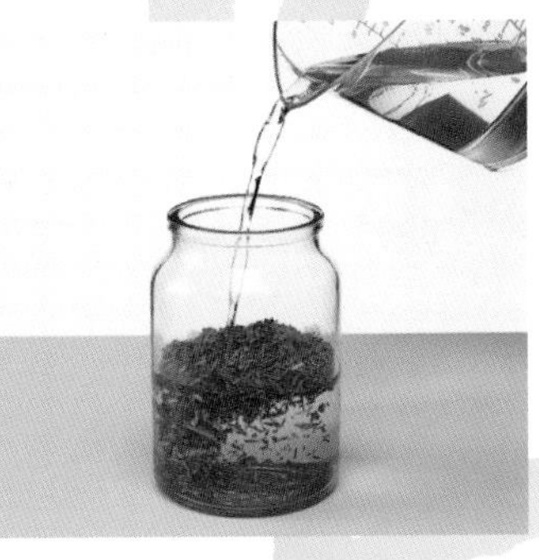

STEP 2 *Pour over 1pt (500ml) of 60 proof (30%) vodka and close the container tightly.*

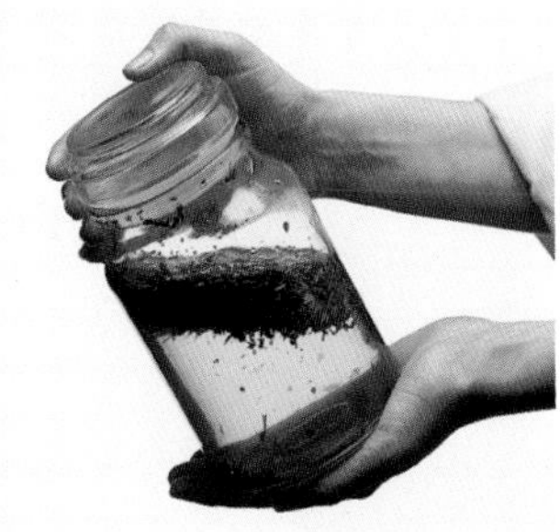

STEP 3 *Keep the container in a warm place. Shake it twice daily.*

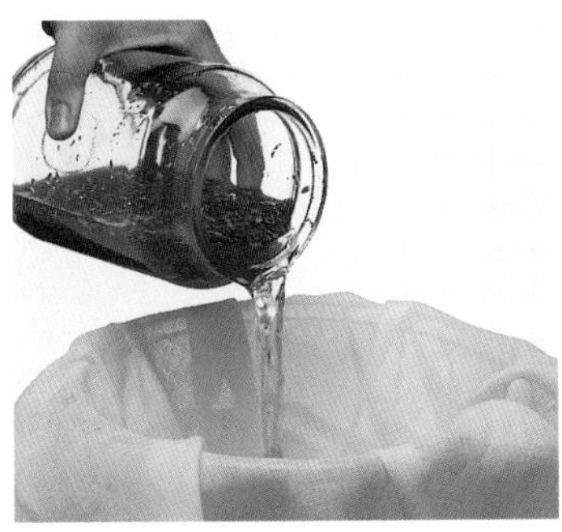

STEP 4 *After six months, strain the liquid through a clean cloth into a bowl.*

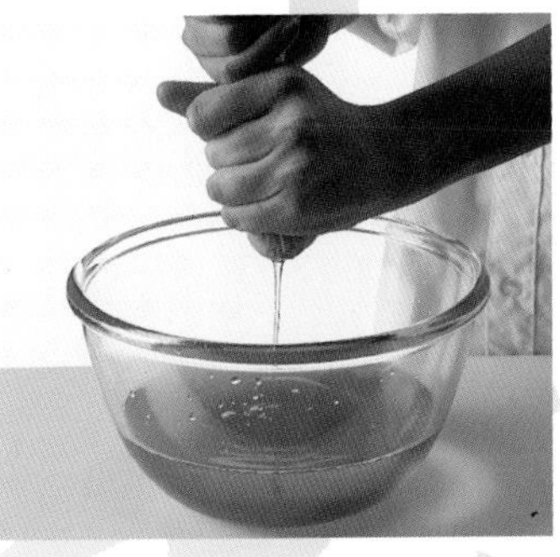

STEP 5 *Wring out the cloth with scrupulously clean hands to extract all the liquid.*

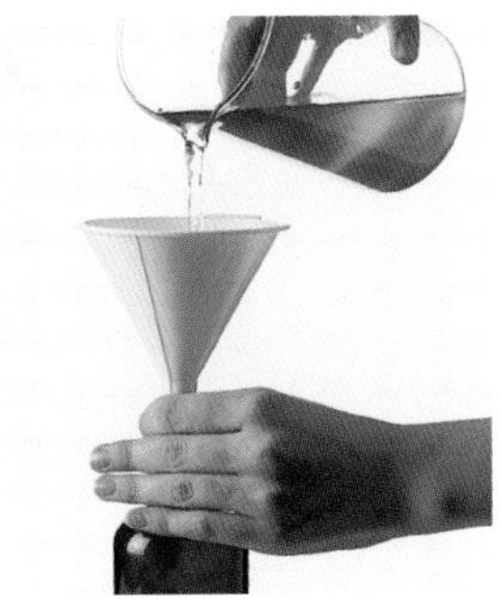

STEP 6 *Transfer the liquid to a dark bottle or pottery container. Keep it well stoppered.*

CAUTION

Do not prepare your own remedies except under the instructions of a qualified herbalist.

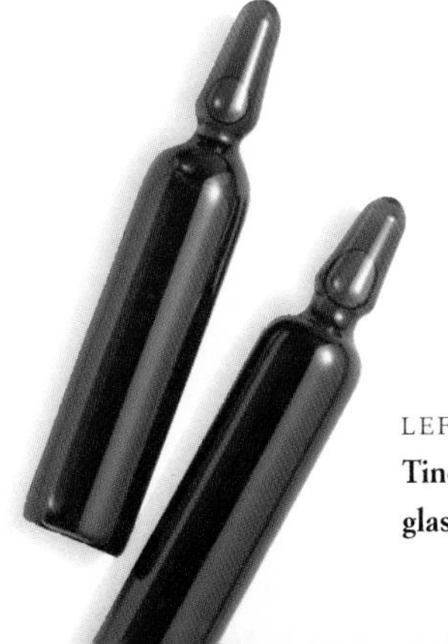

LEFT
Tinctures are stored in glass bottles and containers.

RIGHT
The Chinese herbalist will wish to get a full picture of all aspects of the patient's health.

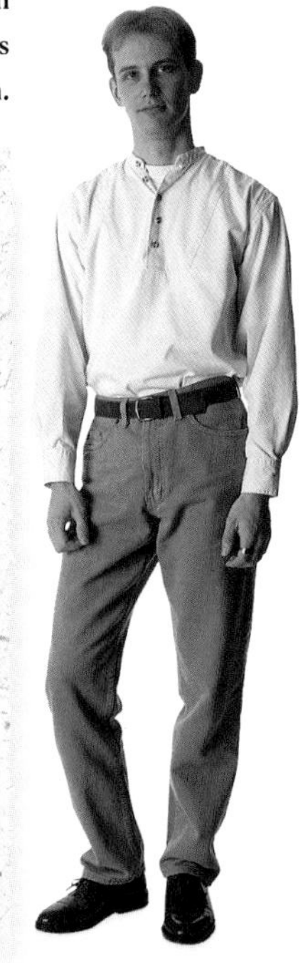

MONITORING TREATMENT

The herbal practitioner will probably see patients a week or so after the first visit and then every two or three weeks. Regular contact is important because prescriptions may need fine-tuning.

CONSULTING A PRACTITIONER

CHINESE HERBS may be used for a full range of problems and disharmonies, and a Chinese herbalist should be able to offer an effective treatment program. Herbal treatment may be combined with other aspects of Chinese medicine, such as acupuncture or massage since these approaches are far from being mutually exclusive. However, this modality also opens up the Chinese approach to people for whom acupuncture is not suitable – either for medical reasons or because they are unable to face needles.

THE DIAGNOSTIC INTERVIEW

THE PROTOCOL for taking a case history is the same as that used for acupuncture *(see pages 138–140)*. In addition, the herbal practitioner may investigate whether there is a Liver problem (some practitioners carry out a Liver function test as a matter of course).

Once the diagnostic interview is complete and the practitioner has discussed the diagnosis and treatment plan with the patient, he or she decides whether raw herbs, powdered herbs, or tinctures would be most appropriate. In acupuncture, treatment takes place in a clinic setting and is under the control of the practitioner, but herbal medicine places a considerable degree of responsibility on patients. They have to be committed to preparing and taking the herbs as prescribed – which, as already discussed, is not always easy.

Once it has been decided in which form the herbs are to be taken, the practitioner usually gives written instructions to make it clear to the patient what is required in terms of preparation and also dosage. Patients are encouraged to get in touch immediately if they have any problem in carrying these out.

Prescriptions take some time to prepare: patients may have to return later to pick them up. Some practitioners have their own herbal pharmacy and dispensing facilities, while others order their prescriptions from a herbal supplier.

Patients are usually advised to stop taking the herbs if they develop a cold or influenza, or if they feel sick or unwell after taking them.

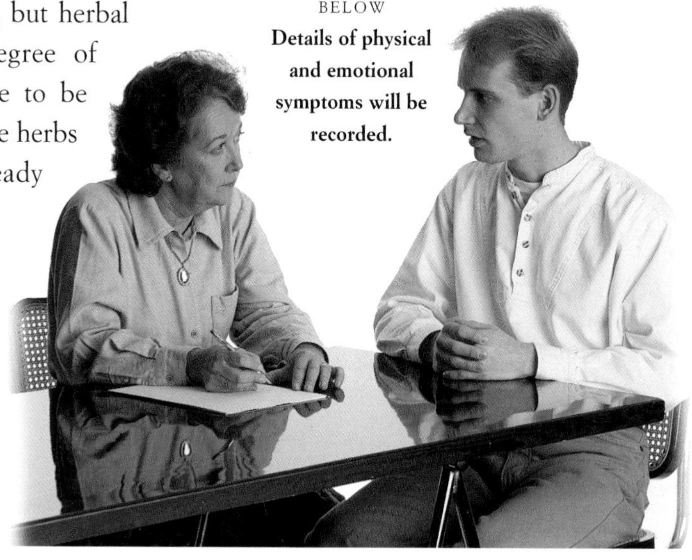

BELOW
Details of physical and emotional symptoms will be recorded.

CASE HISTORY

THE FOLLOWING case history illustrates how Chinese herbal medicine works in practice.

Margaret is 50 years old. She is happily married with two adult children who have both left home. Her husband runs his own business, and Margaret works for him in a secretarial/administrative assistant capacity. The business has expanded quite significantly over the last year and she is finding the work demanding. Within the last year, they have moved to the country, and she is finding the lifestyle quite isolating, although she loves the house. She is well-dressed and immaculately presented and is clearly someone who takes great care with her appearance.

Margaret is seeking herbal treatment for her psoriasis. She has suffered from this for about twenty years, although it has flared up and died down during this time. The parts most affected are her neck, her arms, and the pubic/genital area. Over the last year the psoriasis has become worse, and is now beginning to spread to areas of the body that were previously unaffected.

Margaret feels that the exacerbation of the problem is connected to the house move and the increase in pressure resulting from the expansion of her husband's business. She reports that her digestion is fine and she is trying to stick to what she calls a "healthy" diet – no dairy produce, and plenty of salads and green vegetables. She is not vegetarian. She has experienced severe thirsts in the last year or so and drinks a lot of water. She reports no problems with her bowels or bladder. She has been deaf in her left ear since birth and has begun to experience some slight hair loss in the last eighteen months or so. Her menstrual cycle has been inconsistent. For about four years her periods stopped altogether and she assumed she was entering the menopause. However, her periods then started again, with a light flow of dark blood and some clotting. At the time of the interview she was continuing to have light periods on a relatively regular basis. Emotionally she presents as a very "together" person, but perhaps too controlled. She admits to feeling anxious when she is under stress. Her skin is dry and quite red in the psoriasis patches, and it can be itchy and irritating from time to time. Her tongue is generally pale, with some evidence of purple around the edges. There are some slight cracks, and the tongue body is tooth marked. The pulse is slippery and empty.

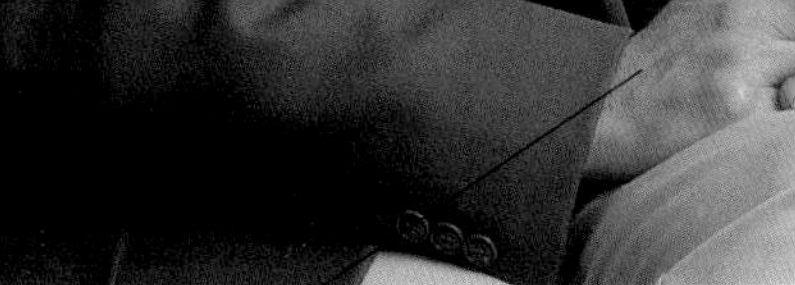

RIGHT
The patient gives an account of her life and symptoms.

TREATMENT

As with acupuncture, a wide range of symptoms responds to treatment with herbal remedies. A patient complaining of a single chronic condition reveals a complexity of symptoms and conditions – both positive and negative – that are all relevant to the case.

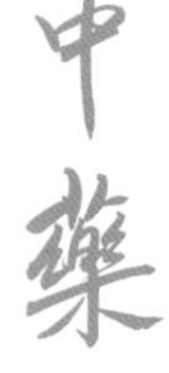

WHAT IS HAPPENING TO MARGARET?

During the diagnostic interview, Margaret gave the impression of being a very "controlled" person. She was anxious to get help for the skin problem but was reluctant to show more than the tops of her arms to the practitioner. In terms of Chinese medicine, Margaret shows evidence of Heart Blood deficiency and a stagnation of Liver Qi. There is also some evidence of an underlying Yin deficiency. When these deficiencies are present, the skin is likely to be dry and flaky because the Yin energy is being consumed and there is a lack of Blood to moisten the skin.

WHAT CAN CHINESE HERBS DO FOR MARGARET?

Initially, the intention was to tonify the Blood and Yin and, later on, to use herbs to move the stagnant Qi. Although the general rule of thumb is to clear an excess condition first, it was decided that it was more important to deal with the underlying Blood and Yin deficiencies in order to improve the psoriasis.

WHICH FORMULA WAS USED TO TREAT THE BLOOD AND YIN DEFICIENCIES?

The formula chosen was Si Wu Tang (Four Materials Decoction) – the classic formula of choice for the tonification and regulation of Blood. It is made up of four ingredients.

- Shu Di Huang nourishes the Yin and Blood.
- Bai Shao tonifies the Blood and preserves Yin.
- Dang Gui nourishes the Yang of the Blood.
- Chuan Xiong invigorates the Blood and moves Qi.

The herbs were given to Margaret in raw form, together with instructions on how to prepare and take them. On her second visit she was somewhat edgy and disillusioned. The psoriasis lesions felt a lot hotter and more uncomfortable, and she expressed disappointment that the herbs did not appear to be working. The practitioner took some time to discuss the nature of herbal treatment and to explain that an initial exacerbation of symptoms is common with such problems. The prescription was altered slightly: Shu Di Huang was replaced with Sheng Di Huang. This form of the herb has a more cooling action on the Blood and the Yin. The other ingredients were retained, and Tao Ren and Hong Hua were added to help move the Blood.

Treatment continued along this line for several weeks. As the lesions improved, the formula was adapted in order to follow the nature of the problem. After three months of herbal treatment the psoriasis lesions had almost totally vanished, and Margaret was feeling much happier and less stressed. She continued to see the herbal practitioner on an occasional basis over the next six months, when contact was then terminated, since by this time the condition was almost completely clear.

DANG GUI

SHU DI HUANG

BAI SHAO

CHUAN XIONG

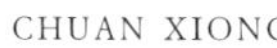

LEFT
Si Wu Tang, the standard formula for tonifying and regulating the Blood, consists of four herbs prescribed in raw form.

PROTECTED SPECIES

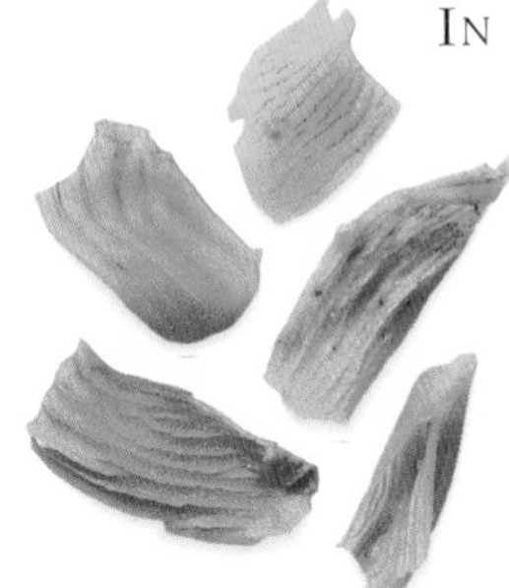

ABOVE
Chicken gizzard (Ji Nei Jin) is used for digestive disorders.

IN CHINESE medicine the concept of herbs includes not only parts of plants but also minerals and animal parts. The use of animals in Chinese herbal medicine is a somewhat contentious issue, particularly in the West. Opinions vary – from a belief that any animal part or product should be used medicinally if it is shown to be beneficial, through acceptance of products from certain species, to insistence that no animal product should ever be used.

The heart of the debate in this area centers on the illegal use of products such as Xi Jiao (Rhino Horn), which was once used to clear Heat from the Blood, and Hu Gu (Tiger Bone), which was used to clear Wind-Damp in the joints – and there are many other traditional ingredients that were derived from what are now endangered species. The points listed below may help to dispel anxiety in anyone considering Chinese herbal treatment. Western practitioners do not stock or use products from endangered species for the following reasons:

- The trade is illegal.
- They would find it morally offensive.
- Such products are obtainable only on the black market.
- The cost would be prohibitively high.
- There are plenty of perfectly acceptable alternatives.

The first of these reasons is in itself enough, but taken together they make a compelling case. Potential patients can rest assured that they will not receive a herbal formula containing endangered animal products from a registered and reputable practitioner.

Individuals who are genuinely concerned about the use of any type of animal product in a Chinese herbal remedy should raise the matter with their practitioner. If necessary, alternatives can be prescribed. (Note: "Tiger Balm," a commonly used and widely available Chinese herbal product, contains no tiger parts.)

LEFT
Scorpion (Xie) is used as a Liver herb, and particularly for Wind-Damp pains.

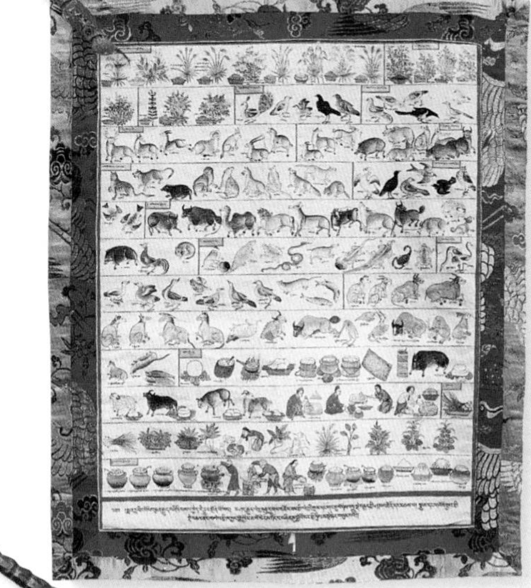

BELOW
Animals used in Tibetan medicine, many aspects of which are derived from China.

LEFT
Centipede (Wu Gong), another Liver herb, is also used to treat snake bites.

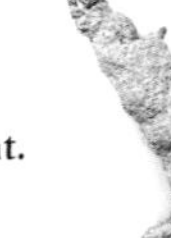

RIGHT
Silkworms are a traditional ingredient.

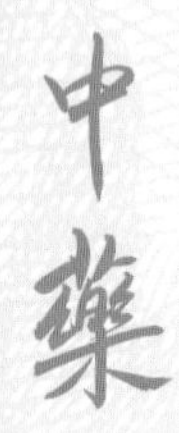

GINSENG, ELIXIRS, AND MAGIC POTIONS

THE DESIRE to seek out instant and "magical" solutions – which, in one swift stroke, will solve all health problems and ensure on-going well-being – seems to be a part of the human condition.

Chinese medicine has not been immune to this trend, and smart marketing has introduced various panaceas in the form of herbs and herbal mixtures into the public domain – but at a price.

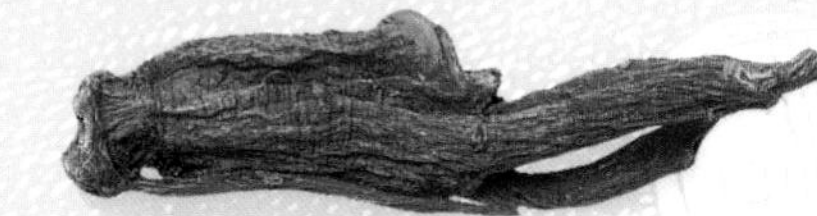

GINSENG ROOT

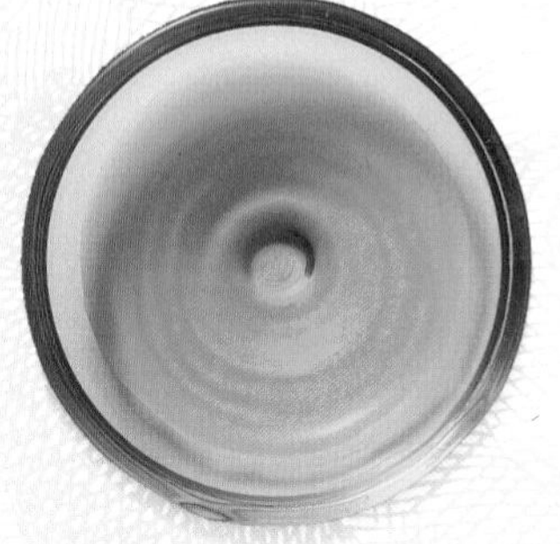

TINCTURE

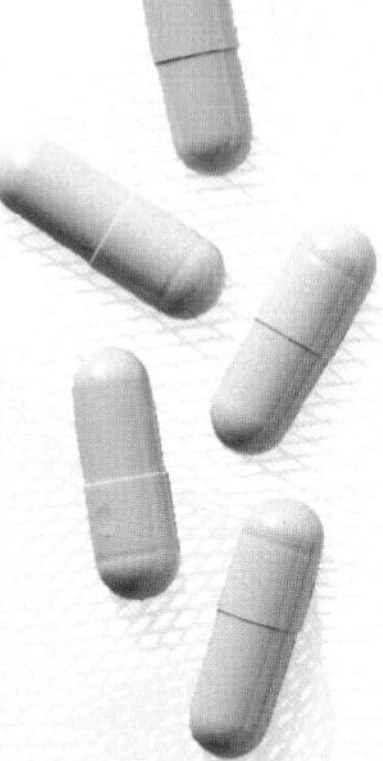

CAPSULES

ABOVE, RIGHT, AND BELOW

Ginseng (Ren Shen) is available in many forms and is sometimes thought of as a cure-all that guarantees physical and mental well-being. Needless to say, it should be used only as prescribed by a qualified herbalist.

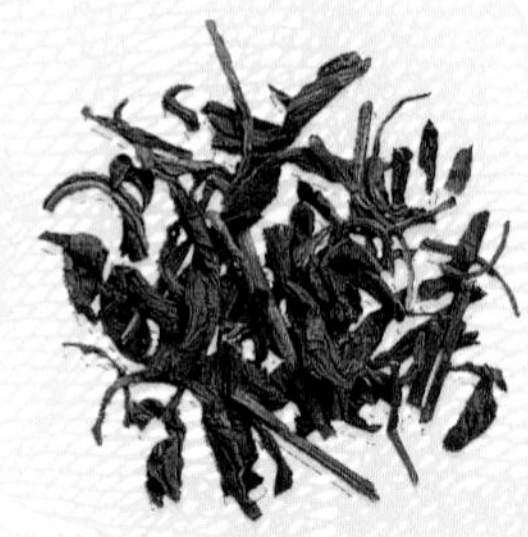

GINSENG LEAF

GINSENG – THE ROOT OF LIFE?

The front-runner in this market is the herb Ren Shen, better known as ginseng. The root of the ginseng plant is greatly valued for its therapeutic properties. In Chinese herbal medicine, Ren Shen is a powerful and important Qi tonic. Its actions are claimed to tonify Yuan Qi and the Lungs, strengthen the Spleen and Stomach, benefit the Heart, and calm the Shen. It is considered an important ingredient in many kinds of Chinese herbal formulae.

Individual herbs are rarely, if ever, given on their own, and Ren Shen is no exception. Qi tonic herbs such as Ren Shen are generally sweet and rich, and this can lead to a feeling of fullness in the chest and diaphragm, and to the development of internal Heat in the body. It is therefore important that these herbs are not used on their own. They must be combined with other herbs, especially those that move and regulate the Qi, in order to avoid a buildup of this cloying effect, which would damage rather than benefit the Spleen and Stomach. Also, if Ren Shen is taken over too long a period of time, headaches, high blood pressure, palpitations, and insomnia can result. Ren Shen is positively contraindicated in patients who show evidence of a Yin deficiency with Heat, or who suffer from high blood pressure.

There are various different types of Ren Shen, and this makes the market even more confusing for the casual browser in the health food store, where the four types of gingseng listed below can usually be found.

- White Ren Shen – neutral – a general Qi tonic.
- Red Ren Shen (usually Korean) – very strong/hot – tonifies Yang Qi.
- American Ren Shen – cooling – tonifies Yin Qi.
- Siberian Ren Shen – a mild Qi tonic.

RIGHT AND BELOW
Ginseng from different sources has different properties. Red Ren Shen (right) is hot, while American Ren Shen (below) is cool.

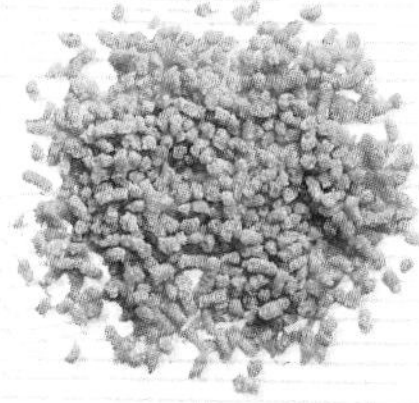
RED REN SHEN

subject to headaches, palpitations, high blood pressure, night sweats, flushing, and other signs of internal empty Heat.

The best advice, as always, is to consult a qualified herbal practitioner, who can diagnose your disharmony and prescribe an appropriate herbal remedy. You may well require a Qi tonic, but alternatives to gingseng can be used. Dang Shen *(Codonopsis* root) is a commonly used substitute; it has very similar properties to Ren Shen – at a fraction of the cost.

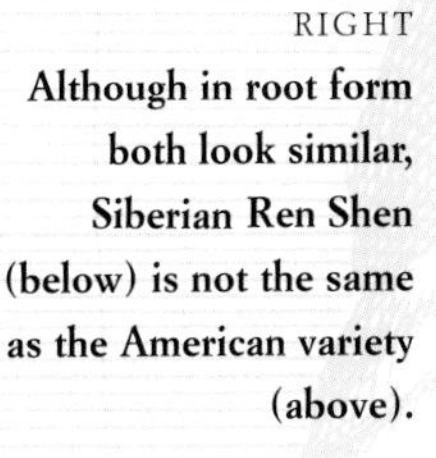
AMERICAN REN SHEN FLAKES

RIGHT
Although in root form both look similar, Siberian Ren Shen (below) is not the same as the American variety (above).

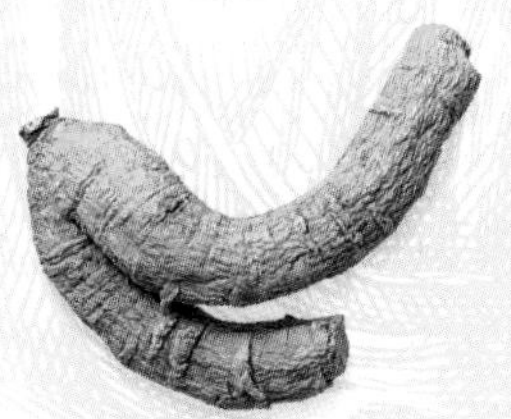
AMERICAN REN SHEN

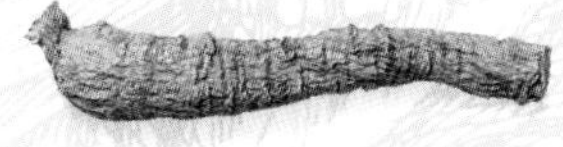
SIBERIAN REN SHEN

These variations in qualities and actions indicate that the use of gingseng is a very complex issue, and it is vital that patients are aware of the potential dangers before spending a lot of money in their search for a "magical" cure. The following guidelines are reasonable pointers to bear in mind:

- In general, Ren Shen should not be taken on its own.
- Ren Shen should not be taken over an extended period of time.
- Ren Shen should not be taken by patients

Elixirs and potions

A disturbing number of generic Chinese herbal potions and remedies are appearing on the market, all claiming a range of wonderful life-enhancing properties. These preparations are usually a tincture form of various well-known – though sometimes more idiosyncratic – herbal formulae. There may be nothing intrinsically wrong with the formulation of these remedies, but anything that takes a "blunderbuss" approach, seeking to deal with a wide range of possible disharmonies, is missing the point. By their very nature, such preparations cannot target specific disharmonies, and they cannot alter and change in response to an individual's reaction to treatment.

The advice is clear – if you feel that you would benefit from Chinese herbs, go to a recognized practitioner and do not waste time and money on attractively presented and vigorously marketed generic herbal preparations that may be, at best, of marginal value and, in the longer term, harmful. This is not the aim of Chinese herbal medicine.

FEATURED MATERIALS BY COURTESY OF THE ACUMEDIC CENTRE, LONDON

RIGHT
The leaves and flowers of the plant may sometimes be used, but it is normally the root that is prescribed.

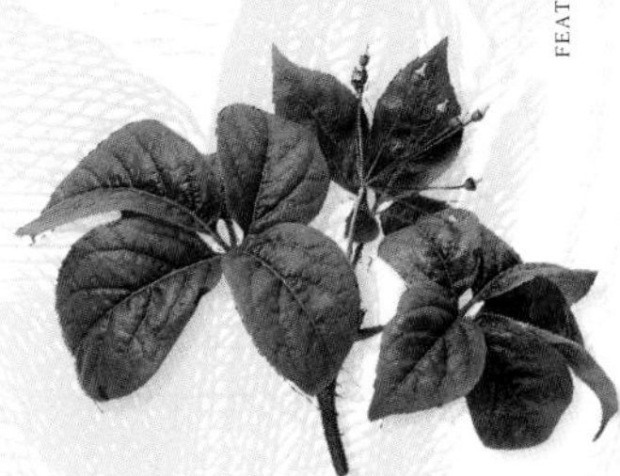
SIBERIAN GINSENG

PLANTS

THE MEDICINAL *use of herbs in China is believed to date back some 4,000 years, to about 2000* B.C.*, when the Emperor Chi'en Nung (also spelled Shen Nong), the "Divine Farmer," is said to have described in a book called the* Pen Tsao *some 300 medicinal plants and their particular curative properties and uses. The Chinese word for herbalism, Ben Cao, is a term which is thought to have come into use about 500* B.C. *Ben means a plant with a rigid stalk, and Cao means a grass-like plant. As this name suggests, at this stage of development herbalism still meant the use of plants, although, as we have seen, the concept now also covers animal and mineral ingredients.*

Until about this time, it seems that the plants were generally used singly, but during the period 450–220 B.C. *combinations of herbs came into use. From this time onwards, herbs were generally combined, sometimes also with animal and mineral ingredients, to form preventive and curative treatments.*

Historically, the main body of written knowledge of plants and their uses originated from the sixteenth century A.D.*, when Li Shih-chen (also spelled Li Shizhen) published the findings of his many years of systematic research into the medicinal effects of herbs. The book gives details of almost 2,000 herbs, and prescribes some 10,000 ways in which they can be combined. Many of the herbs used in this materia medica are still used in Chinese herbalism today. There is also a very long folk tradition in the use of plants in China and a huge body of traditional knowledge has been passed down from generation to generation within families.*

Many of the remedies and methods of Chinese medicine spread to Japan, and in the late eighteenth century some of the plants used became known in the West through this source. Rhubarb, licorice, aconite, and ginger are some of the Chinese plants that came into use in Western medicine in this way.

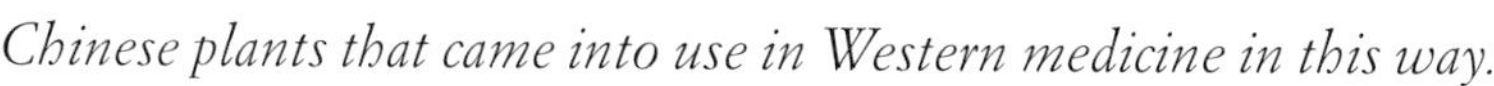

Every possible part of a plant can be used – root, seed, bark, flowers, buds, leaves, stems, and stalks.

ZHI ZI
Gardenia

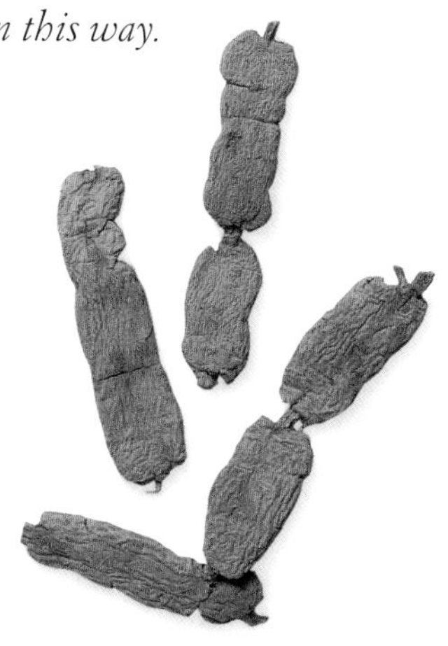

BA JI TIAN
Morinda Root

MU DAN PI
Tree Peony Bark

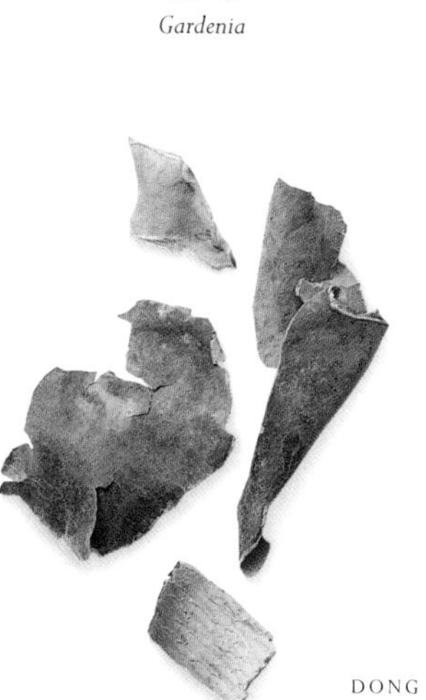

DONG GUA PI
Water Melon Skin

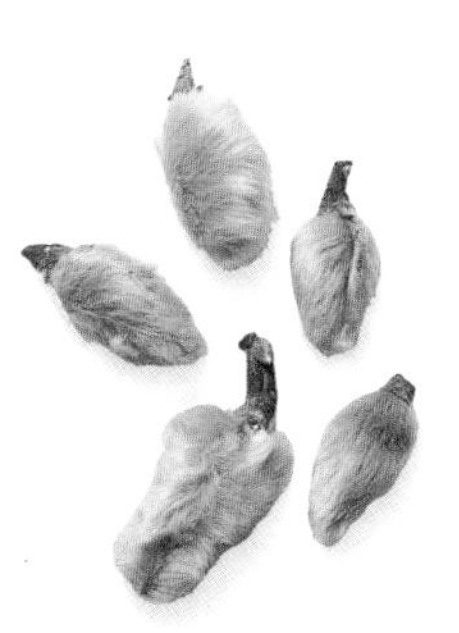

XIN YI HUA
Magnolia Buds

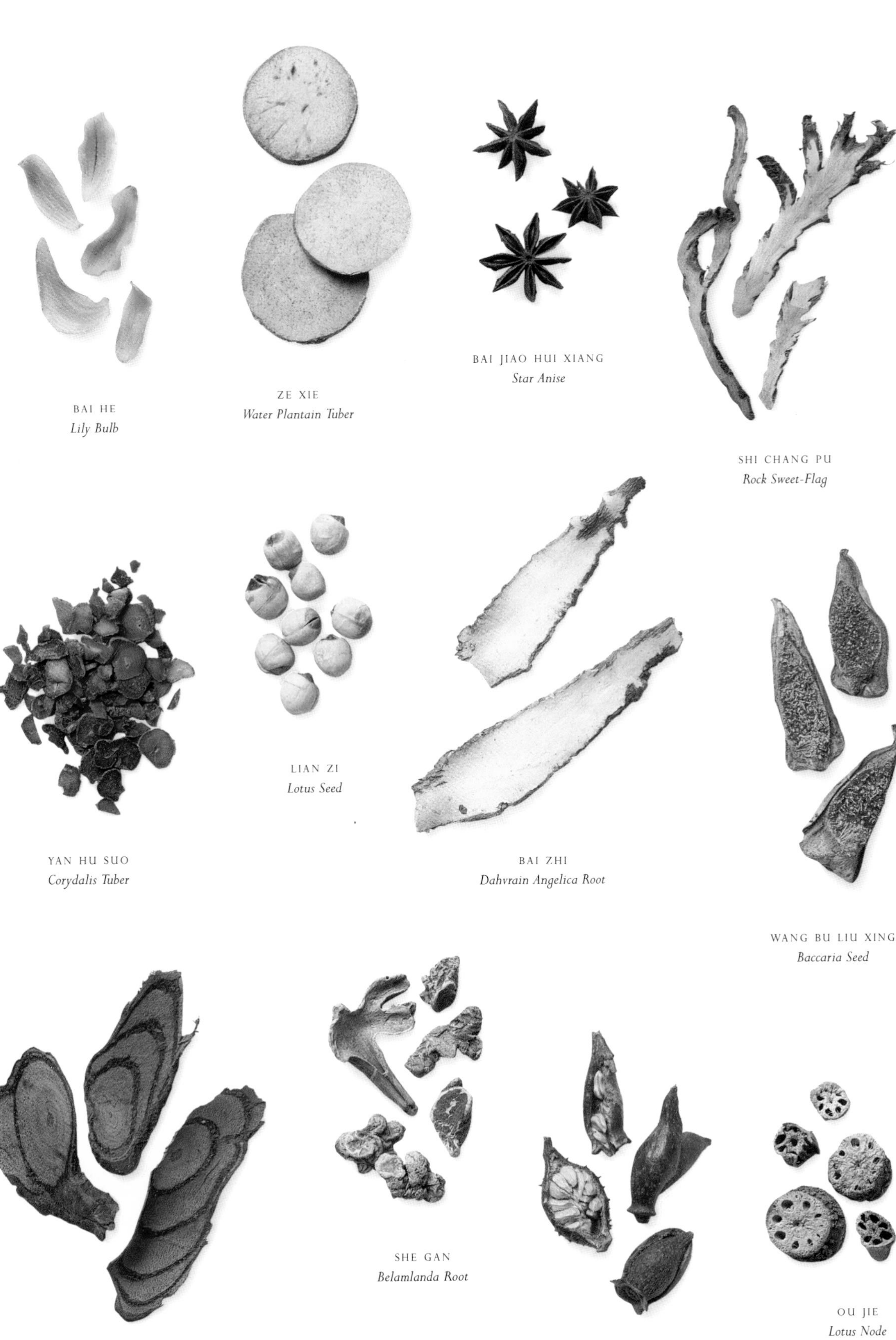

BAI HE
Lily Bulb

ZE XIE
Water Plantain Tuber

BAI JIAO HUI XIANG
Star Anise

SHI CHANG PU
Rock Sweet-Flag

YAN HU SUO
Corydalis Tuber

LIAN ZI
Lotus Seed

BAI ZHI
Dahvrain Angelica Root

WANG BU LIU XING
Baccaria Seed

JI XUE TENG
Millettia Stem

SHE GAN
Belamlanda Root

JIN YING
Rosehip

OU JIE
Lotus Node

ANIMALS

ANIMAL INGREDIENTS have been used in herbal remedies since at least 100 B.C. This is related in part to the importance of diet for Chinese medicine. A balanced diet helps to keep one healthy, and a corrective diet is one of the ways to restore good health in illness. Foods were, and still are, classified as cold or hot and used to treat heat or cold in the body. For example, a herbal soup of salted fish heads, classified as mild, would be prescribed for fever; crab or pork, classified as cold, would be given to counteract heat in the body; while a broth of pork with watercress, classified as hot because of the hot plant ingredient, would be given to remedy colds.

Sympathetic magic and symbolism also play their part in the use of animal ingredients. The chief characteristics of the animal concerned would be thought to be transferred to the patient, or the ingredient would be used for its obvious symbolism – staghorn as a restorative of masculine vigor, for example. Various parts of the animal, such as liver, heart, and so on, would be taken in the diet as a tonic for the same part of the human body.

However, the therapeutic uses of ingredients were also put to the test. For example, it was known in the seventh century A.D. that remedies based on deer and lamb thyroid with seaweed (all now known to be iodine-rich) could cure goiter – the enlargement of the thyroid gland now known to be caused by iodine deficiency.

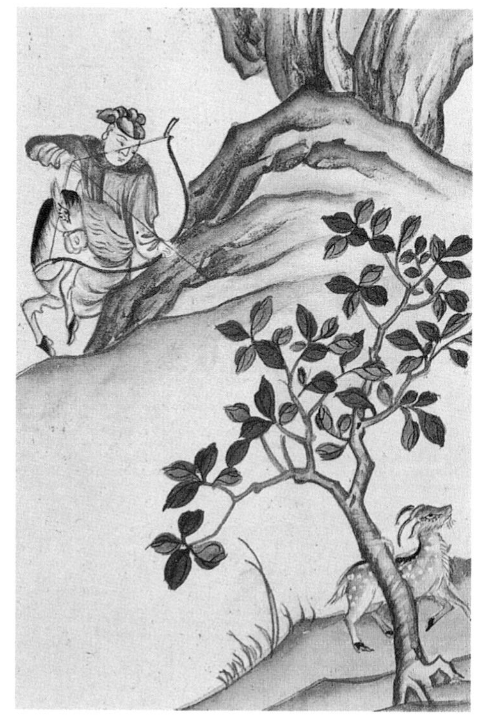

ABOVE
Hunting provided important dietary and medicinal ingredients, as well as recreation.

Not all ingredients of animal origin come from living animals. Shells and egg cases are used, as well as exotically named dragon's teeth and bones, which are really fossilized bones.

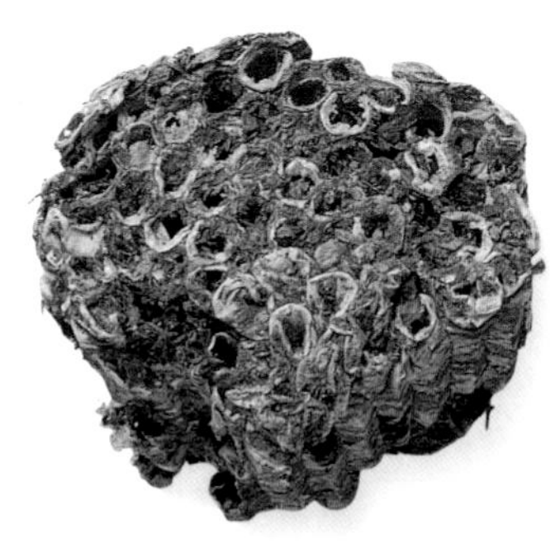

FENG FANG
Hornet's Nest

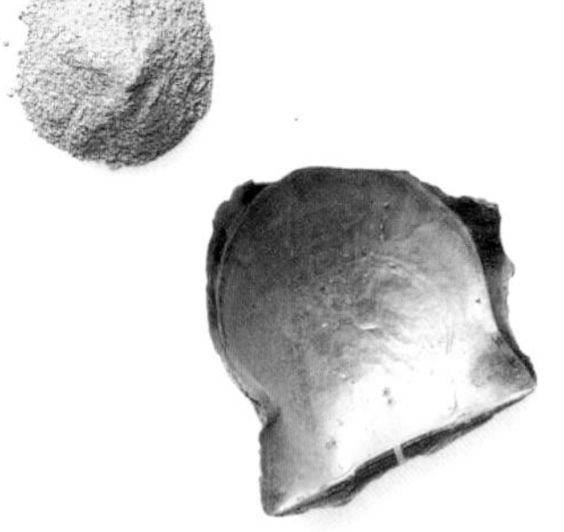

ZHEN ZHU MU
Mother-of-Pearl

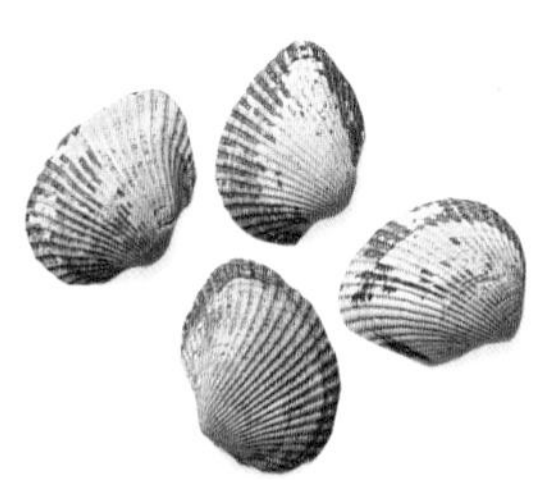

WA LENG ZI
Cockle Shell

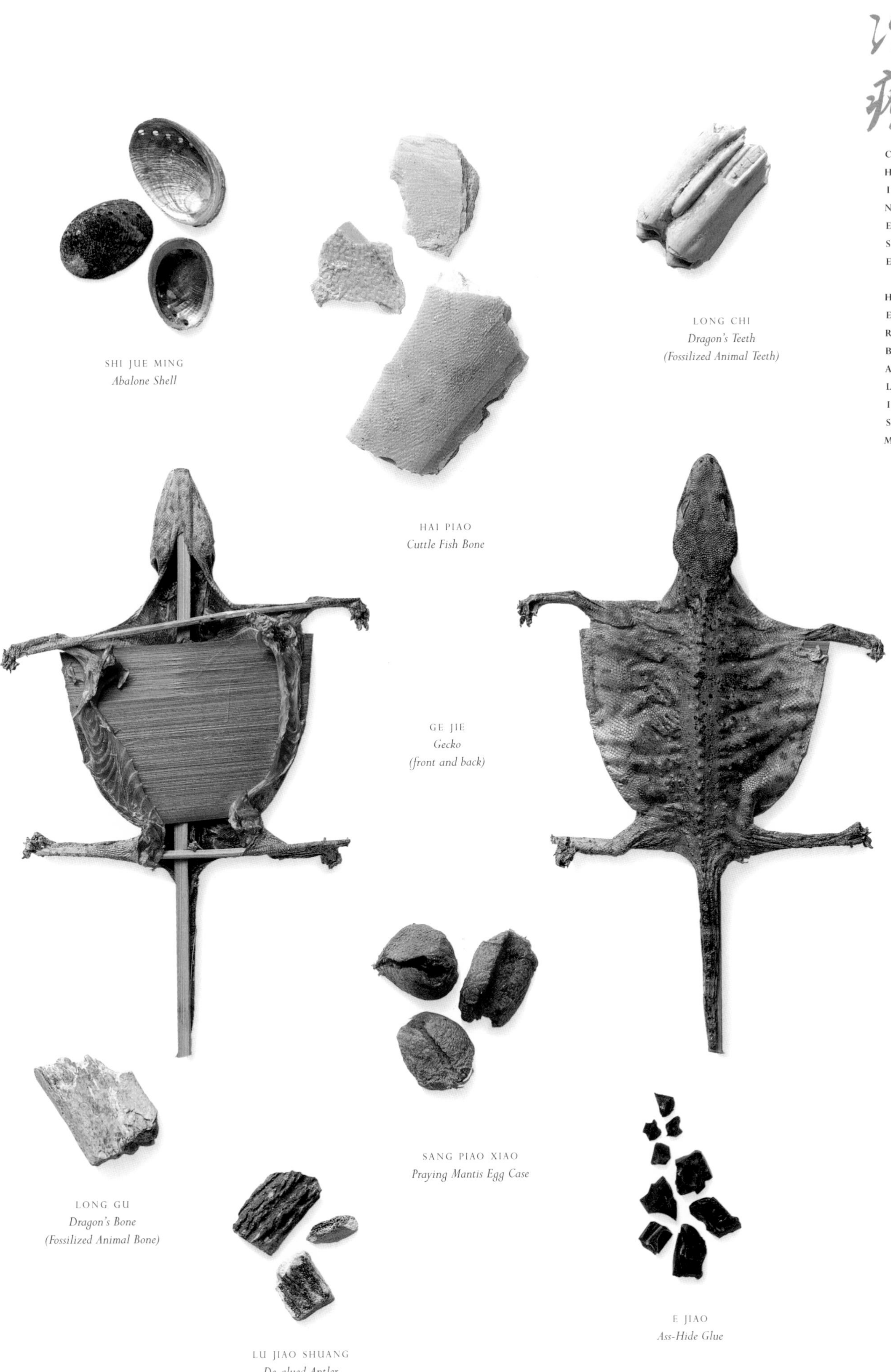

SHI JUE MING
Abalone Shell

HAI PIAO
Cuttle Fish Bone

LONG CHI
Dragon's Teeth
(Fossilized Animal Teeth)

GE JIE
Gecko
(front and back)

SANG PIAO XIAO
Praying Mantis Egg Case

LONG GU
Dragon's Bone
(Fossilized Animal Bone)

LU JIAO SHUANG
De-glued Antler

E JIAO
Ass-Hide Glue

MINERALS

FROM A Western point of view, the importance of minerals and what are called trace elements in the diet, including metals such as zinc and copper, is now well recognized. Western medicine also fully acknowledges the link between some forms of disease and lack or surfeit of minerals, either because of a poor diet or because of the body's inability to metabolize these ingredients. (Anemia is linked to low levels of iron, goiter is linked to lack of iodine, fluid retention and high blood pressure are linked to too much salt, for example.)

We all need small quantities of essential minerals in our regular diets but these are usually obtained from secondary sources: calcium (dairy products and green vegetables), iron (meat, oatmeal, treacle), sodium (salt), potassium (milk, potatoes, fruit, and vegetables), magnesium (various foods, especially vegetables), zinc (pulses, meat, whole grains, some nuts), iodine (seafood, seaweed, some vegetables, depending on where they were grown).

The success of some plant and animal ingredients is perhaps partly due to their mineral content, but Chinese medicine also uses some mineral ingredients in their own right. In Chinese medicine these ingredients are prescribed according to their cold/hot and ascending/descending qualities and according to their particular affinities.

BELOW
The itinerant herbalist would have his own stock of animal, vegetable, and mineral ingredients.

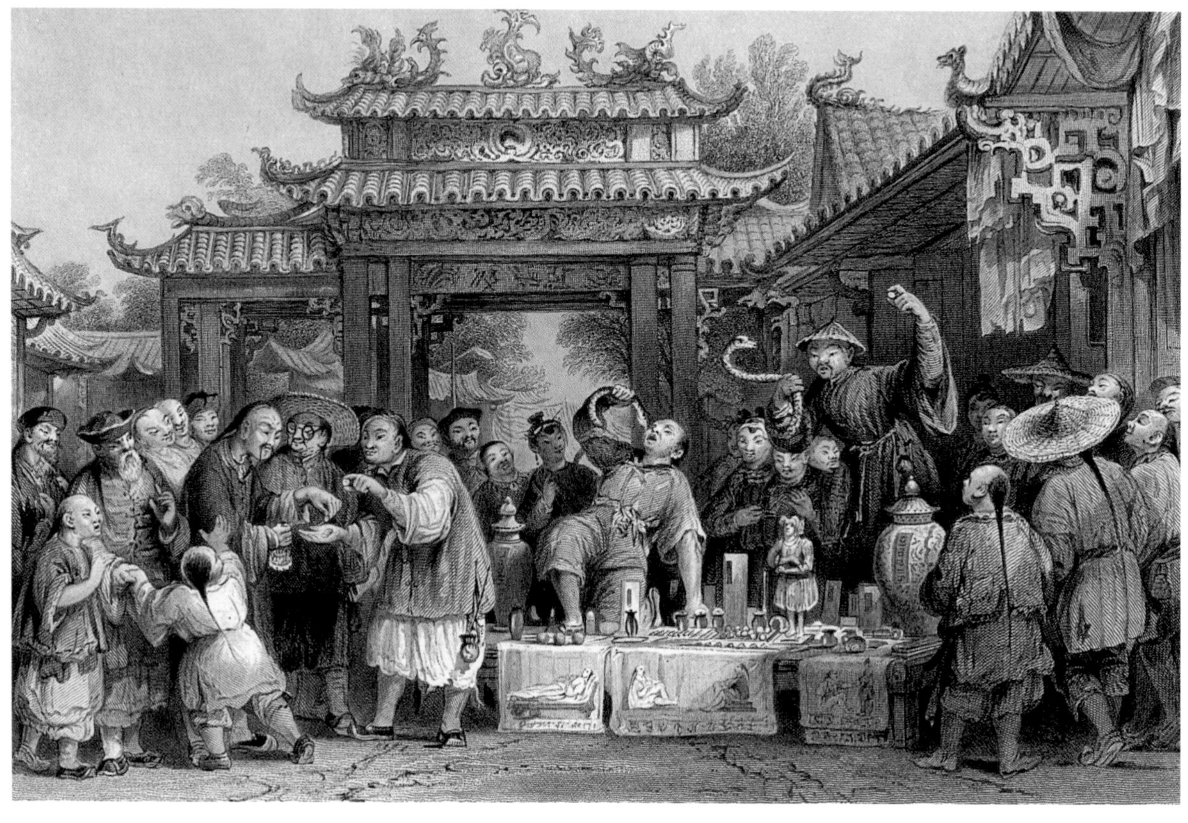

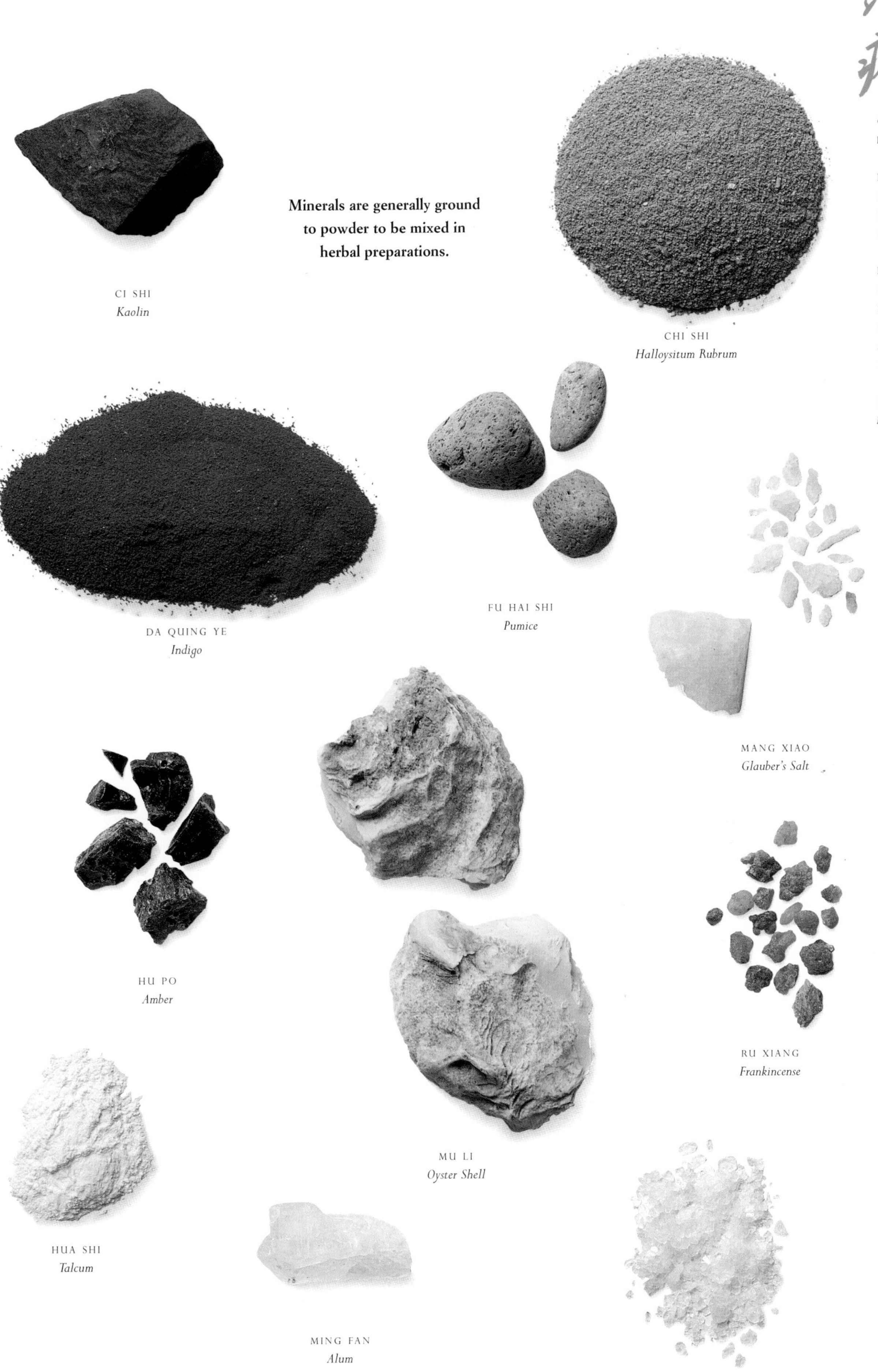

Minerals are generally ground to powder to be mixed in herbal preparations.

CI SHI
Kaolin

CHI SHI
Halloysitum Rubrum

DA QUING YE
Indigo

FU HAI SHI
Pumice

MANG XIAO
Glauber's Salt

HU PO
Amber

RU XIANG
Frankincense

MU LI
Oyster Shell

HUA SHI
Talcum

MING FAN
Alum

BING PIAN
Borneol

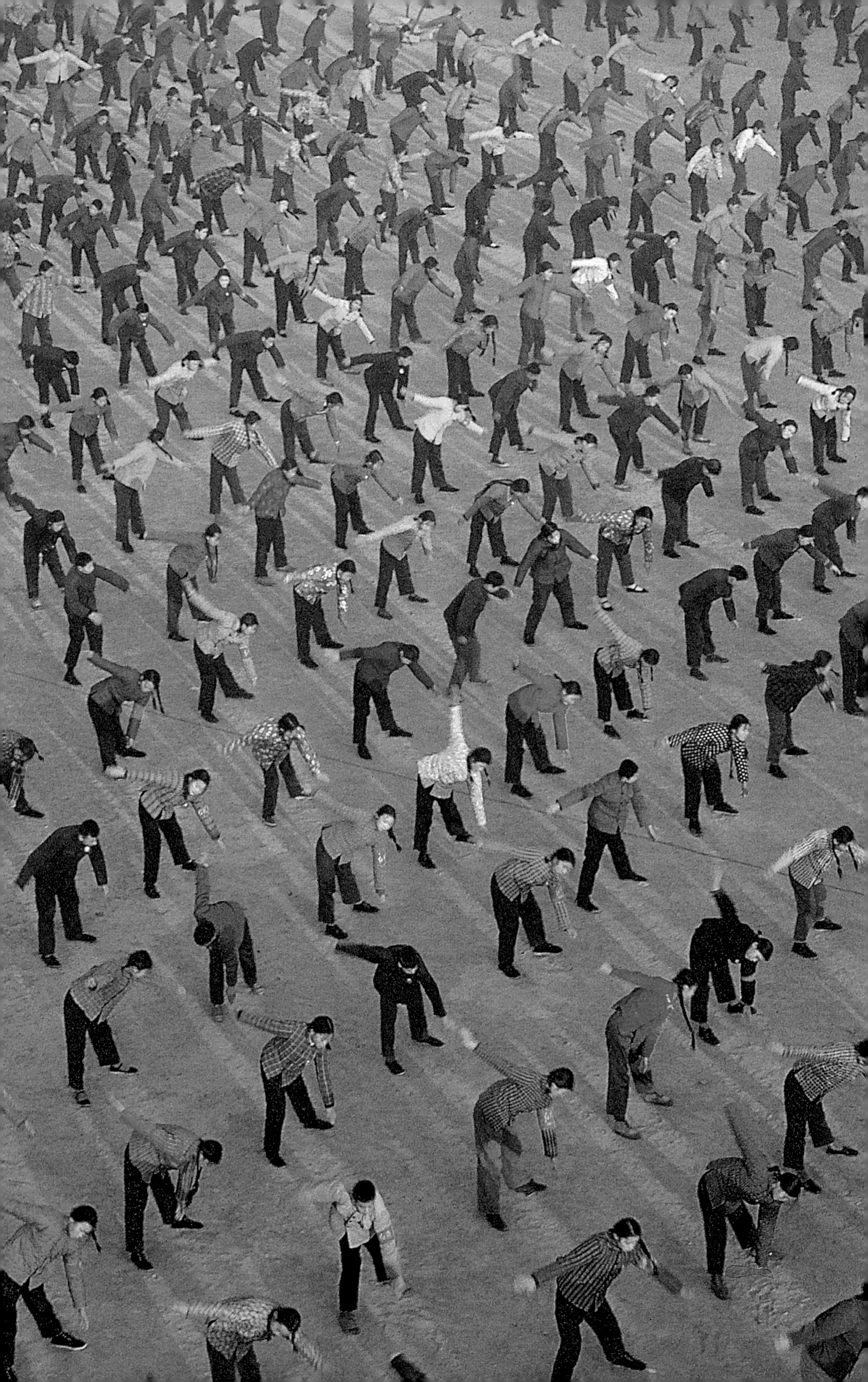

QIGONG

AT 5:45 A.M. *the streets of Beijing are already alive with the myriad activities that accompany Chinese daily life. A significant part of this early morning activity takes place in the hundreds of parks scattered across the city – some large, many small – and it is there that thousands of ordinary Chinese people prepare for the day to come.*

By 6 a.m. the parks are pulsating with movement and people: some on their own, some in loosely organized groups, some in tightly regimented groups. The common thread that runs through all this activity is "Qi" – the vital life energy responsible for the healthy functioning of the body. Qi is absolutely central to Chinese thinking and governs everything from diet and medicine to life attitudes, even how to organize living and working space. "Good" Qi is taken in through the air we breathe and the food we eat; "bad" Qi is then expelled and ultimately recycled as part of the endless cosmic round. The early morning is the best time to take in Qi, and the best place to do this is in close proximity to nature. Even in the most crowded and polluted urban settings, great care is taken of, and reverence is shown to, natural spaces, however small, in order to promote their good Qi.

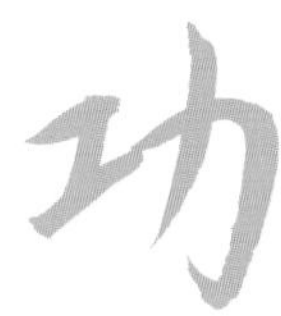

ABOVE
The Chinese characters for Qi and Gong.

The picture in the Beijing park is one of either movement – graceful, slow, and rhythmical – or balanced, rounded stillness. Every day, thousands of ordinary people practice the flowing movements of various Taiji forms, the focused stillness and flexibility of Qigong postures, and the peaceful clarity of meditation. The objective of all these exercises is to enhance the movement of Qi through the meridians and collaterals of the body so as to achieve maximal physical stamina and flexibility, and a clear and calm state of mind. Qigong is thus the traditional physical and psychological antidote to the difficulties of daily life – no more or less stressful in China than in any other part of the world.

By 7:30 a.m. the park is empty again, except for groups of elderly people who stay to talk and play chess, or young mothers chatting and playing with their children. The daily ritual of "moving the Qi" is over again until the early evening, when the same people return to the park and once again employ Taiji and Qigong skills in their endless but beautiful and rewarding search for physical and psychological health and well-being.

LEFT
Qigong exercises are part of daily life in China.

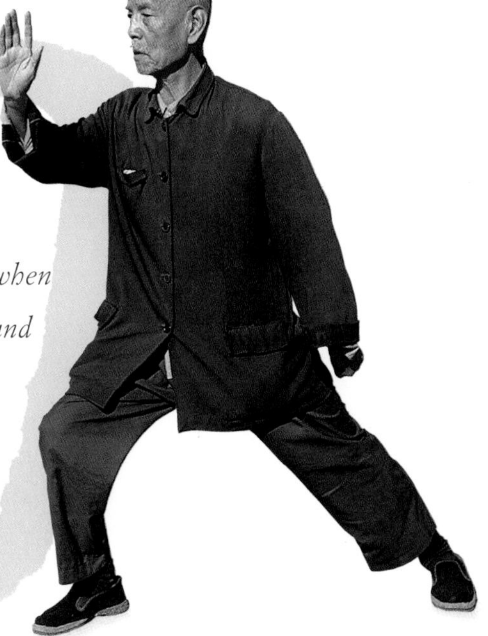

RIGHT
Qigong exercises cultivate a strong energy system.

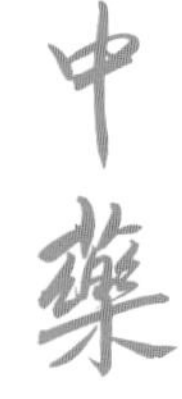

C H I N E S E M E D I C I N E

BACKGROUND

ABOVE
Comfortable clothes and soft shoes should be worn for Qigong.

THE TERM Qigong is often thought to mean "the development of Qi," but this somewhat loose translation is rather misleading since it tends to suggest that Qi is not naturally present and must be developed. This misses the essential point – that Qi is everywhere all the time: flowing, permeating, and energizing everything in the universe, including our bodies. A better translation that more readily captures the essence of Qigong is "energy cultivation." This implies that the practice can help to maximize the efficiency and effectiveness of how we store, move, and use Qi to enhance our health and well-being.

The scene in the park emphasizes the extent to which these practices, described under the umbrella of "Qigong," are an essential part of Chinese cultural life, as they have been for many thousands of years.

Only in the last twenty to thirty years has Qigong practice begun seriously to appear in a Western context. The apparent simplicity of many of the postures and movements initially led to a dismissive attitude, but the effectiveness of Qigong in helping to cure illness and maintain health has now been thoroughly proven, and it is essential that any discussion of Chinese medicine stresses the importance of these practices.

Archeological evidence illustrating the use of Qigong includes the "Jade Pendant Inscription on Qigong," an engraving dating back to the Zhou dynasty (*c.*600 B.C.), which discusses Qigong theory and practice. One of the most famous discoveries, the "Dao Yin Illustrations," a silk painting dating from the Han Dynasty (which spanned the centuries just before and after the beginning of the Christian era), depicts a series of Qigong postures accompanied by short descriptions referring to the therapeutic benefits to be gained.

Generally speaking, Qigong practices were handed down through families, or through the monasteries where they were practiced regularly by Daoist and Buddhist monks. Various different schools developed with different emphases, but ultimately the thousands of Qigong postures and movements all share the common principles that underpin the practices of Chinese medicine – reinforcing and tonifying depleted Qi; clearing blocked or excess Qi; and strengthening both internal and external (or defensive) Qi. Some of the exercises strengthen and harmonize the essential internal Qi of the body, insuring that all the Zangfu systems work efficiently and

BELOW
Qigong exercise strengthens and rebalances the Qi.

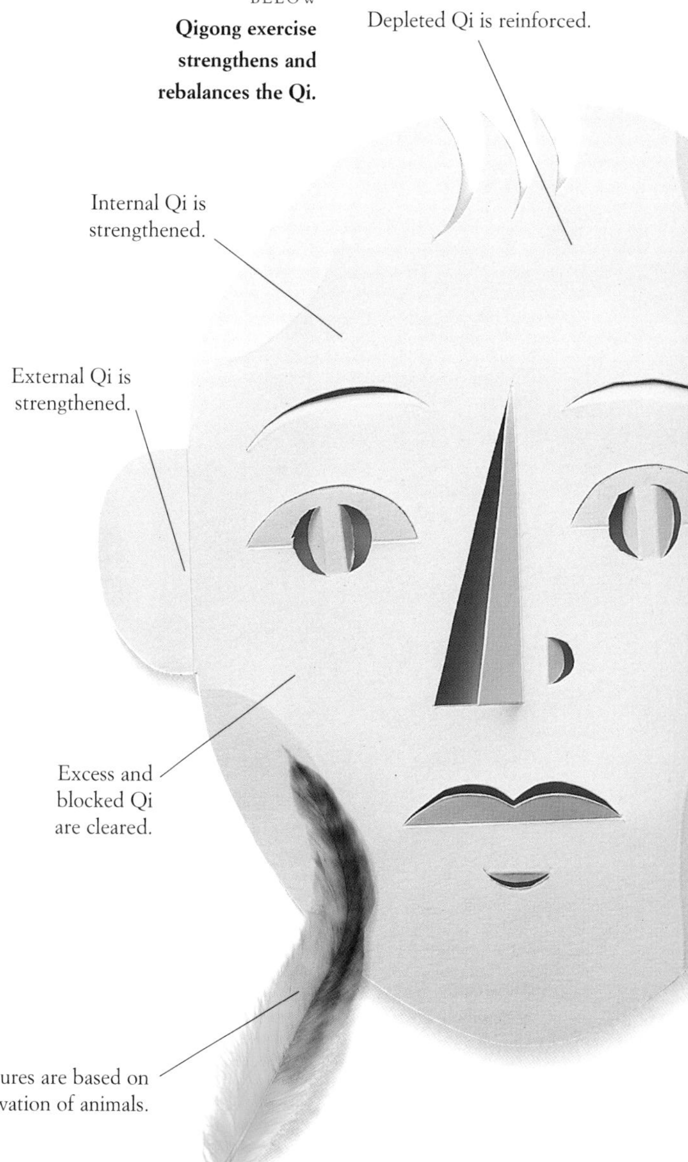

effectively, while others emphasize building up the more external manifestations of Qi in order to protect the body. The former are known as Nei Dan (the "inner elixir" of life), the latter as Wei Dan (the "external elixir").

Wei Dan exercises enable the practitioner to demonstrate apparently amazing feats of external muscle strength – the ability to resist a direct and powerful blow to the abdomen or chest from a sharpened spear, for example. The less dramatic Nei Dan practices are designed to strengthen the internal Qi of the body and hence promote excellent health and longevity.

Over the centuries Qigong masters have come and gone, and some traditions have flourished while others have died away; but we are now at a point where Qigong is not confined to the Chinese traditions but is accessible to the whole world. Over the last twenty years or so, as Chinese masters have traveled west to the United States and Europe, they have introduced Qigong practices to a wider and more eclectic audience. They have gathered "disciples" who, in time, have developed skills to a level where they can teach others. A growing number of very competent and committed Western practitioners are now insuring that Qigong practice is given a cultural context that "works" with overstressed Westerners, helping them to strengthen their immune systems and overcome disharmonies.

As the understanding of Qigong grows and the number of reliable practitioners increases, connections with other branches of Chinese medical practice also develop. More and more people are beginning to appreciate that acupuncture or herbal treatment can be greatly enhanced by Qigong, and that in the long run the practice may even render such interventionist treatments unnecessary.

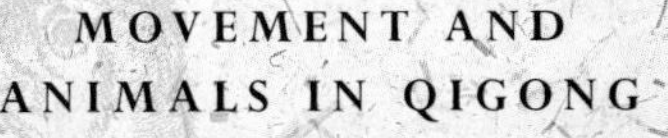

MOVEMENT AND ANIMALS IN QIGONG

Qigong exercises can consist of static postures or of movements that flow smoothly from posture to posture. Some of the sets of movements are relatively simple but some consist of more dynamic forms inspired by animals. These include the Dayan (Wild Goose) Qigong, and the Swimming Dragon Qigong.

There is no recognized training in Qigong, which can make the process of finding a suitable teacher difficult. However, it is vitally important to emphasize that the full benefits of Qigong practice can only accrue from, expert tuition. Many teachers have, at best, only a scant knowledge of Chinese medical principles and are not well-placed to integrate Qigong practice with any disharmonies of the body's energy system.

When seeking a Qigong teacher, ask yourself the following questions:

- Does this practitioner know and understand the principles of Chinesephilosophy and medical practice?
- Does this practitioner teach in a large, impersonal hall or gymnasium with a large number of impersonal students, or in small, manageable groups that allow for personal dialogue and teaching?
- Does this practitioner give the impression of running these Qigong classes merely as a money-making exercise?
- Do I feel comfortable with this teacher and his or her approach?

In the end, use your intuition and go with what your heart tells you.

Unlike Taiji, for which a teacher is essential, and which cannot be learned effectively from a book, to a certain extent Qigong practices can be self-taught from a book or video; but it should be remembered that there is no substitute for a good teacher, although books and videos can be a helpful complement. In this general spirit, the following simple and straightforward exercises are offered to give an indication of what Qigong has to offer.

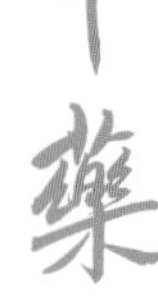

SELF-HELP PROTOCOLS

PREPARATION FOR PRACTICE

CHINESE MEDICINE

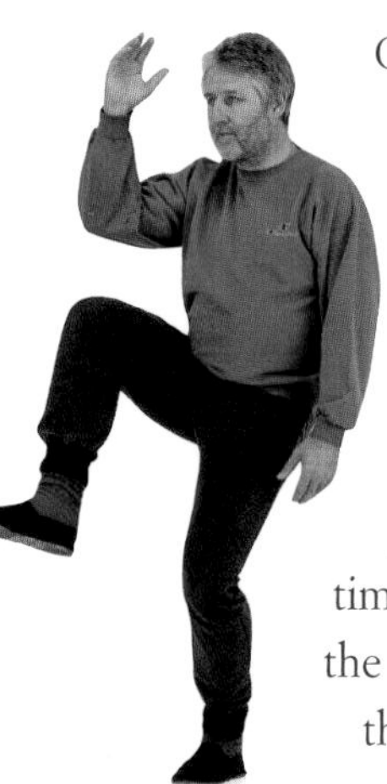

ABOVE
The exercise known as "golden rooster stands on one leg."

QIGONG IS not something that should be rushed into. Setting the scene and thorough preparation are essential to maximize the potential benefit. Many of the following preparatory points are self-evident, but at times it is appropriate to state the obvious in order to reinforce the message.

- Decide clearly how much time you are going to give to practice before you start.
- Insure that you will not be disturbed for the duration of your session (by the telephone, family members, and so on). If you cannot be reasonably sure that you will not be disturbed, consider postponing your practice to a more suitable time.
- Wear loose and comfortable clothing – contrary to popular myth it is not necessary to wear any kind of "uniform," as in Karate, for example. However, what you do wear must be comfortable and capable of keeping you either warm or cool (depending on the temperature). There is an argument that says that since Taiji and Qigong are essentially Yin in nature (compared with Karate, which is more Yang), it is appropriate to wear black, a more Yin color. (In Karate, the color of choice is usually white, which is relatively more Yang.) There is some validity in this idea, but not to the extent that it defines a uniform. You may wish to consider this point when choosing clothing, but comfort should take precedence.
- Take a few minutes just to "be" in the room, or outdoor space, before you turn your attention to any form of practice.
- Be confident that the temperature is comfortable – neither too hot nor too cold. It is especially important when practicing outside to insure that it is not too windy, too hot, too cold, or too wet. The additional benefits that can flow from outdoor practice may be totally nullified if the weather is too harsh. Invasion by external pathogenic factors is a major cause of disease and disharmony in Chinese medicine. If you are practicing outside, make sure that you dress for the environment as it is, not as you would like it to be. Indoors, it is important to insure that the room is well ventilated, and neither too hot nor too cold. Avoid gas or electric heaters if this is at all possible.

ABOVE
This exercise is known as "snake creeps down."

LEFT
The symmetrical posture known as "the horse stance."

THE FIRST FIVE MINUTES

AS WITH any form of exercise, it is important to "warm up" properly. When following any Qigong protocol, you are not only gently stretching and moving the body; you are also aiming to calm the mind in order to focus mind intent and attune to the Qi of the surrounding environment. With this in mind, the following protocol is suggested here as a five-minute warm-up before commencing any form of Taiji or Qigong routine.

- *Spend approximately two minutes gently stretching and moving the body – in any way that works for you – in order to get the blood flowing and the muscles warmed up. Do not overstretch or strain yourself: this will lead to a local Qi or Blood stagnation. Follow whatever simple routine feels comfortable.*

- *After you have completed the initial stage of physical warm-up, locate the spot in the room or outdoor space where you feel most comfortable. This may at first seem an odd thing to do, but the more you become aware of your surroundings, the more sensitive you will become to the "energetic ecology" of places – feeling more comfortable in certain spots, less so in others.*

- *Once you have located your spot, adopt the classic Taiji opening posture – Wu Chi or "Emptiness." This stance is characterized as follows:*

1. *Stand with your feet approximately shoulder-width apart and parallel to each other; the feet should be facing directly forward, neither turned in nor out.*

2. *Allow your knees to bend slightly, but not too much. A good rule of thumb is to bend the knees to the point where you can still just see your big toe over the end of the knee. If you can see the whole foot, your knees are not bent enough; and if you cannot see any part of your feet, your knees are bent too much.*

3. *Let the hands fall loosely to the side, as if weights on the ends of the fingers are pulling them to the ground.*

4. *Round the shoulders slightly, but make sure that the trunk follows the curvature of the spine as naturally as possible.*

5. *Allow the abdomen to expand – do not hold it in tightly. You should be able to feel the abdomen gently expanding on the in-breath and gently contracting on the out-breath.*

6. *Hold the head erect, as if a string were running to an imaginary support from the Baihui point on the top of the head.*

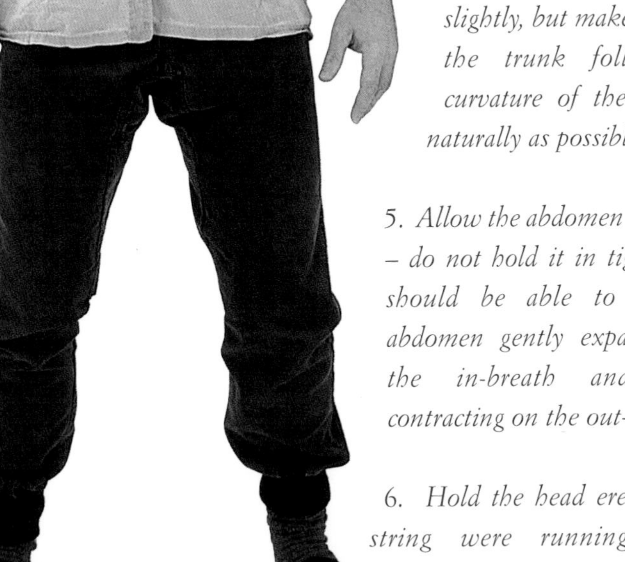

ABOVE
The opening posture in Qigong is known as Wu Chi or "Emptiness."

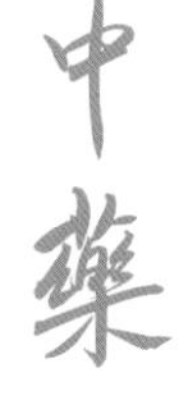

STANDING POLE

THIS SET of five static, standing postures is often considered one of the classic Qigong protocols. It is relatively simple, yet the benefits that can accrue from its regular practice are substantial. (Elements of Standing Pole are among the most commonly practiced postures in Chinese daily routine.) Initially these postures are all held for two minutes. After extended practice, the time can be increased to five minutes. Prepare for the exercise as described on page 193.

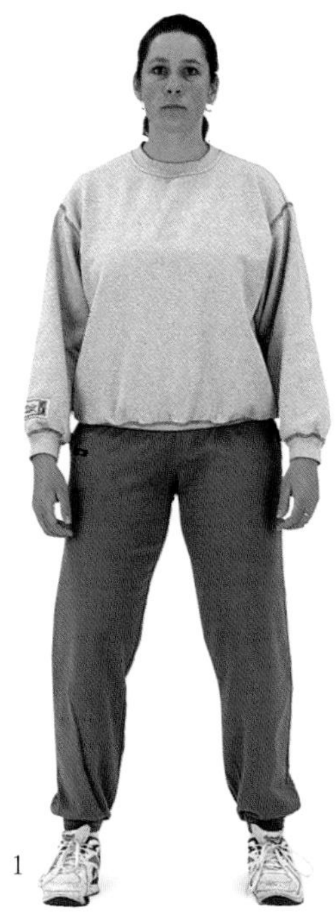

POSTURE 1

Assume the classic Wu Chi posture described on page 193. Hold for two minutes.

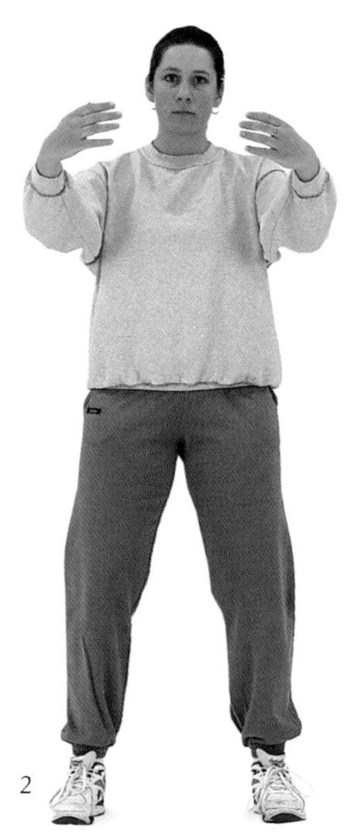

POSTURE 2

Bring the arms up to approximately upper chest height as if holding a large soft ball against the chest, with your gently bent arms resting on the ball. Hold this position for two minutes.

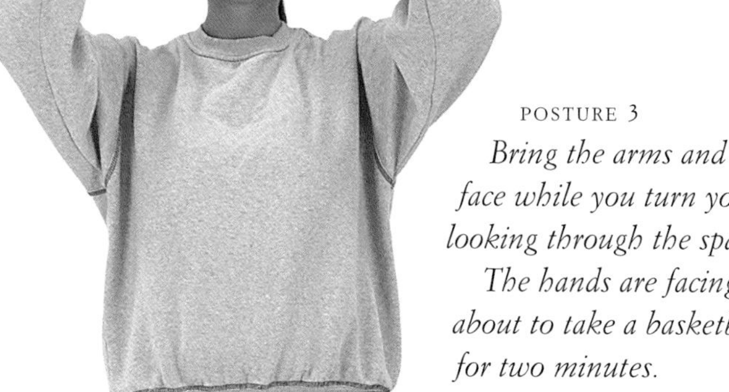

POSTURE 3

Bring the arms and hands up in front of the face while you turn your head slightly upward, looking through the space between the hands.

The hands are facing away from the face as if about to take a basketball shot. Hold this position for two minutes.

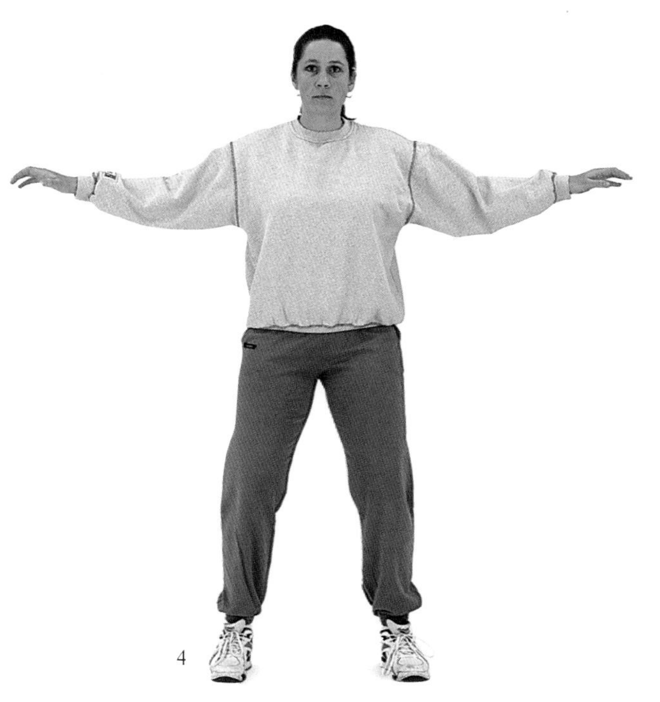

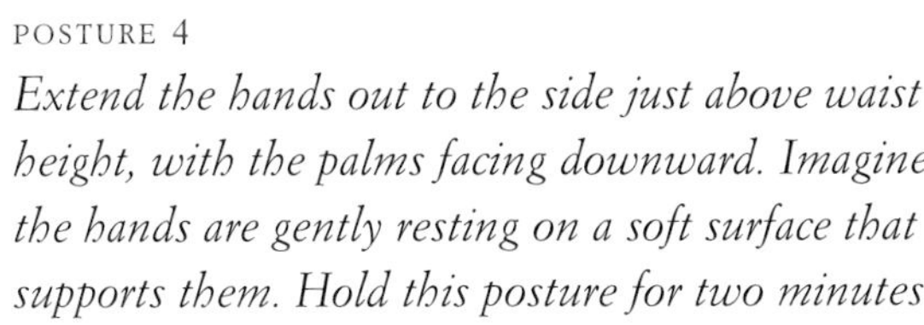

POSTURE 4

Extend the hands out to the side just above waist height, with the palms facing downward. Imagine the hands are gently resting on a soft surface that supports them. Hold this posture for two minutes.

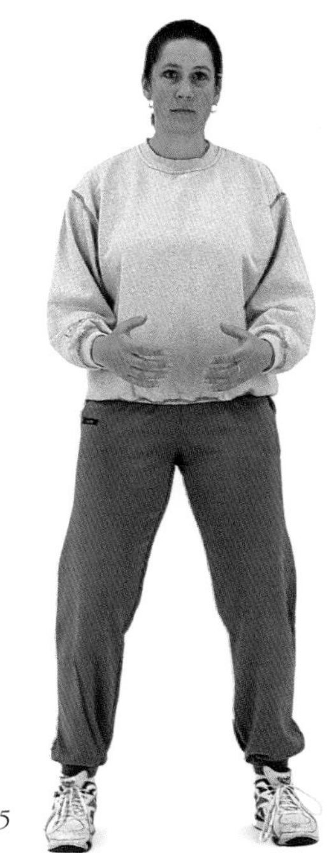

POSTURE 5

Place the hands as if holding a small ball of energy – about the size of a soccer ball, or slightly smaller – in front of the Dantian area (see "General points" below). Hold this posture for two minutes.

General points

As you go through the postures, focus your mind on the lower Dantian area – about two inches (5cm) below the umbilicus and three inches (7.5cm) beneath the surface. This area, known as the "Sea of Qi," is one of the major areas of the body where Qi is stored. Throughout the exercise, breathe naturally and slowly "through the Dantian" – letting the lower abdomen gently expand on inhalation and then gently contract on exhalation.

If at any point you find any of the postures becoming a strain, do not persevere. Simply hold the postures for as long as is comfortable and gradually build up your time. There is nothing to be gained from straining the body: indeed, this can easily result in problems of Qi depletion and local Qi stagnation.

The apparent simplicity of these postures often misleads people into thinking that they must be easy; this is most emphatically not the case, and you should always be sensitive to your own capabilities as well as your stage of development when practicing.

In order to benefit from such a sequence, it is vital to practice the postures regularly – every day if possible. The occasional venture into Standing Pole is of little benefit.

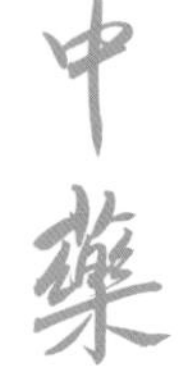

STANDING FORM BROCADE EXERCISES

THIS SET of exercises is based on the Ba Dua Jin, which literally translates as the "Eight Sections of Brocade." The concept of eight sections is highly symbolic in Chinese thought (for example, the Yi Jing consists of 8 x 8 hexagrams). Jin (brocade) is a symbol of great beauty in Chinese thought. This set of eight postures dates from the Southern Song Dynasty (1127–1279) and is undertaken in a standing position.

Begin the set of exercises with a period of quiet preparation as described on page 193, warming and loosening, settling into your spot, then taking up the Wu Chi posture. Begin this posture with focused and regular breathing.

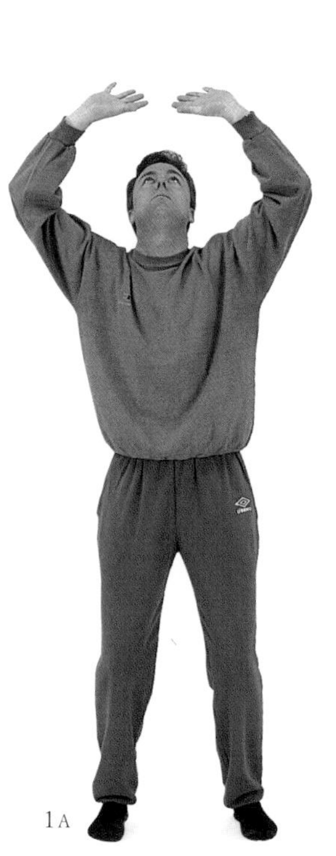
1A

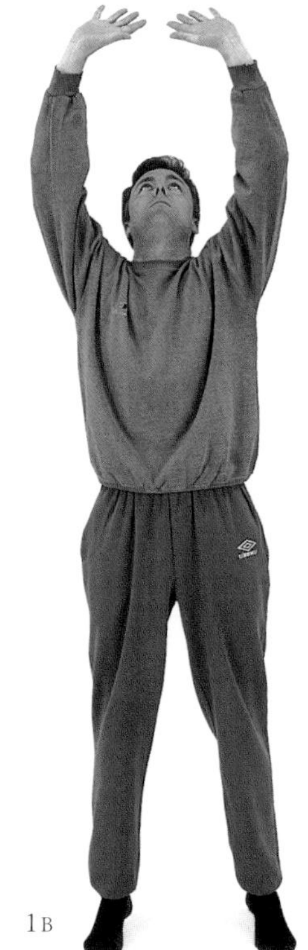
1B

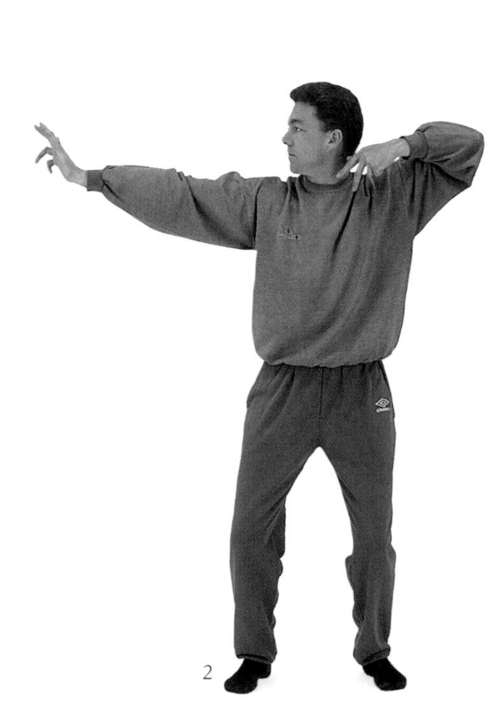
2

POSTURE 1

Hold up Heaven to Benefit the San Jiao

Raise both hands above the head with the palms facing upward, as if holding up the heavens (1A). The eyes should follow the hands over the head.

Then stretch up on the toes (1B) and hold the posture for a few seconds before gently returning to the starting position. Inhale through the nose while bringing the arms up, and exhale through the mouth when bringing the arms down. Repeat the posture up to eight times. This posture is said to benefit the flow of Qi through the San Jiao or "Triple Heater."

POSTURE 2

Draw the Bow to Benefit the Lungs

From the Wu Chi posture, draw the hands up and pull as if drawing a bow to the right. On the full draw, extend the hand and arm.

Return to the center of the body and repeat, drawing the bow to the left as shown.

Repeat the sequence four times on each side, inhaling through the nose while drawing the arms up, and exhaling through the mouth while extending the bow. Focus the eyes over the raised fingers at the end of the bow.

This posture is said to benefit the Lungs.

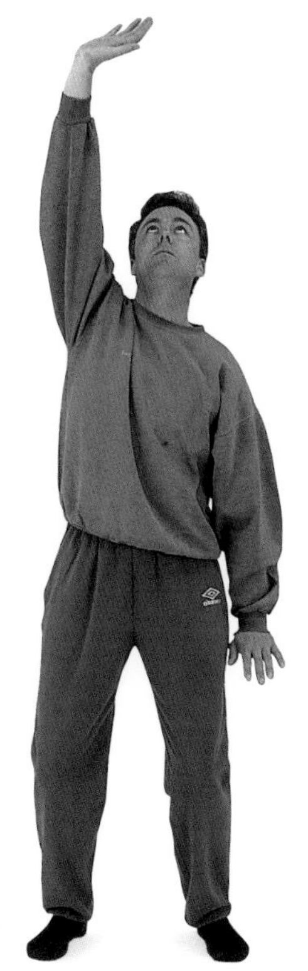
3

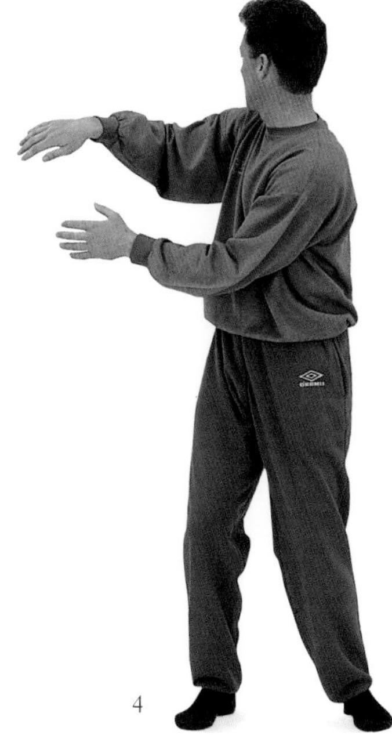
4

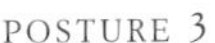
POSTURE 3

Press to Sky and Earth to Benefit the Spleen and Stomach

From the Wu Chi posture draw the right hand up to the sky with the palm facing upward, and the left hand downward with the palm facing the earth. On the extension, straighten the legs.

Inhale through the nose in the Wu Chi posture and exhale through the nose or mouth on the sky press.

This posture is said to benefit the function of the Spleen and also the Stomach.

POSTURE 4

Cow Turns to Face the Moon to Benefit the Kidneys

This posture is similar to the section of the Taiji form known as "Fair Ladies Weave Shuttles." Starting from the Wu Chi posture, turn the body to the right with the hands pushing away. The gaze should follow the turn of the waist.

Return to the center and repeat the posture to the left side. Repeat four times on each side. Inhale through the nose at the starting point, and complete the exhalation through the nose or mouth at the end of the turn.

This posture is said to benefit the Kidneys. It also stretches the muscles of the upper torso and focuses the eyes.

POSTURE 5

Side Bend to Benefit the Heart

Start from the Wu Chi position and bring the right arm up, arched above the head; then bend to the left. Return to the opening position and repeat by turning to the right with the left arm arched over the head.

Inhale through the nose on the opening position, and exhale on the side stretch.

This posture is said to benefit the function of the Heart by clearing excess Heat.

5

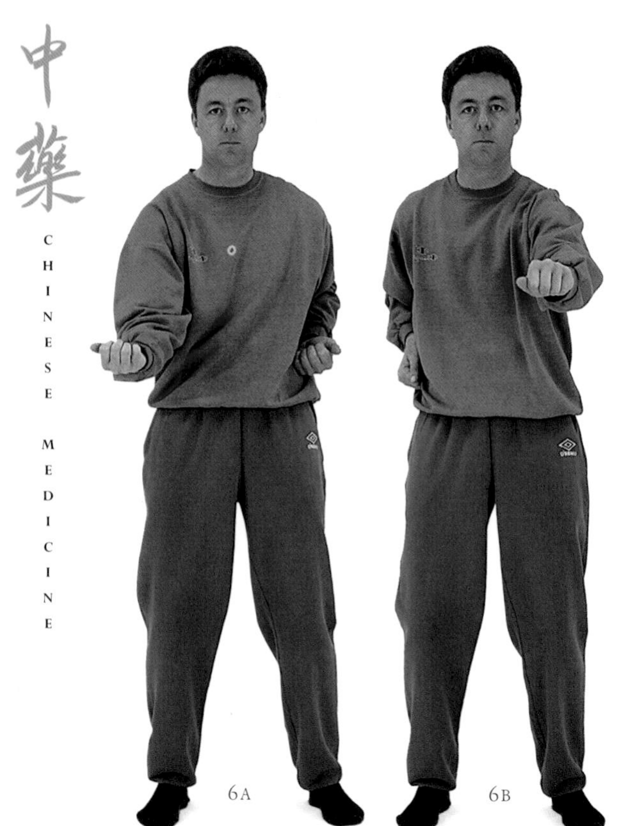

6A 6B

POSTURE 6

Clench Fist and Punch to Regulate the Liver

From the standing Wu Chi posture, clench the right fist, draw it back and punch through while drawing back the left arm (6A). Repeat on the other side by clenching and punching with the left arm (6B). Repeat with four punches to each side.

Inhale through the nose on the opening posture, and exhale powerfully through the mouth on the punch. Imagine any pent-up anger being released through the punch.

This posture is said to promote the smooth flow of Qi from the Liver.

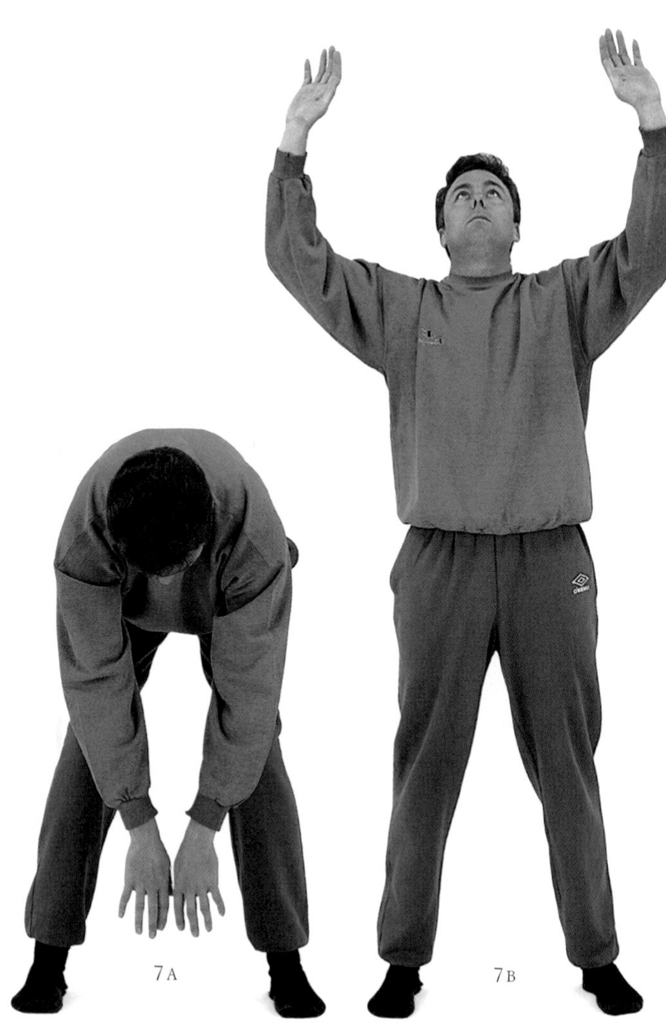

7A 7B

POSTURE 7

Sink Down and Rise to Benefit the Kidneys

Starting from the Wu Chi posture, bend over with the legs straight (7A). Allow the backs of the hands to touch, and draw up together.

Then separate the hands above the head (7B) and circle the arms around to return to the opening posture. Repeat this movement eight times.

Inhale through the nose at the start, and complete the exhalation as the arms are at the top of the circle.

This movement is said to benefit and strengthen the Kidneys.

CAUTION

Pregnant women should avoid these exercises, which in extreme cases may result in miscarriage.

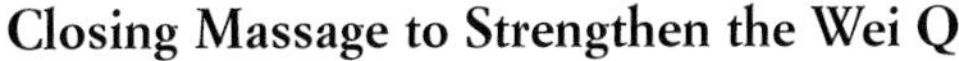

Closing Massage to Strengthen the Wei Qi

At the end of the eight postures, move around freely and gently tap, with the tips of your fingers, or with a loosely closed fist, the meridians running up and down the arms, legs, trunk, and head. This stimulates the flow of the external and protective Wei Qi, and helps the body to build its immune system and ward off illness. If you are working together with a partner, you may perform this closing massage on each other.

Several of the Brocade postures focus on tonifying and strengthening the Kidneys. This is essential from the perspective of Chinese medicine, given that the Kidneys are the source of all the Yin and Yang energy in the body; they thus support the function of all the other Zangfu systems.

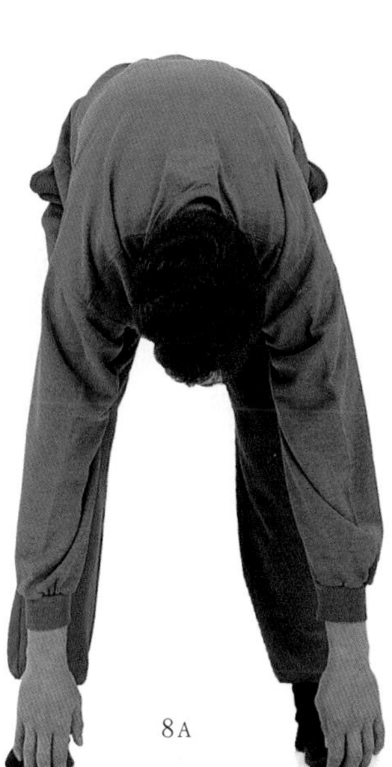

8A

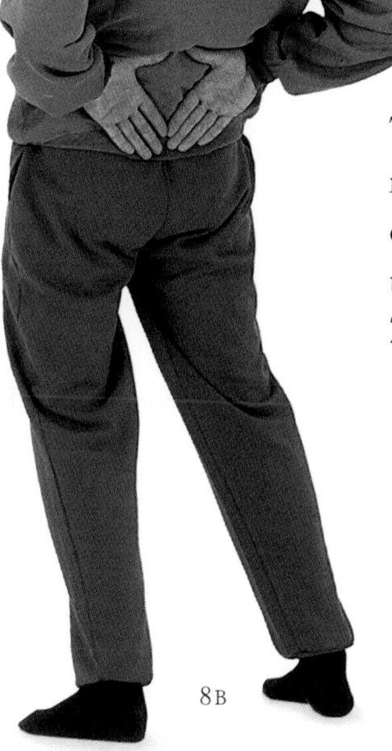

8B

POSTURE 8

Bending and Stretching to Strengthen the Kidneys

From the Wu Chi posture, bend forward with the legs straight and touch the ground (8A). Return to the center and then, with the hands placed in the small of the back, bend backward and stretch as far as you can (8B).

Inhale through the nose at the start of the bend and exhale through the mouth at the end. Inhale again at the opening position, and exhale again during the back stretch. Repeat the sequence eight times.

This posture is said to strengthen and benefit the Kidneys.

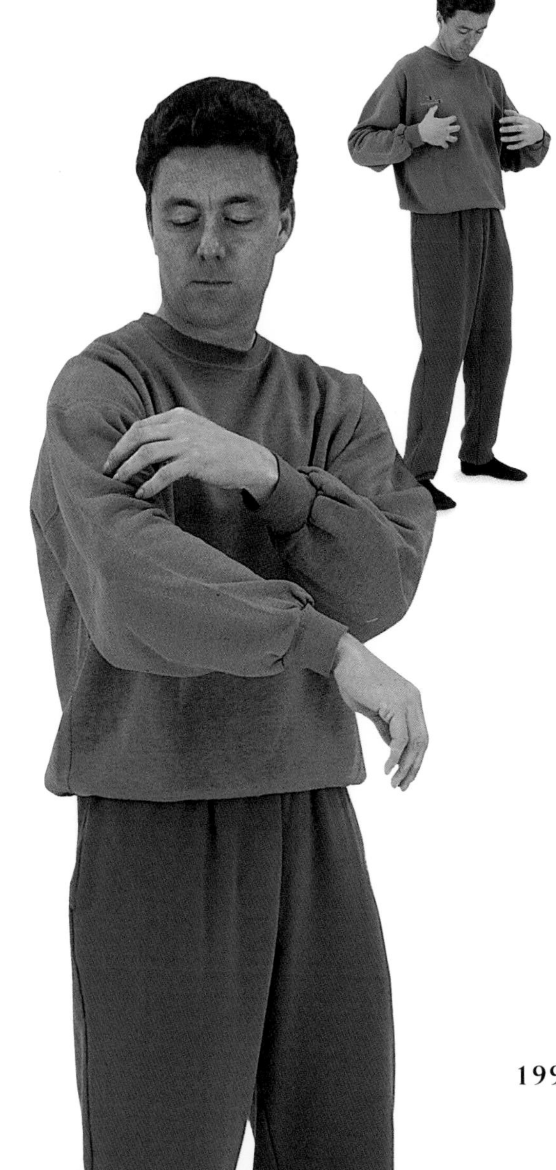

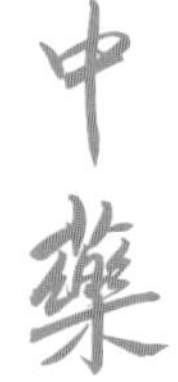

SITTING FORM BROCADE EXERCISES

THIS SEQUENCE of six Qigong exercises performed in a sitting position, originates in the Ming Dynasty (1368–1644).

Each of the movements is performed in order to strengthen a particular internal Zangfu system of the body.

FORM 1

Strengthen the Heart

Sit comfortably on a chair or stool with the feet firmly on the floor, about shoulder-width apart. Pound the arms and the body 30 times (step 1), then raise the right hand above the head with the palm upward, while the left faces downward to the earth (step 2). Tap the teeth together a total of 30 times, then gargle any collected saliva before swallowing (step 3).

Meditate quietly at the end of this sequence (step 4). This form is said to help cure palpitations and generally strengthen the Qi of the chest.

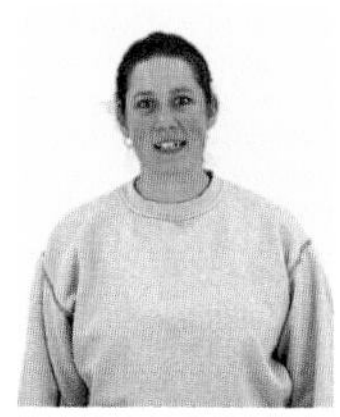

STEP 3

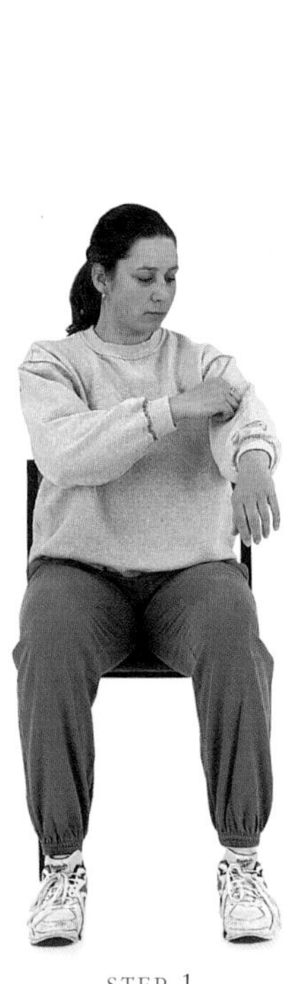

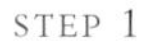

STEP 1

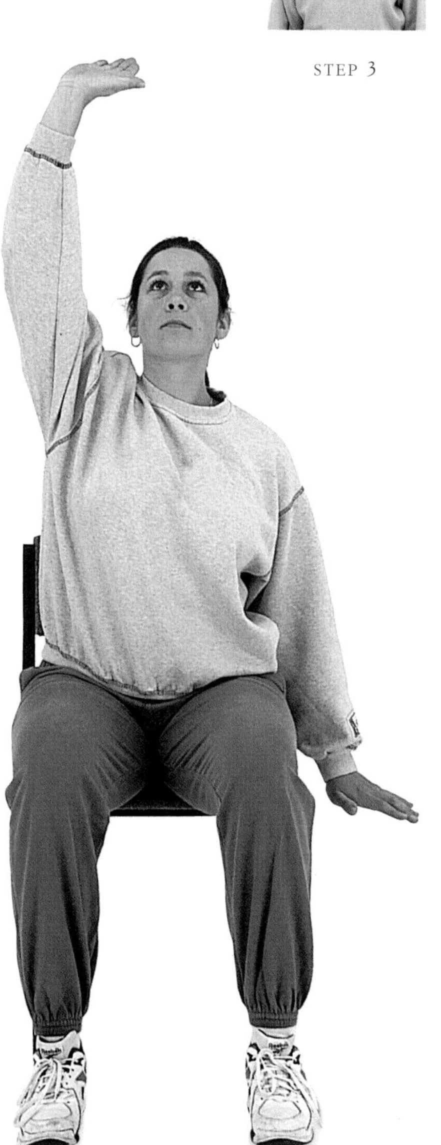

STEP 2

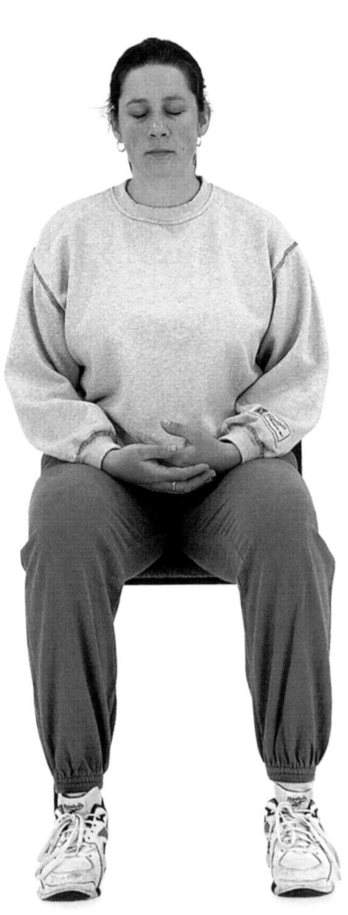

STEP 4

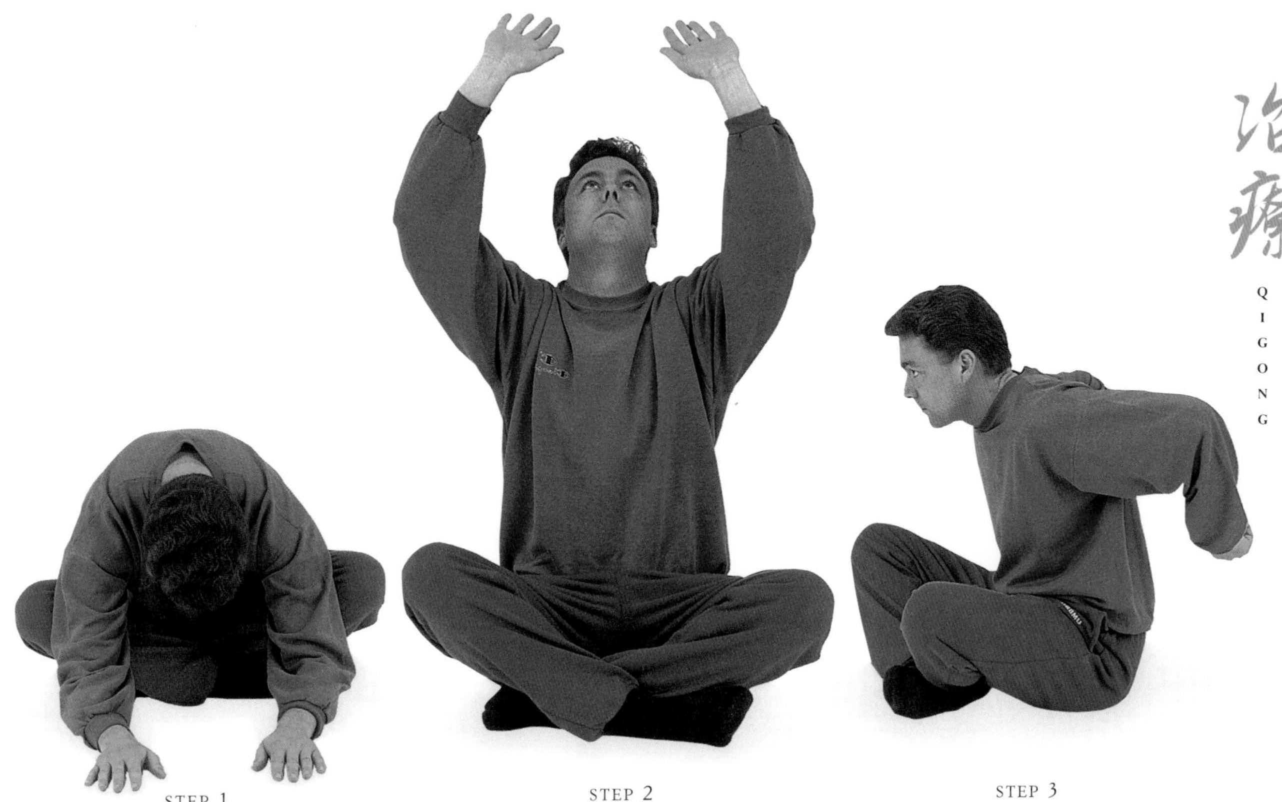

STEP 1 STEP 2 STEP 3

FORM 2

Strengthen the Lungs

Sit on the floor with the legs crossed. Bend forward until the outstretched arms touch the floor (step 1). Then raise the arms upward as the trunk comes back to the upright position, and stretch toward the sky with the palms facing upward (step 2). Repeat three times, then pound the upper and lower back 32 times with your fists (step 3). Strike the teeth together 30 times, then gargle and swallow the saliva.

Meditate quietly at the end of the sequence. This form is said to clear the Lungs of an invasion of pathogenic Wind.

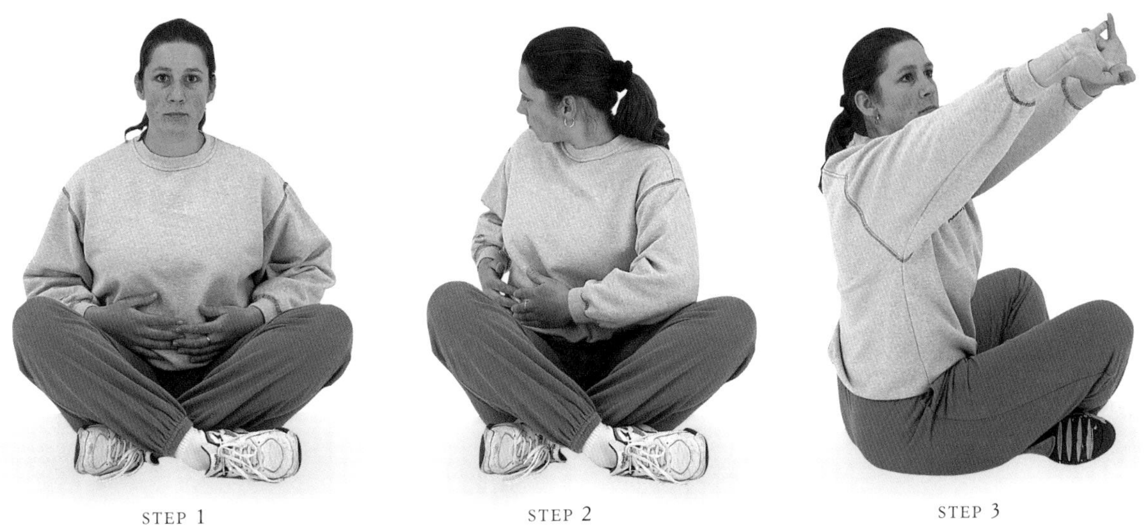

STEP 1 STEP 2 STEP 3

FORM 3

Strengthen the Liver

Sit upright with the legs crossed. The palms should be held inward toward the Dantian (step 1). Turn the trunk to the left and right 15 times (step 2). Interlock the fingers and turn the hands to face away from the body; push outward eight times (step 3). Strike the teeth and swallow the saliva. Finish by meditating quietly.

This form is said to clear internal pathogenic Liver Wind.

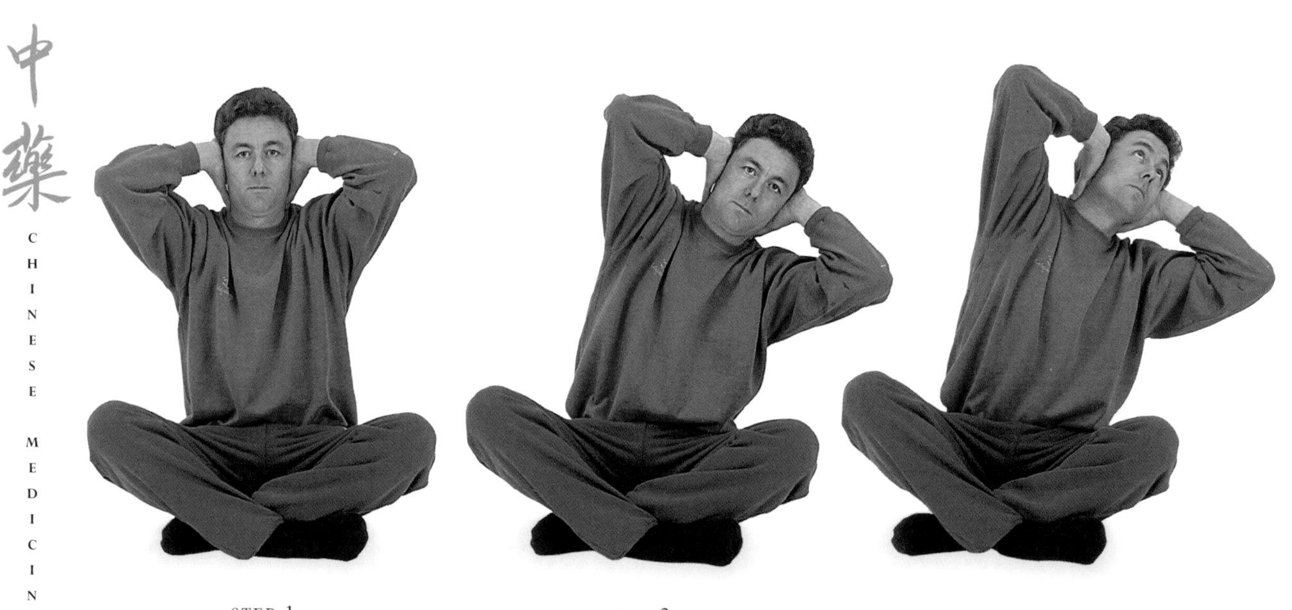

STEP 1 STEP 2 STEP 3

FORM 4

Strengthen the Kidneys

Sit upright with the legs crossed. Place the hands over the ears with the elbows facing outward (step 1). Bend left and right five times (step 2).

Then push up the arms, with the hands still covering the ears, first left then right, 15 times each (step 3). Strike the teeth and swallow saliva. Meditate quietly. This form is said to strengthen the Kidneys and the Bladder.

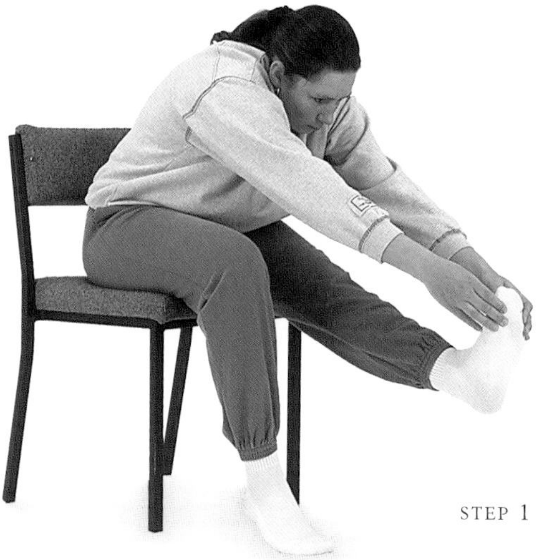

STEP 1

FORM 5

Strengthen the Gall Bladder

Sit upright on a comfortable straight chair or stool. Hold the left foot with both hands and move it from side to side 15 times (step 1). Repeat the sequence with the right foot.

With the hands resting on the chair seat, push the body forward and arch the back as far as you can, holding the fully extended position for a few seconds (step 2). Repeat 15 times. Strike the teeth, and swallow saliva. Meditate quietly. This form is said to balance the Qi flow in the Gall Bladder.

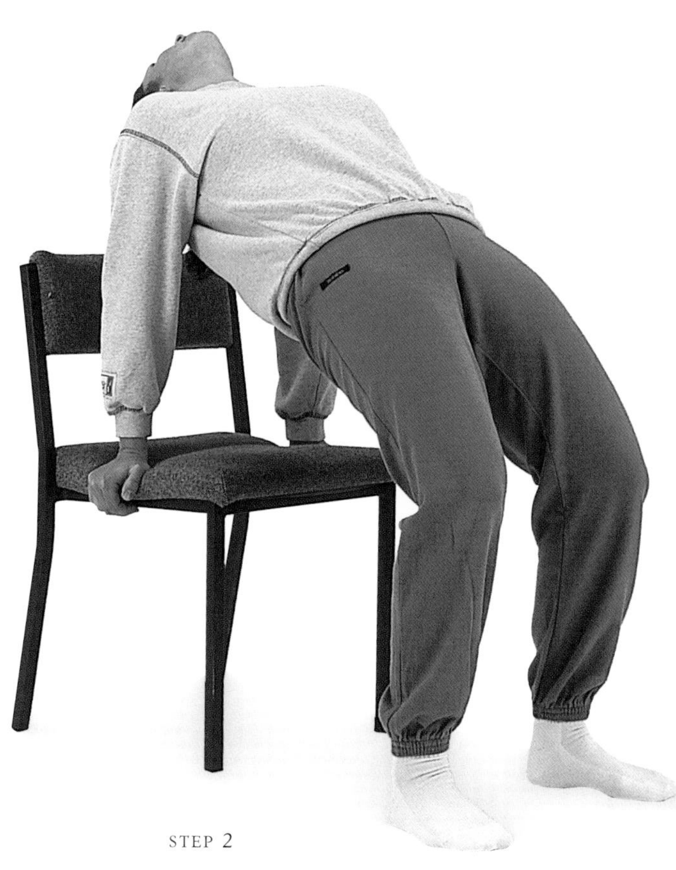

STEP 2

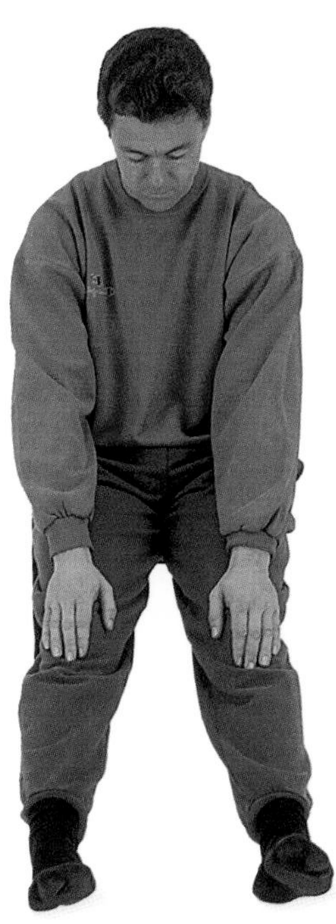

STEP 1

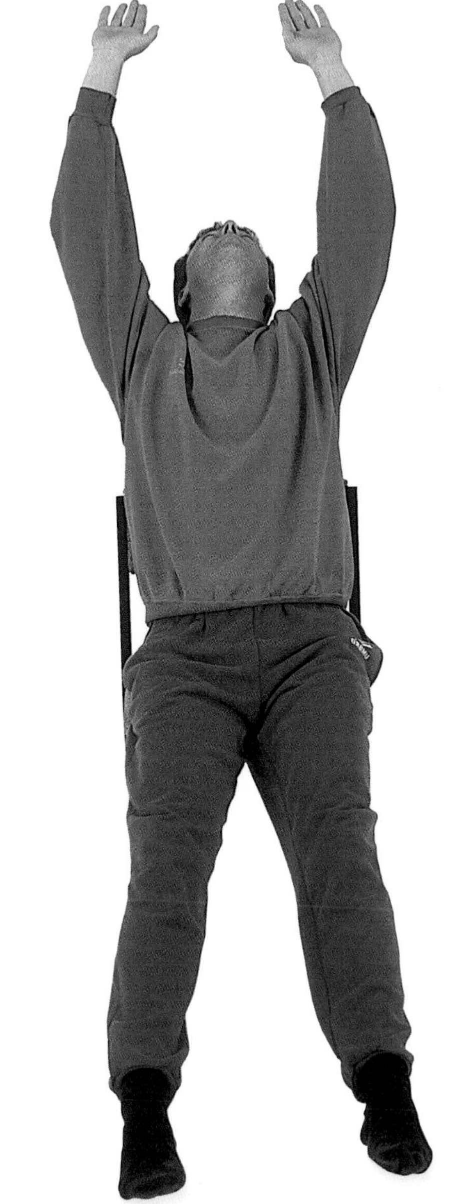

STEP 2

FORM 6

Strengthen the Spleen

Sit upright on a straight chair or stool. Stretch out the legs and rest the palms of your hands on your knees (step 1). Raise up the arms with the palms facing upward, and stretch the back in an arch as far as you can go (step 2). Hold the extended position for a few seconds and then return the hands to the knees.

Repeat five times and then kneel on all fours on the floor. Turn the head to the left and right, looking over each shoulder – five times on each side (step 3). Strike the teeth, and swallow saliva. Meditate quietly. This form is said to benefit the Spleen and aid digestion.

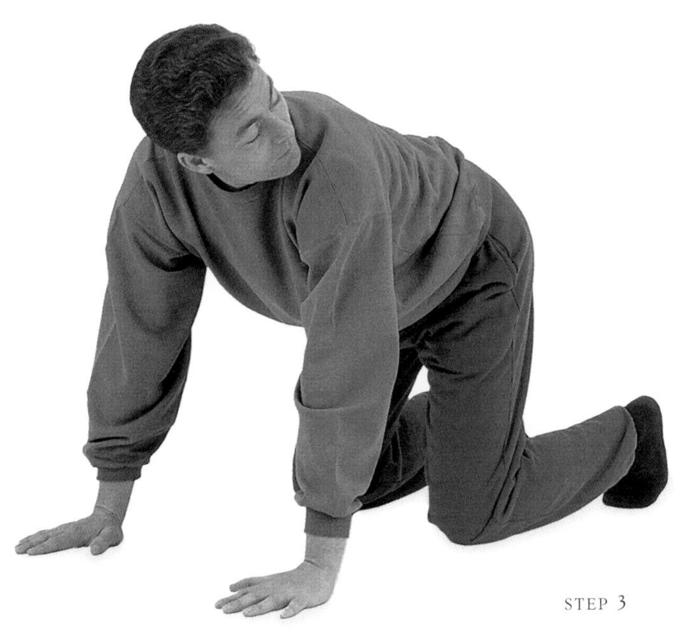

STEP 3

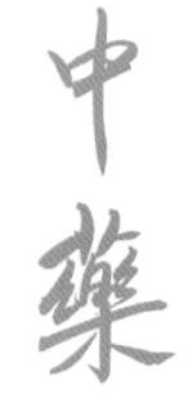

TAIJI QIGONG SEQUENCE

THE FIVE ELEMENTS

This short, flowing-movement exercise has the same qualities as a Taiji sequence, but it is much shorter and more easily learned. This beautiful sequence is based on the Five Elements of Chinese thought (*see page 26*); it thus offers not only a relatively simple introduction to the flow of a movement exercise but also a link to one of the most powerful sets of symbolism in Chinese medicine. Regular practice of this sequence develops flexibility and suppleness by encouraging balanced Qi flow through the body.

Start in the classic Wu Chi posture (stage 1) and hold your hands in front of the lower Dantian. Imagine that you are holding a ball of fire in between your hands (stage 2). Hold this posture and focus your imagination for a couple of minutes – you are now ready to begin the Five Elements sequence.

Draw the ball of fire into the Dantian. The fire evaporates the water, which rises up to the heavens (stage 3). The water then forms into clouds and condenses (stage 4), falling as rain (stages 5–7). The rain nourishes the earth (stage 8) from which spring the seeds of the tree (stage 9). The tree grows tall and strong and moves in the wind (stages 10–12). Eventually the tree dies and the organic matter returns to nourish the earth (stage 13). This decaying matter eventually forms minerals and metals that are drawn from the right side (stage 14) and the left side (stage 15). The full cycle of the elements is completed as you open out to embrace the whole universe (stages 16 and 17), and return the universe to your own Dantian (stage 18). The sequence ends in Wu Chi (stage 19).

These sequences and protocols will, it is hoped, provide some insight into the wonderful world of Qigong and perhaps encourage you to find a teacher and begin to integrate some very simple Qigong sequences into your lifestyle.

Among the thousands of Qigong sequences, postures, and protocols, it is often said by the Chinese themselves that the simple Standing Pole exercises represent the "royalty" of Qigong. If you practice these diligently, the benefits to your health and well-being will be remarkable.

Qigong exercises are begun by adopting the classic opening posture. They rehearse in stages the story of the five elements transforming into each other in the cycle of the universe. A ball of fire evaporates the water, which rises to form clouds of rain to nourish the earth. Trees grow, move in the wind and die, yielding to minerals and metals. The strength from the universe is drawn inward and the sequence ends as it began.

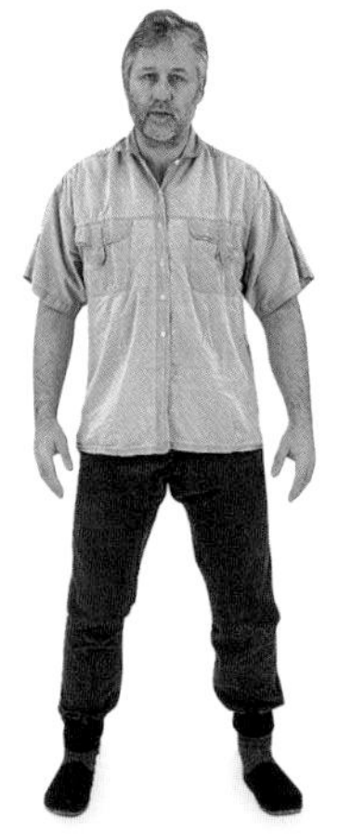

STAGE 1

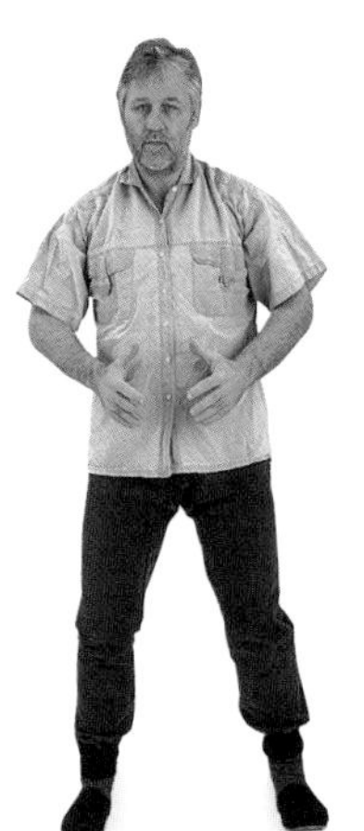

STAGE 2

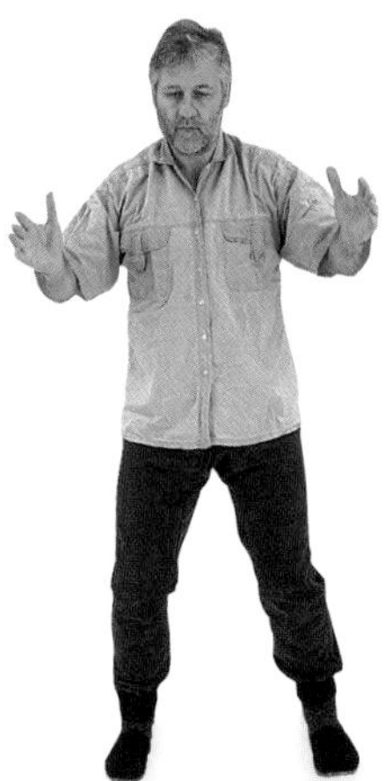

STAGE 3

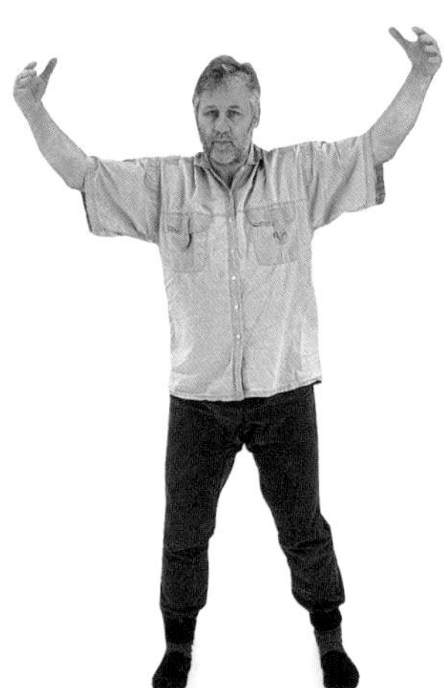

STAGE 4

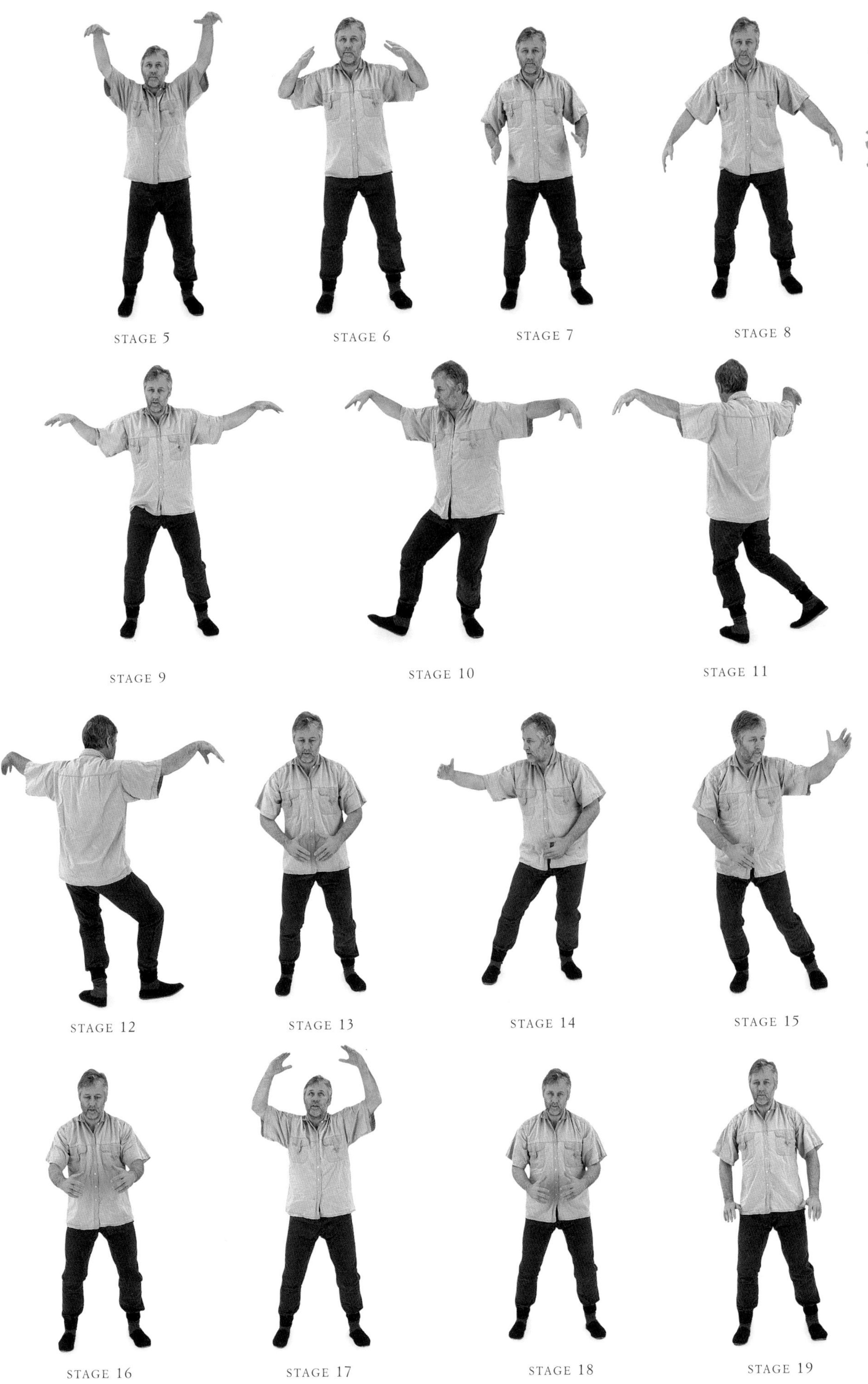

STAGE 5

STAGE 6

STAGE 7

STAGE 8

STAGE 9

STAGE 10

STAGE 11

STAGE 12

STAGE 13

STAGE 14

STAGE 15

STAGE 16

STAGE 17

STAGE 18

STAGE 19

TAIJI AND TAIJIQUAN

MANY PEOPLE in the West are better acquainted with the graceful, flowing movements of Taiji forms than with the more static Qigong forms. However, the two share a common philosophical background, and both can contribute to the development and maintenance of health and well-being. In essence, the forms that are seen performed as Taijiquan (literally, the "supreme ultimate fist," or "supreme ultimate boxing art") can be conceptualized as a dynamic form of Qigong, or "energy cultivation," and a way of regulating the system and preventing disease.

At its roots, Taijiquan is a powerful and effective martial art, but behind the martial applications lie the same Daoist principles: the development of perfect harmony between the Yin and Yang energies of the body, the promotion of smooth and uninhibited flow of Qi throughout the body, and the maintenance of maximal health.

BACKGROUND

THE ORIGINS of Taiji or Taijiquan are unclear, but it is likely that Daoist martial practices were in existence well over 2,000 years ago. Conventional mythology links the origins of these martial arts to the Indian monk Bodhidharma, who was reputed to have taught the Zen boxing that developed more fully into Kung Fu to the monks of the Shaolin temple in the fifth century. It is generally believed that Taijiquan as a fighting art can be traced back to the Daoist monk Chang San Feng in the 14th century. He is said to have dreamed about a fight-cum-dance between a bird and a snake and developed a set of thirteen movements from his dream. The forms have evolved and changed over time, mainly within the context of family lineages, up until the present day. Numerous styles of Taiji are practiced in China today, but among the most commonly taught styles in the West are

- *Yang – long and short forms*
- *Wu*
- *Sun*
- *Chen*
- *Wudang.*

Each style has its own postures, sequences, and moves, but they all share the same basic Daoist principles that link them firmly with the more general practice of Qigong.

To pursue Taiji practice as an operational martial art requires a level of commitment – in terms of training, discipline, and time – that is rarely attained by the average student whose aim is to keep fit and healthy. With this in mind, it is more appropriate to drop the word "quan" ("fist") and use the more descriptive name "Taiji" (the "supreme ultimate"). Anyone who has taken the time to learn Taiji as a movement form will readily attest that, in terms of balancing the Qi flow of the body, calming the Shen or mind, and promoting the fullest form of internal and external health, it is certainly the "supreme ultimate" form of exercise.

LEFT
Taiji practice is based on Taijiquan, linked to martial art.

TAIJI AND CHINESE MEDICINE

TO LEARN Taiji properly it is necessary to seek the supervision and support of an experienced and knowledgeable teacher. While it is quite possible to learn the basics of simple Qigong postures and forms from a book, it has to be stated that Taiji cannot really be learned in this way, nor from any other indirect medium such as a video. When looking for books on Taiji, bear in mind that the usefulness of any book is in direct proportion to the number of illustrations showing how to perform the Taiji forms.

In terms of health, Taiji practice promotes flexibility and strength in the limbs and trunk; it develops the most appropriate upright posture; it clears areas of Qi stagnation in the channels and the collaterals; and it establishes a healthy balance of flow between the Yin and Yang Qi throughout all the internal Zangfu systems.

It is also important to appreciate that the subtleties and complexities of the Taiji form require that you embark on a process that never really ends. Suffice it to say, once you start on this road, you will find that Taiji opens up a level of experiential understanding of the energetics of the human being that no other practice appears to do, and results in a physical, emotional, and spiritual grace – and flexibility of the highest order.

SNAKE CREEPS DOWN

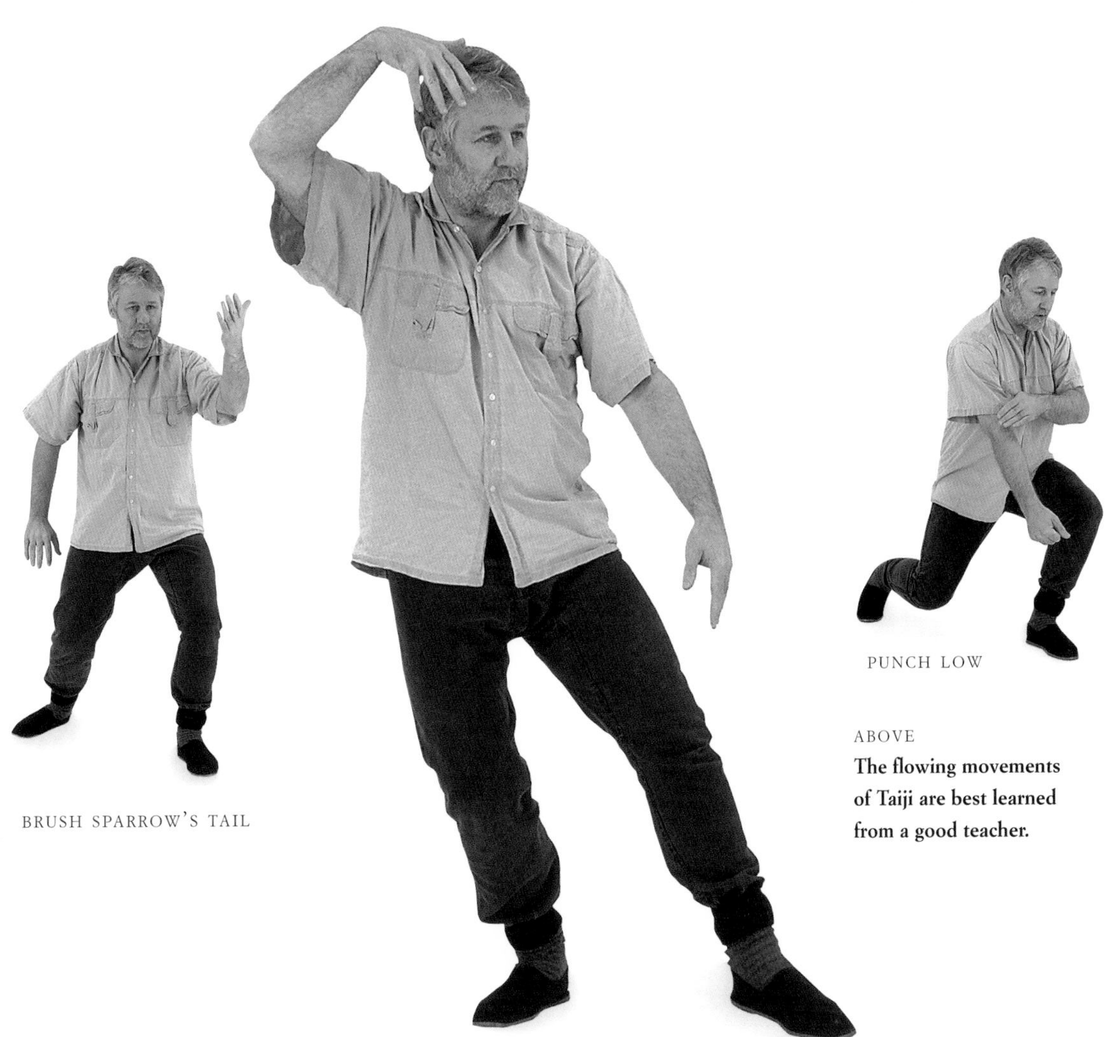

BRUSH SPARROW'S TAIL

PUNCH LOW

WHITE CRANE SPREADS WINGS

ABOVE
The flowing movements of Taiji are best learned from a good teacher.

QIGONG HEALING

QIGONG HEALING is a fascinating and altogether more controversial area of Chinese medical practice. In this process, the practitioner guides his or her own Qi, emitted through key acupuncture points in the body, to enhance Qi flow in the patient. In most instances, this is done without any physical contact. Central to Qigong healing is the practitioner's own strong and robust energy system, which will have been developed by practicing many of the Qigong exercises and postures already discussed. There is a growing body of literature and evidence from China regarding the emission and guidance of Qi and how this can be focused onto the patient in order to facilitate his or her Qi balance and redress any apparent disharmony.

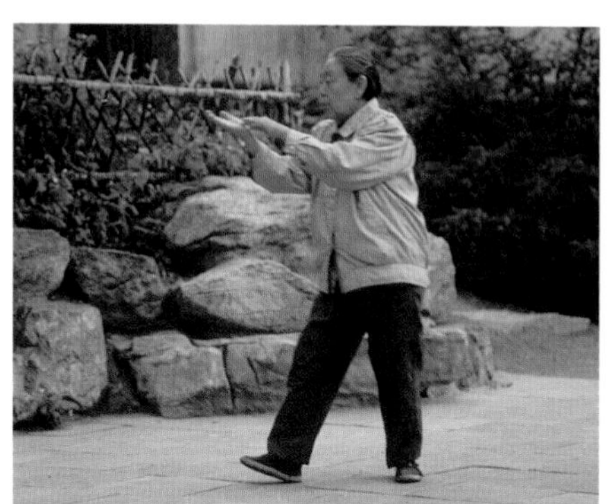

ABOVE
Many people claim to have been helped by Qigong healing, usually performed without physical contact.

Many Chinese hospitals have a Qigong department where techniques (often akin in style to what may be termed the "healing hands" approach in the West) are used to treat a whole variety of problems. Qigong healing techniques are also commonly used on patients in acupuncture clinics in order to enhance the effectiveness of the treatment.

In most large public parks in the major Chinese cities, there are usually several Qigong masters offering healing and Qigong exercise classes. One notable exponent, whom I had the privilege to see in action, had a regular group of cancer patients who visited daily for a combination of Qigong exercises and healing.

While it is not yet possible to offer any statistical data, it is clear from anecdotal evidence that many of the patients benefited greatly from the treatment. One particular woman who had been coming every day for about eighteen months, pointed out that, two years previously, her doctor had told her that she had only two or three months left to live. Although she was not yet clear of the cancer, her general health was much more stable, and she was able to do things that she had not been able to do for a considerable period of time.

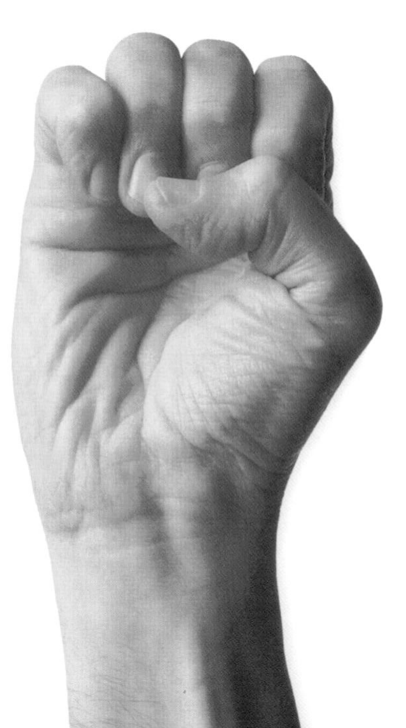

LEFT
Five Thunder Fingers, one of the hand gestures through which a Qigong healer emits Qi.

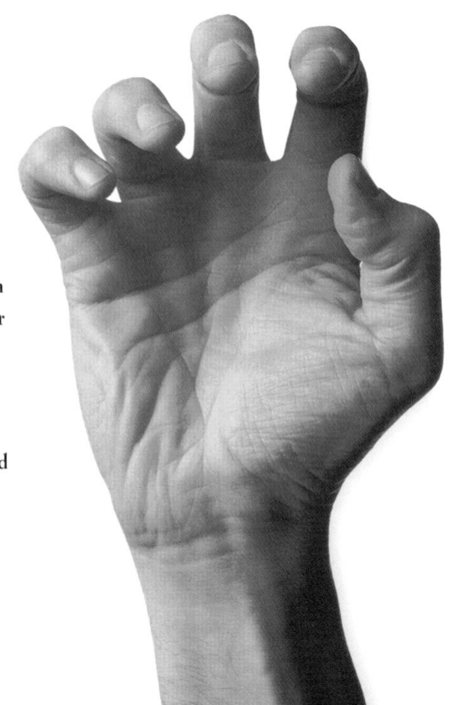

RIGHT
The Spreading Claw hand gesture, also used by Qigong healers.

Several quite specific hand gestures are used in order to emit Qi – including the "Five Thunder Fingers" and "Spreading Claw" techniques *(shown on page 208)*.

Qigong healing practices are only now becoming better known in the West, and to some individuals – even to some practitioners of Chinese medicine – they represent an extremely challenging conceptual shift. A lot more research and training is required before such practices become an accepted part of the treatment offered by practitioners outside China.

It seems highly possible that many of the techniques ascribed to the "laying on of hands" or "distance healing" (in a Western context) can be attributed to a process of energetic transfer between practitioner and patient, which balances the underlying Qi flow and helps clear disharmonies. Chinese medicine offers the most comprehensive theoretical articulation of what happens during this process.

As has already been emphasized, Chinese medicine operates at an energetic level and produces changes at a physical level. No one reading this book should be in any doubt that Qi emission and guidance are real. The corollary of this is that these healing techniques require a deep understanding of Chinese medicine, specific training, and supervised experiential practice.

When considering Qigong healing, it is important to remember that powerful energetic forces are involved; consequently, you need to feel confident about the qualifications and experience of the practitioner you choose.

Qigong as a specific therapeutic approach is only now developing in the West, but it has the potential to stand beside acupuncture and herbal medicine as a major pillar of Chinese medicine. In the meantime, many health benefits can be acquired by the regular practice of simple Qigong exercises. Such a self-help approach is of far more value than waiting until the system breaks down and medical intervention is necessary.

Conclusion

In many ways, Qigong and Taiji represent the paradox that is central to the whole way of thinking in Chinese medicine. These practices are so gentle and apparently effortless, yet they are in fact inordinately powerful and bring tremendous benefit to anyone who adopts them as part of a regular healthcare strategy.

LEFT
Some teachers of Taiji and Qigong exercise also practice a form of Qigong healing.

HEALING HANDS

Massage is a part of many cultures and has its roots in fundamental instinctive behavior. Qigong therapy includes a form of massage and laying on of hands, and appears to enable a transfer of Qi to take place from the therapist to the patient. Even though it is open to quackery, in some cases it seems to have spectacular results.

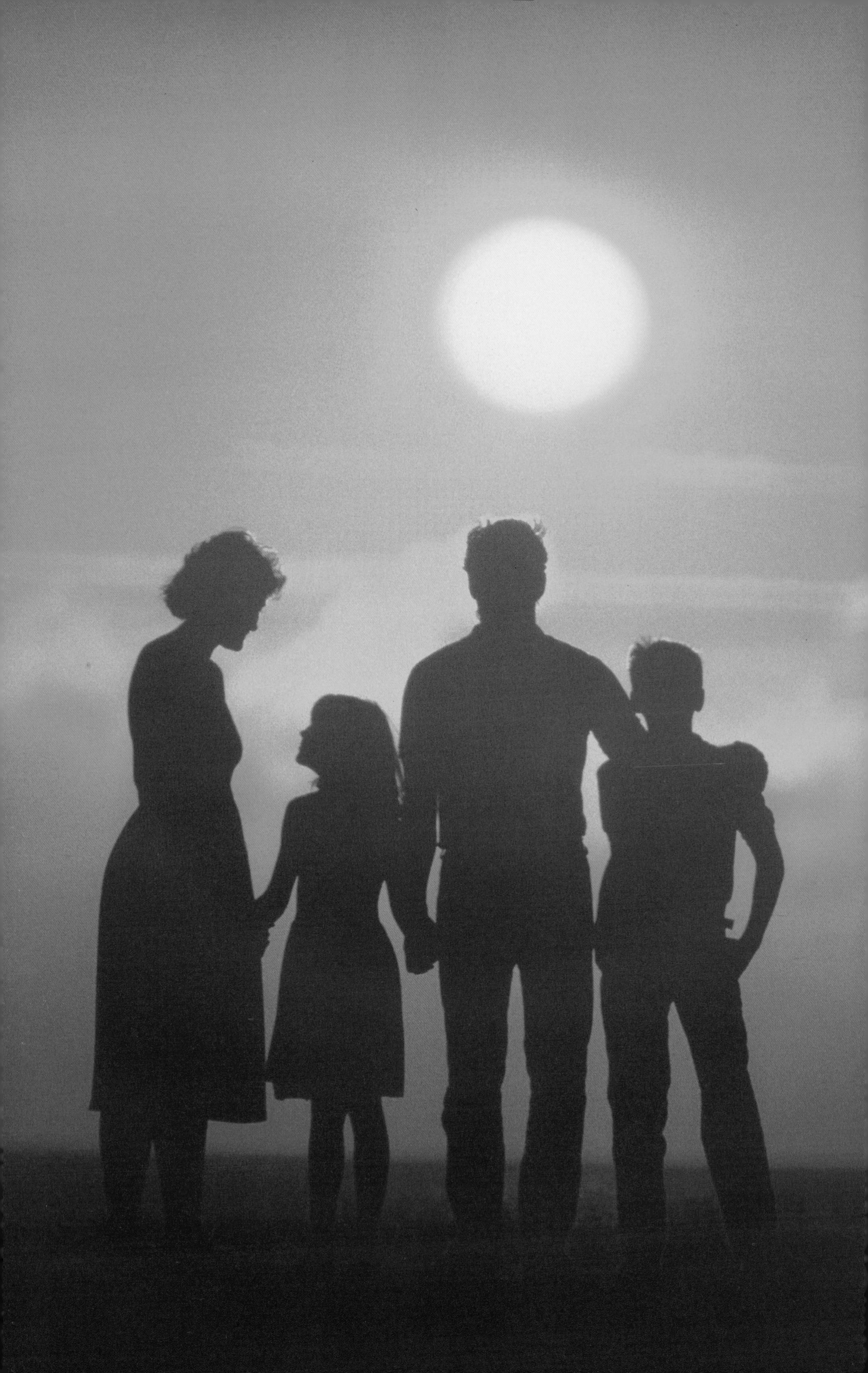

LIFESTYLE

WE ARE *constantly bombarded with conflicting advice – eat this, don't eat that, do this kind of exercise, play this sport, drink a little alcohol, don't drink any alcohol, and so on. Sometimes the advice appears to be common sense, at other times it appears contradictory and confusing; but it all points to the fact that we instinctively recognize that our habits and lifestyles are of vital importance in trying to stay fit and healthy.*

There would be little disagreement that in order to maintain a healthy and vital body, mind, and spirit, it is essential to have a general lifestyle that supports rather than undermines this aim. The problem for most of us is sorting out what it is we need to do. The Chinese medicine approach to health-care is no different from the general philosophy of Western approaches. It considers that appropriate exercise, diet, relaxation, social relationships, and habits all play a part in promoting or inhibiting the healthy flow of Qi in the body. Where the Chinese model may differ is in the area of what is considered "appropriate." Its emphasis on the importance of dynamic balance of Yin and Yang in everything we do, leads to approaches that do not favor extremes – of exertion or diet, for example. Balance and the "middle way" are everything, and while little is ever totally ruled out, nothing is ever considered to be totally dominant.

ABOVE
We need balance in every aspect of our lives.

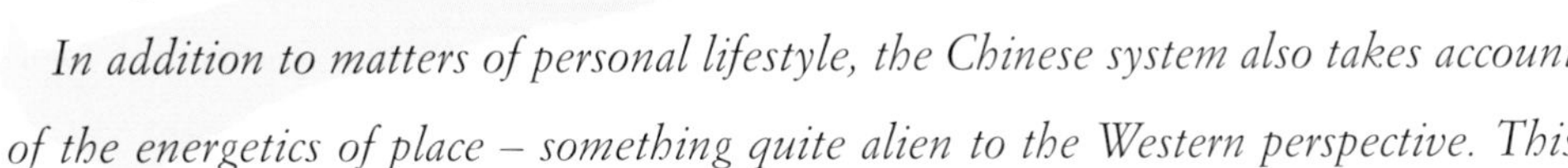

In addition to matters of personal lifestyle, the Chinese system also takes account of the energetics of place – something quite alien to the Western perspective. This understanding of the role of our physical surroundings in the promotion of health and well-being is termed Feng Shui (pronounced "fung shoy"). The following sections explore some of these issues, looking at how the energetics of lifestyle and place give a vital context to our understanding of disease and disharmony.

LEFT
The way we live naturally affects our health and vitality.

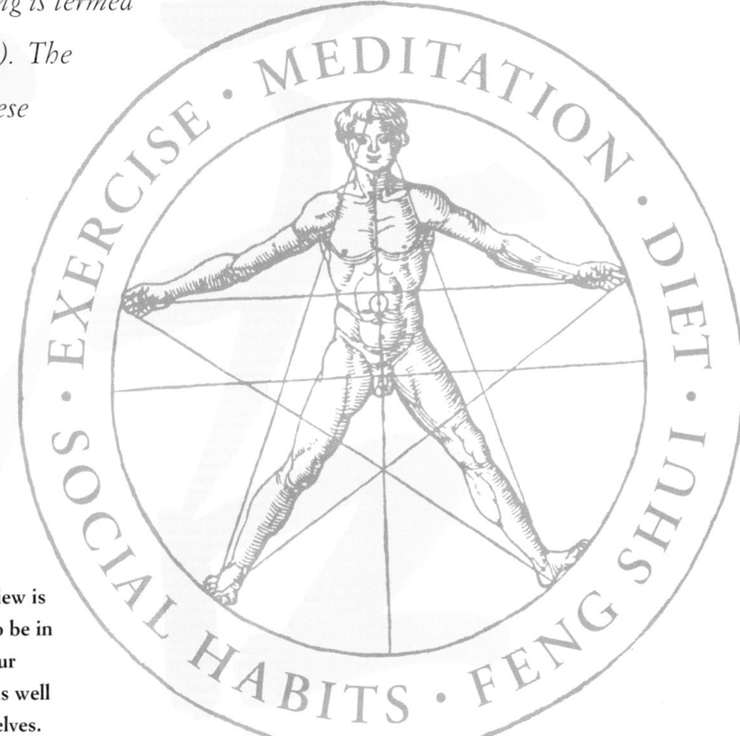

RIGHT
The Chinese view is that we have to be in balance with our surroundings as well as within ourselves.

EXERCISE

PHYSICAL EXERCISE, or the lack of it, can be very important to the way in which a disharmony is developed and maintained. Generally speaking, moderate physical activity is considered an excellent way to move Qi and Blood around the body so that they can protect and nourish all the vital energetic systems. Lack of moderate physical activity can lead to sluggishness and may result in Qi stagnation or deficiency, but too much vigorous activity can be weakening.

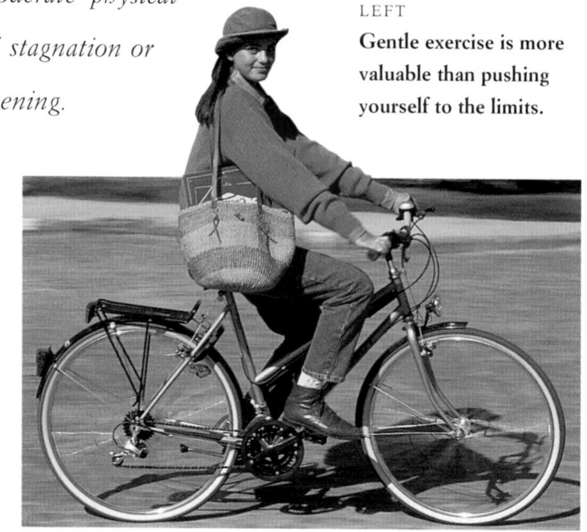

LEFT
Gentle exercise is more valuable than pushing yourself to the limits.

It is quite remarkable to watch the Chinese partake in their daily exercise routines in the parks and gardens of every village, town, and city. The tapestry of different approaches and levels of personal competence may be confusing to the Western eye, but invariably the most arresting feature is the fact that all these exercises appear assiduously to avoid straining the body – no sweating, no panting, no red faces; just grace and flow. Contrast this with the typical image of physical exercise in the West, where so often there is a tendency to push the body to its limits, believing that nothing has been achieved unless the body is on the verge of collapse! Granted, this is an extreme image, but it does highlight the essential difference between the Western and Chinese view of physical exercise.

The Chinese system emphasizes the gentle flow and movement of the body, encouraging the smooth flow of Qi that is necessary to maintain health, harmony, and well-being. Regular practice of Taiji and Qigong can help to attain this balance and insure an on-going healthy lifestyle. Some simple exercises are highlighted in the Qigong section (*see pages 193–203*), and other suggestions are referred to in the Bibliography.

However, not everyone will be attracted to Taiji or Qigong and, even for those who are, good qualified teachers are often hard to find. The practice of Taiji or Qigong is not a prerequisite of a balanced-energetic lifestyle, although it is certainly very good in this regard. It is no coincidence that the Chinese who practice their characteristic forms of exercise enjoy good health and vitality into old age, whereas the Western approach to exercise – in athletics, for instance – often creates injury, sometimes to a chronic degree. Long-distance runners may develop an efficient Heart/Lung system, but very often they become chronically Qi deficient, leaving themselves open to minor illness and injury. The hypersensitivity to injury of top-class athletes attests to this phenomenon.

In any activity, an awareness of the general principles of gentle and rhythmic movement can bring tremendous benefits. The following guidelines provide a healthy and balanced approach to exercise from a Chinese medicine perspective.

- Be cautious with any activity that pushes the body to the very limits of its capabilities.
- Be careful with activities that put sudden and dramatic stresses on the body – for example, weight lifting, and squash.
- Be sensitive and sensible about the climate when doing any activity out of doors. Wrap up well, especially when it is cold or damp. Failure to do so renders the body highly susceptible to an invasion by Wind-Cold-Damp, leading to a range of disharmonies.

If you remain alert to these general pointers, you can safely take part in any physical activity you choose. However, certain sports and leisure activities and forms of exercise are more consistent with the principles of the Chinese system than others. These include

- *walking*
- *gentle jogging*
- *swimming (although care must be exercised if there is evidence of internal Damp, which may be exacerbated by prolonged periods of time in the water)*
- *cycling*
- *yoga.*

Other activities may need to be modified by applying the guidelines given on page 212 in order to avoid problems. Vigorous and physically robust team sports such as soccer and football are fine for younger people, provided they balance these activities with a regime of more gentle and Qi-enhancing exercise. If injuries do occur, however, it is important to allow time for complete healing.

Minor injuries are the result of a local stagnation of Qi, and more serious injuries of a stagnation of Blood. Unless care is taken with recovery, stagnation is likely to recur in the future at these damaged sites – many soccer players, for example, develop arthritis in the knees later in life. It may well be possible that if these players had practiced Taiji and/or Qigong on a regular basis, such disabilities would not have developed, or would certainly be of a minor nature.

In summary, physical activity and exercise are highly desirable from the perspective of Chinese medicine, but there are limits within which the most effective energetic outcome is achieved.

BELOW

Unfortunately, cycling or running to work has gone out of fashion in the West as the car has taken over.

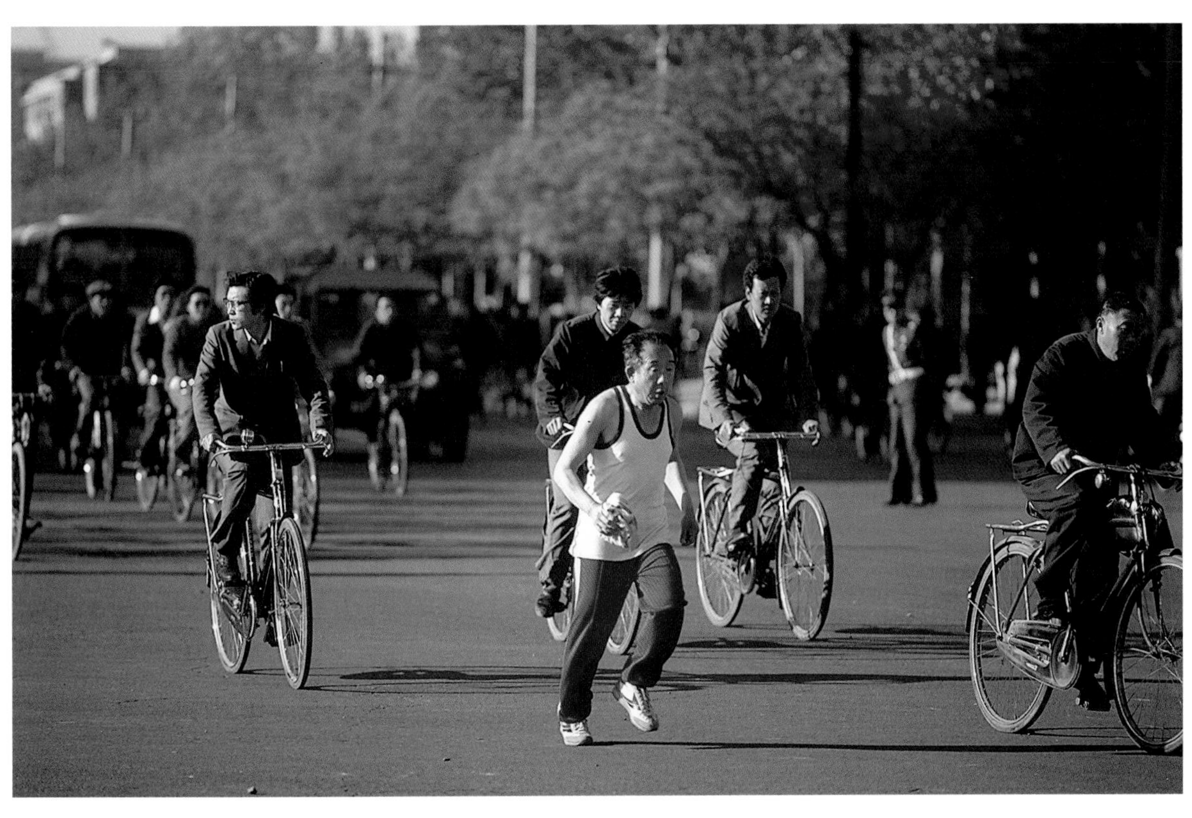

MEDITATION

BACKGROUND

FUNDAMENTAL TO Daoist thinking and Qigong practice is the concept that Qi follows the mind intent. It is said that when the mind is confused, the mind intent disperses and becomes unable to focus. When the mind intent is dispersed, the Qi of the body tends to become weak and insubstantial. The corollary of this, as stated in Qigong literature, is that, in effect, when the Qi sinks to the lower Dantian (the area at the Qihai point on the Ren meridian, about two inches (5cm) below the umbilicus and three inches (7.5cm) beneath the surface), the mind intent becomes strong and focused and the mind becomes tranquil. Qigong theory thus sees these three aspects of the body – the mind, the mind intent, and the Qi – in a state of mutual equilibrium and support.

To insure overall health and well-being it is important to settle the mind and focus the mind intent. The various techniques that are used to do this are not unique to Daoism and Qigong, but the structure that links them together provides a unique insight into how the Chinese perceive the body-mind connection. The meditation techniques are described on pages 215–217.

ABOVE
Keeping the mind clear and calm is linked to the health of the body.

MEDITATION PRACTICES

THERE ARE many different meditation practices and they do not always involve going into a trance, or even keeping still – indeed, the practice of Qigong and of Taiji in effect involve developing a meditative state while standing or sitting in a static posture or even while in motion. Spending about half an hour a day in meditation is calming and strengthening. It is advisable to set aside the same time each day, and to make sure that you will not be disturbed. Wear comfortable, loose clothing, and insure that you are warm enough. If you can, practice meditation outside in the fresh air, early in the day; avoid meditating within an hour of eating. Breathing is all-important and harmonizes the flow of Qi.

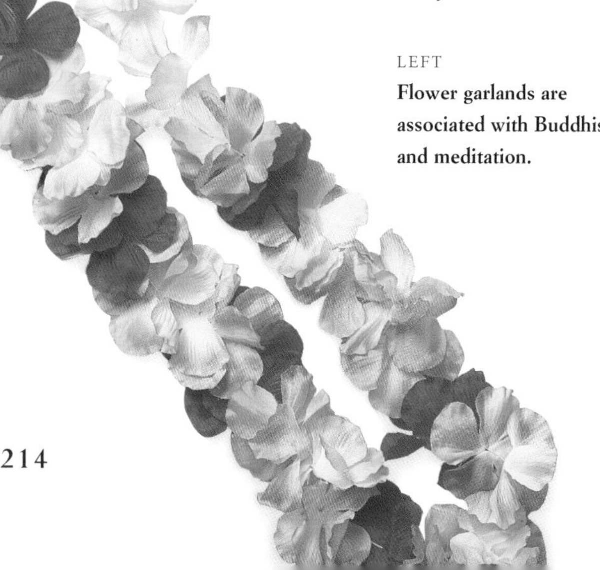

LEFT
Flower garlands are associated with Buddhism and meditation.

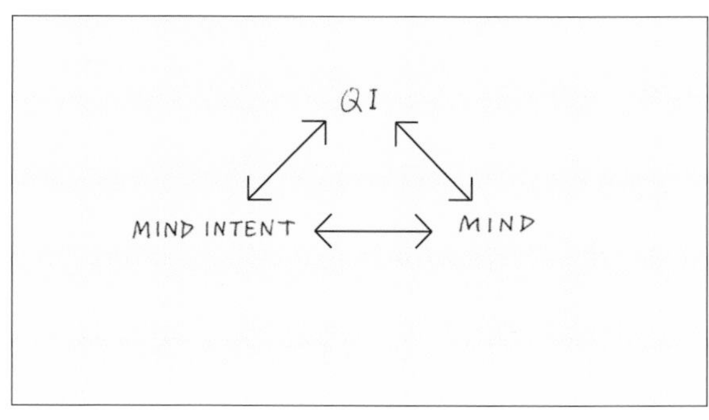

ABOVE
The mind, mind intent and Qi – three aspects of the body – should exist in mutual equilibrium.

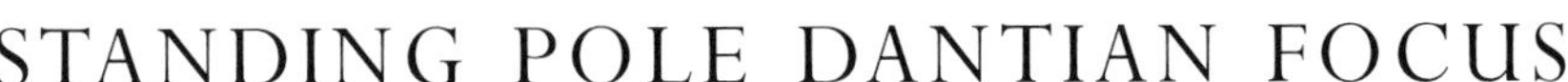

STANDING POLE DANTIAN FOCUS

WU CHI STANDING

This meditation can be performed in any classic static Qigong posture, or when seated comfortably with the back erect and the Baihui point at the top of the skull aligned with the heavens. Here, it is shown performed while standing in the basic Wu Chi posture.

Commence the meditation by adopting the Wu Chi stance (*see page 193*) – body erect but not stiffly upright, legs shoulder-width apart, feet parallel, legs slightly bent at the knee. This posture is fundamental to Taiji and Qigong practice, and there is a lot to be gained from using it for this simple meditation.

Once you have settled comfortably in the basic posture, begin to become aware of your breathing. As you breathe in through your nose, be aware of your abdomen expanding; and as you breathe out – either through your nose or through your mouth – be aware of it contracting. Focus your mind on the area of the lower Dantian (*see page 214*). This area – the Qihai or "Sea of Qi" – is the major reservoir of Qi in the body and links into the main distribution channels – the Ren Mai and the Du Mai.

As you breathe in, imagine fresh Qi from the universe entering your body and flowing into the Qihai. On the out-breath, imagine the spent Qi leaving the body and reuniting with the universe, where it will ultimately be renewed. Hold that image for at least ten minutes and be aware of the power of the Qi you are storing in your body. At the end of the meditation, simply allow your focus to leave the Dantian and return gently to an awareness of the rest of your body.

As with all these meditations, if you cannot manage ten minutes at first, simply meditate for as long as you feel comfortable and then gradually extend the time. With practice, it is quite possible to stand in this meditative state for up to half an hour, or even longer.

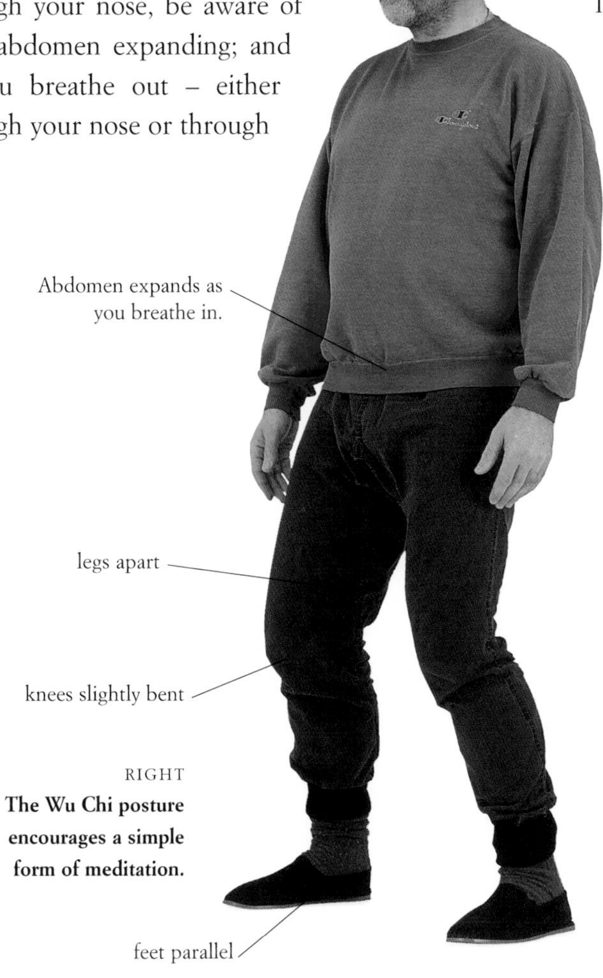

RIGHT
The Wu Chi posture encourages a simple form of meditation.

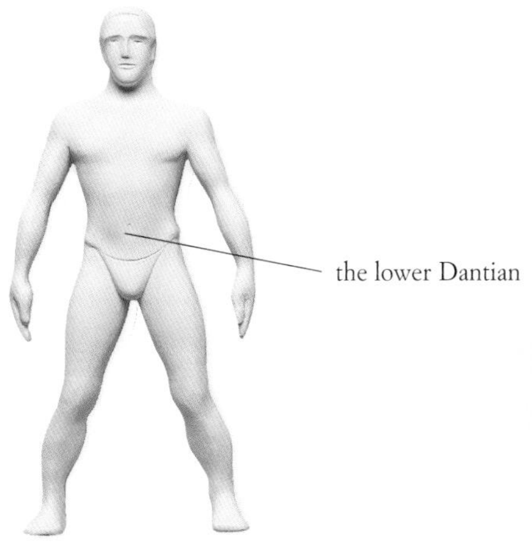

ABOVE
Breathing gently in and out is the key process.

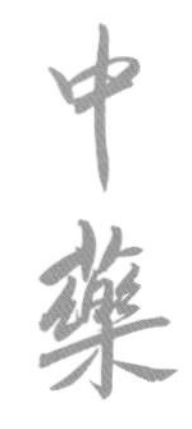

QI-FLOW MEDITATION

THIS MEDITATION is a simplified variation of more esoteric meditations that seek to allow you to experience the sensation of Qi flow through the body – the meditations on the microcosmic cycle, for example.

In this simple meditation you adopt one of the basic Standing Pole Qigong postures and then allow your mind to become aware of the sensation of Qi, wherever it arises in your body. The aim of the meditation is to progress from an awareness of the random and uncontrolled nature of your Qi flow, to an ability to bring it under the control of your mind intent.

Adopt the Wu Chi posture (*see page 193*) and hold for a minute or so. Once you have settled, bring your hands up to a position in line with the upper chest, as if you are holding a large beach ball against you. The length of time that you can hold this posture will depend on practice, but work toward about ten minutes if possible. If you practice daily for a couple of months, this goal should be quite achievable. Your breathing should be slow and rhythmical, as in the previous "Dantian" meditation.

After a minute or two you should become conscious of sensations in your body – especially in your arms and the palms of your hands. Become aware of these sensations for a few minutes without focusing on any particular one. After about five minutes of this meditation, focus your mind on an area where you are particularly aware of the Qi activity – it may feel warm, tingly, itchy, cold, and so on. There are no "right" or "wrong" indications of this activity, so simply be aware of what it feels like for you. As you focus your attention more and more, be aware that you are bringing your mind intent to bear on the Qi flow. Your mind intent is directing the Qi to flow smoothly through the meridians, nourishing every part of the body. With every in-breath you are directing the Qi along the meridians, and with every out-breath you are drawing it forward, thus creating a coherent flow between the in-breath (where the Qi from the universe floods into the body) and the out-breath (where the stale and spent Qi leaves the body and returns to the universal source).

Allow yourself to maintain this focus for as long as possible, and as you end the meditation and draw your arms back to the Wu Chi position, simply hand over the control of Qi through your body to the perfect mind intent of your higher self. This can be a very energizing and powerful meditation, building on the realization that the Qi flow is the life-blood of not only your body but of the whole universe as well.

ABOVE AND RIGHT
The Standing Pole posture is conducive to energizing meditation.

THE FIVE YIN COLOR MEDITATION

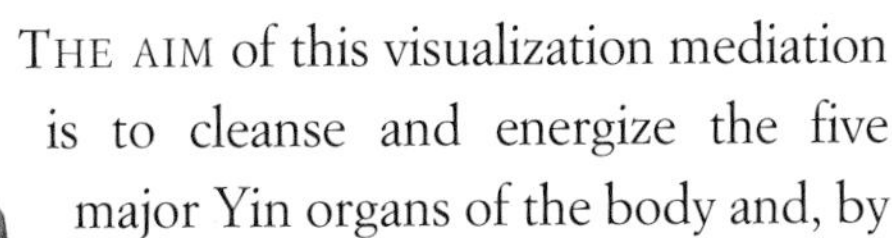

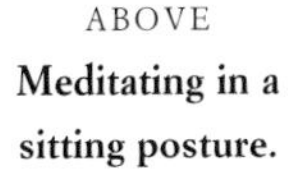

ABOVE
Meditating in a sitting posture.

THE AIM of this visualization mediation is to cleanse and energize the five major Yin organs of the body and, by association, their five Yang counterparts. The meditation is built around the correspondences of the Five Element sequence and recognizes that each of the Zangfu systems has its own energetic frequency, which can be energized by visualizing the appropriate color.

For this meditation adopt a sitting posture – either upright on the edge of a straight seat or cross-legged in the classic meditation posture – whichever you feel most comfortable with. Hold your hands in your lap facing upward, with the back of the right hand resting lightly on the palm of the left hand.

Begin by allowing your mind to focus on the lower Dantian area and coordinate your in-breath and out-breath, as you did in the first meditation. Once you feel quite calm and centered, begin the meditation by focusing on the uppermost Zang organs – the Lungs.

Imagine a bright white light entering the Lungs on each in-breath. This light is so intense that it cleanses every part of the Lungs, promoting the full function of the Lung system. It also floods the Large Intestine, the paired Fu organ of the Lungs. Hold the image of the white light flooding in, and on the out-breath imagine you are expelling a dull, stale light that takes with it all your negativity. It also takes any unresolved Grief (the emotion associated with the Lungs), which may be blocking your Lung function, and gently returns it to the universe. Maintain this image for about three to five minutes.

Continue in exactly the same way for the other four Zangfu systems. In each case, focus on the dominant color of that system and imagine it in the most powerful way that you can. On the out-breath visualize the dull, stale light taking all your negativity and the negative aspect of the characteristic emotion. Work through the Zangfu in the order below.

Once you have been through all five systems, allow your attention to return once again to your lower Dantian, and imagine all five colors coursing through your body, from the top of your head through the point that is most immediately "earthed" (which will depend on your posture). Slowly return to the outside world.

As in the literally hundreds of other forms of meditation, the object of the Five Yin Color meditation is to work toward a balance between the Qi, the mind, and the mind intent. In that equilibrium comes health.

ORGAN	COLOR	EMOTION
Lungs	*white*	*Grief*
Heart *(Small Intestine)*	*red*	*Joy*
Spleen *(Stomach)*	*yellow*	*Pensiveness*
Liver *(Gall Bladder)*	*green*	*Anger*
Kidneys *(Bladder)*	*deep blue*	*Fear*

LEFT
This form of meditation is good for expelling Grief and negativity.

DIET

INAPPROPRIATE AND *imbalanced dietary habits are among the most significant causes of energetic disharmony in the West, and an understanding of food from the perspective of the theory of Chinese medicine can be of tremendous benefit in working toward a more healthy lifestyle. Sun Si Miao, a famous Chinese physician who lived and worked around* A.D. *800, is quoted as saying: "Those who are ignorant about food cannot hope to survive."*

The Chinese system takes food very seriously, and the balance of energies and tastes reflects the same attention to detail that is apparent in its understanding of the energetic properties of herbs. While, in general, food is consumed to sustain the Qi of the body and promote good health and vitality (rather than for therapeutic purposes of a more specific nature), the parallels with ingesting herbs (where the purpose is dictated by an energetic disharmony) are obvious. Just as selected herbs have energetic qualities, so, also, does food. If we can approach food selection, preparation, and consumption with this firmly in mind, we will begin to see how important diet is for our energetic health.

The middle Jiao is the area of the body responsible for digestion. The Spleen extracts the Gu Qi (literally, "grain Qi") from ingested food and sends it upward to the Lungs. In order to perform this job efficiently, the Spleen itself needs to be healthy. It may be useful to consider some key points with regard to diet from the perspective of Chinese medicine.

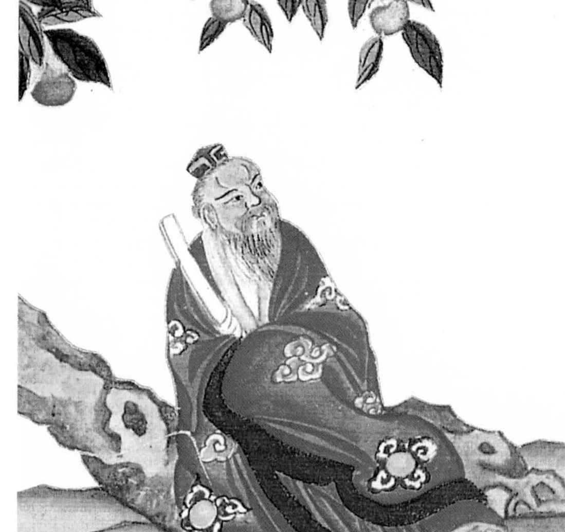

RIGHT
A Chinese sage sits in contemplation beneath a peach tree.

only small quantities of hot foods
a good variety of fresh vegetables
pulses and wheat products (pasta)
grains

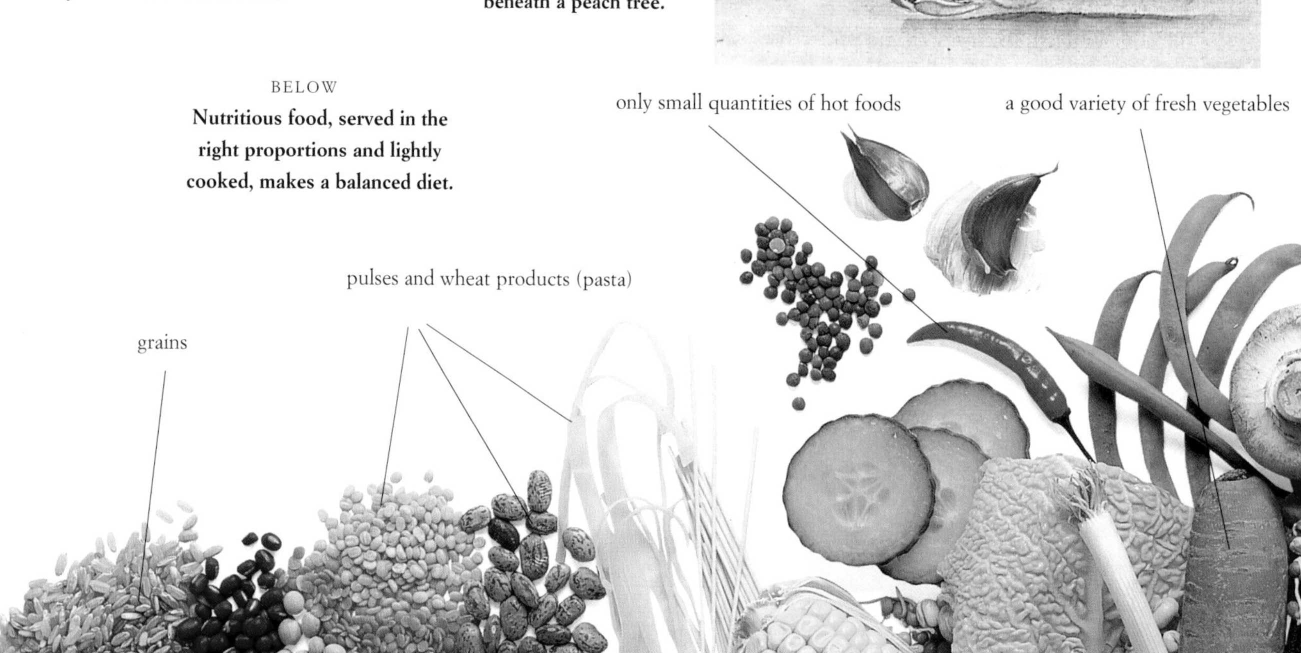

BELOW
Nutritious food, served in the right proportions and lightly cooked, makes a balanced diet.

RAW OR COOKED FOOD?

CHINESE MEDICINE views digestion (associated with the Stomach and the Spleen) as a process of internal cooking. The digestive process "cooks" the food in order to allow its essence – the Gu Qi – to rise up to the Lungs. Thus, the cooking of food is seen as an important process in aiding the subsequent digestive "cooking" that has to take place. The Chinese system emphasizes the importance of cooking food lightly. This makes digestion much simpler, and the energetic Gu Qi qualities of the food are better retained. Overcooking, or cooking in too much oil or fat, can lead to an accumulation of internal Phlegm and Damp, which damages the Spleen's ability to carry out the digestive function. The Spleen also needs to be warm, but not too hot: thus it is felt that the overconsumption of cold, raw foods damages the Spleen by cooling it.

SOME DIETARY RULES

- Cook food lightly and serve warm.
- Avoid cooking in heavy fats and oils.
- Consume cold, raw foods sparingly.
- Chew food well and digest without undue haste.
- Use energetically hot and spicy foods sparingly.
- Do not cook and warm food in a microwave: this can seriously upset its energetic balance.

IS A VEGETARIAN DIET BETTER?

THERE ARE many different views on this. Some people argue that it is important to take a moderate amount of animal products in order to ensure adequate and balanced nutrition; others argue that a predominantly vegetarian diet is more appropriate. Whichever type of diet is followed, bear in mind the following points:

- It is vital to eat plenty of lightly cooked grains and vegetables.
- Small amounts of meat and dairy produce can be highly nutritious, but there is a danger of Phlegm developing in the Spleen if animal products are eaten to excess.

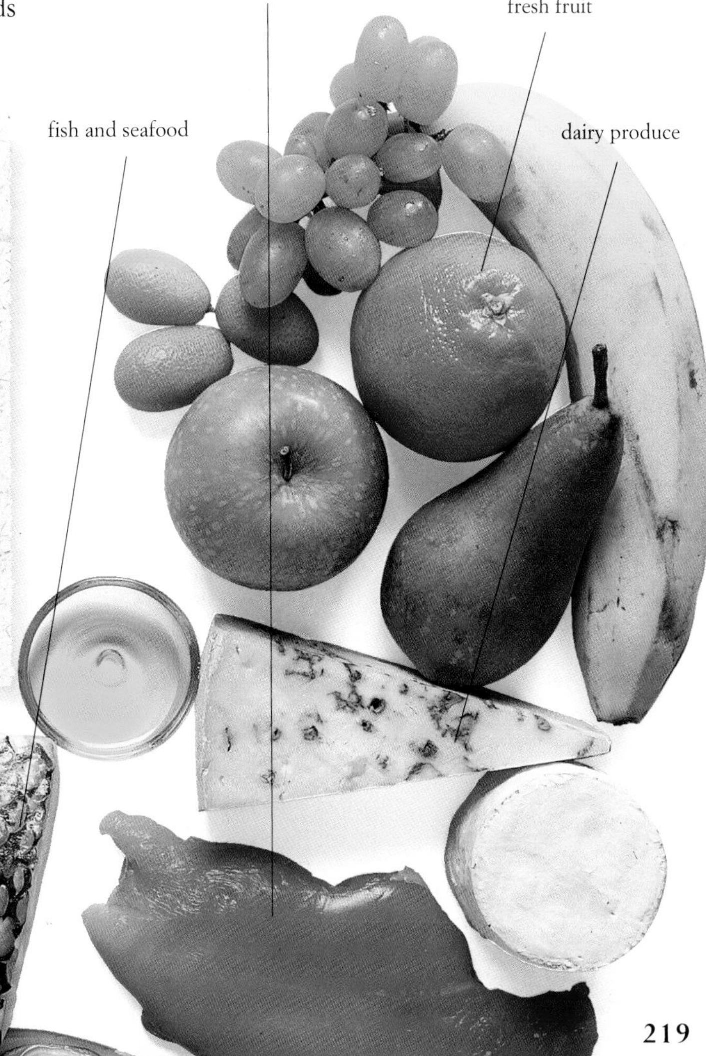

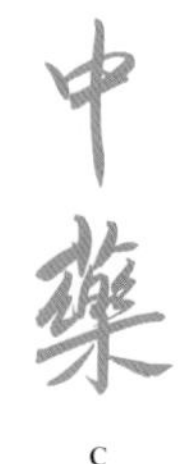

THE HARMONY OF THE FOUR ENERGIES AND THE FIVE FLAVORS

As in Chinese herbal medicine, a balance of the energetic qualities in the food we eat is essential. In herbal formulae the balance is designed for a particular energetic and therapeutic effect, but in our normal food consumption a principle of generalized balance is applied.

Overconsumption of hot and spicy foods impairs the original Qi of the body, consumes the Body Fluids, and ultimately damages the Yin. On the other hand, too much cold and raw food damages the Qi of the Spleen and the Stomach and leads to problems with the digestive process. In terms of flavors, the most healthy diet reflects all five – sweet, sour, salty, bitter, acrid. This insures that the Qi and Blood flow smoothly, and the Zangfu system functions efficiently and effectively. Overemphasis of any one flavor leads inevitably to disharmony. For example, in many Western diets the tendency to eat too many sweet foods can lead to problems of internal Heat and impairment of the Spleen function. It also impairs the function of the Kidney Qi, which can have a follow-on effect throughout the whole Zangfu system. Similarly, any excess in terms of the five flavors is likely to lead to levels of energetic disharmony.

Thus, the ideal diet should aim for a sensitive balance between temperature and taste in order to avoid Qi impairment.

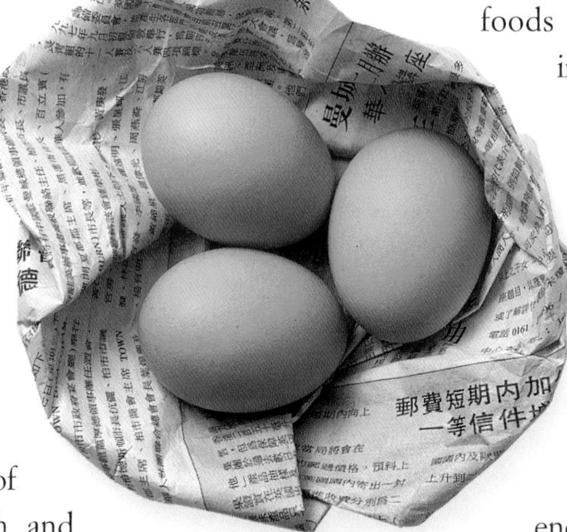

ABOVE
The size of a meal should depend on the time of day.

THE IMPORTANCE OF GOOD EATING HABITS

Walk fifty yards or so to the south of Tiananmen Square in Beijing and you can choose between McDonald's, Pizza Hut, and various other Western fast-food chains. In addition to the food itself, the practice of "in, out, and get-it-down" stands in stark contrast to the discipline of a traditional Chinese meal. Eating the right amount at a regular time and in a disciplined manner is considered crucial if maximum benefit is to be gained from the food. The maxim "eat when you are hungry and drink when you are thirsty" sums up the Chinese approach, with the added caveat that you should eat to only about 75 percent of your capacity. If you do this you will allow adequate digestion to occur.

The Chinese system considers that the functions of the body are locked into a regular rhythm; consequently, it is felt that eating should also follow a clear and regular pattern. It is suggested that meals are taken at regular intervals, and that they decrease in size as the day progresses, insuring all food is fully digested before sleep. It is also believed that you should eat slowly, chew food thoroughly, and avoid eating if you are unable to concentrate fully on the meal. In eating, as in Qigong, the mind intent and the smooth flow of Qi are fundamentally related; so being focused is vital. A corollary of this is that if you are in any way emotionally upset, the scattered mind will result in unhealthy Qi flow.

From the viewpoint of Chinese medicine, moderation, discipline, and balance are the fundamental concepts to bear in mind when considering eating. Be aware of the flavors and the temperature of the food; be aware of a disciplined approach to quiet and reflective eating; and be aware of the body's natural daily rhythms. It is not necessary to eat Chinese food in order to follow these basic principles, but it has to be said that the manner of preparation, the methods of cooking, the mixture of ingredients, and the disciplined approach of a Chinese meal serve as a powerful role model.

To insure that your dietary habits support the balance of your body energies, try where possible to follow these rules.

- Use fresh, organic produce.
- Use foods local to your area.
- Use seasonal fruit and vegetables.
- Prepare and blend foods with an awareness of the need for energetic balance.
- Prepare, serve, and eat food in a quiet and disciplined way.

Good Yin tonic
Can help with fluid retention.
Menu
Chicken & Egg Drop Soup
~
Tuna with Tomato & Pepper
~
Stir Fry Vegetables
(Spinach and Leek)
~
Steamed Rice
~
Fresh Fruit
~
Green Tea
Tonifies the Spleen.
Harmonizes the function of Middle Jiao and aids digestion.

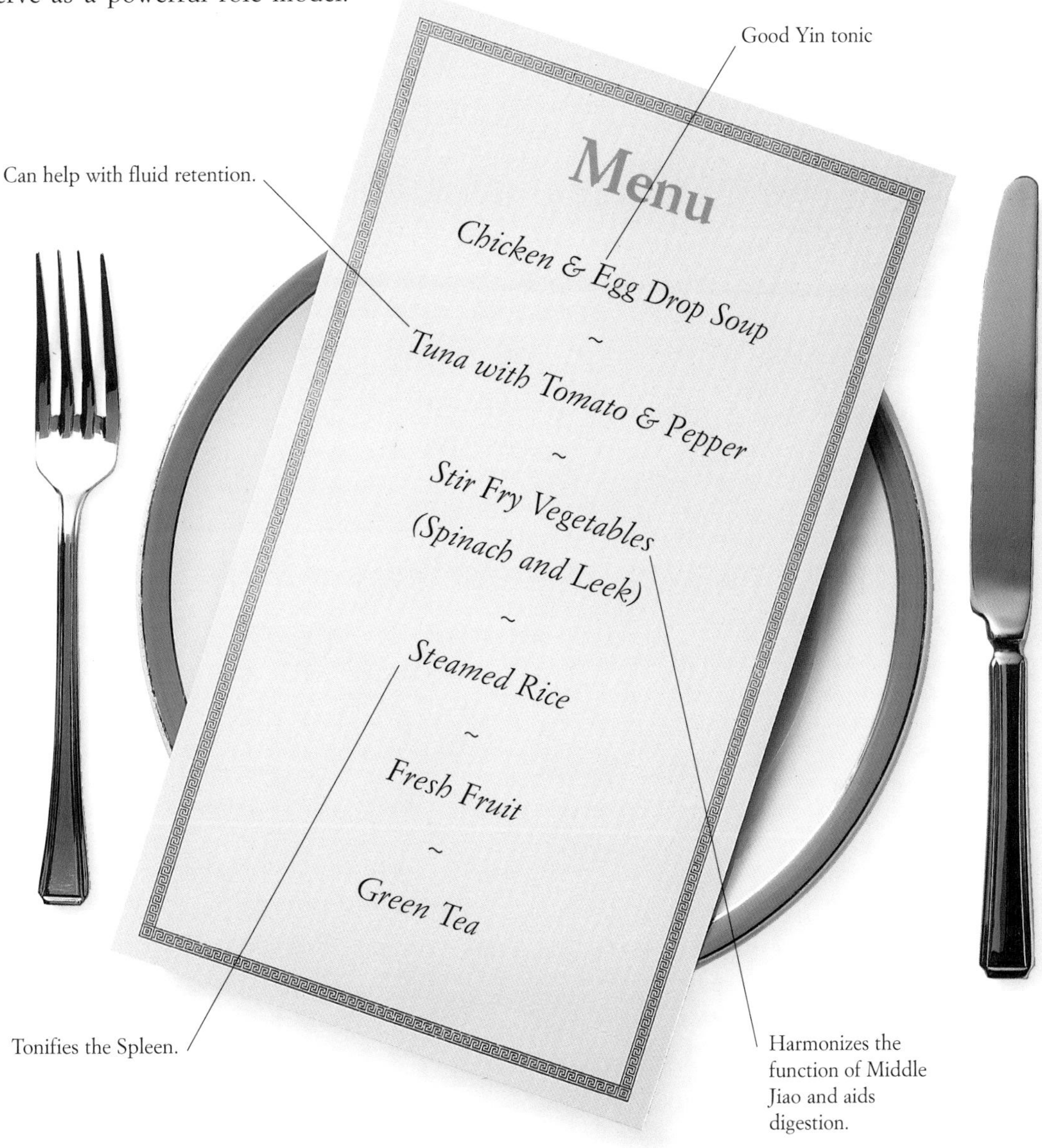

ABOVE
It is important to create space and time for your meals. The menu shows examples of foods that mix to make a balanced diet. They can be spread out through the day and there is no particular order in which they must be served.

SOCIAL HABITS

UNFORTUNATELY, MANY of our patterns of social behavior in the West do us no favors when it comes to maintaining our health and well-being. In addition, our legal and illegal pleasures can do us absolute or relative harm. In particular, cigarette smoking, overconsumption of alcohol and prescribed or prohibited drugs, and unthinking dissipation of sexual energy are all harmful. Some of the more common issues are discussed from the perspective of Chinese medicine.

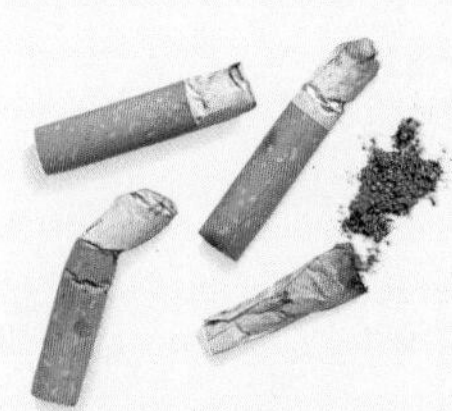

SMOKING

TOBACCO SMOKE is energetically Hot and puts Heat into the body – most notably the Lungs. In the short term there can be some apparent benefits from this.

For example, many smokers find that a cigarette relaxes them – this is because the Heat of the inhaled smoke moves any stagnant Qi, thus producing a short-term beneficial effect.

However, this effect is only temporary and Qi stagnation will more than likely recur. The need to move the Qi is then reinforced and the vicious cycle leading to addiction is set up. In the long term, the Heat will damage the Yin of the Lungs and there will be an escalation of serious disharmonies.

ABOVE
Cigarette smoking is seen to cause damage to the Yin of the Lungs.

EFFECTS ON QI

Stagnant Lung Qi may be moved but the stagnation soon returns. Eventually craving sets in and serious Lung damage is caused.

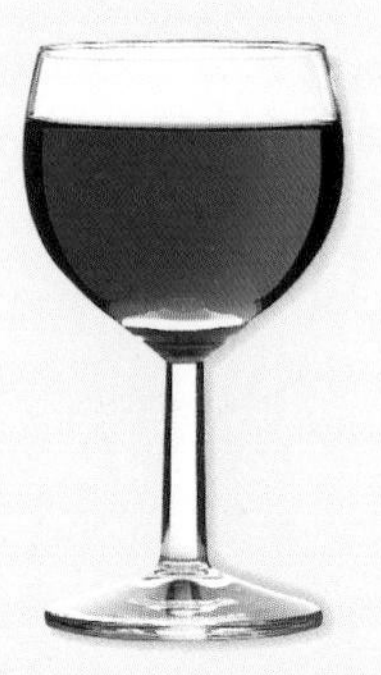

ALCOHOL

ALCOHOL IS another energetically Hot and also Damp substance, and in many respects its effects are similar to those of cigarettes.

However, it is accepted that a little alcohol can be beneficial, especially in the winter and in cold climates. As ever, the key word is moderation, allied with an understanding of the energetic qualities of alcohol.

ABOVE
A glass or two of wine from time to time can be a valuable tonic to the Blood and circulation. Too much alcohol, however, is damaging to the Liver.

EFFECTS ON QI

Stagnant Qi can be temporarily moved by alcohol but the stagnation soon returns.

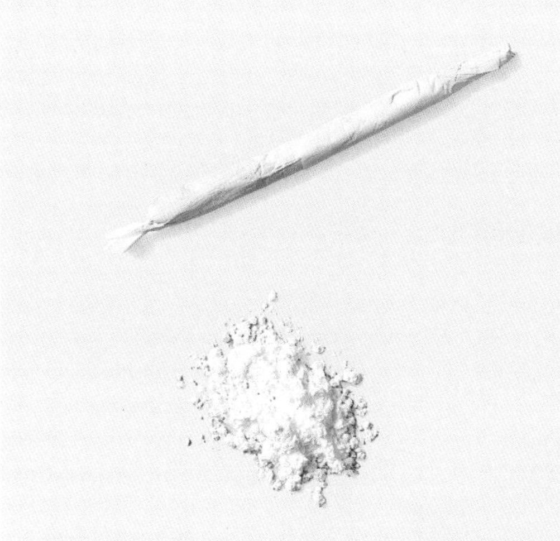

DRUG ADDICTION

THE WHOLE area of addiction is too complex to discuss here in detail; suffice it to say that the long-term abuse of drugs causes a range of serious energetic disharmonies. While Chinese medicine may be able to help with the disharmonies related to addiction, it is not a magic wand and cannot automatically effect a cure. When treating an addiction using Chinese medicine, the attitude and willingness of the patient to address the problem are essential if any success is to be achieved.

ABOVE
A complexity of inter-related disharmonies may result from drug-taking.

EFFECTS ON QI

Drug addiction can cause deficiency of Qi as well as leading to a whole range of disharmonies.

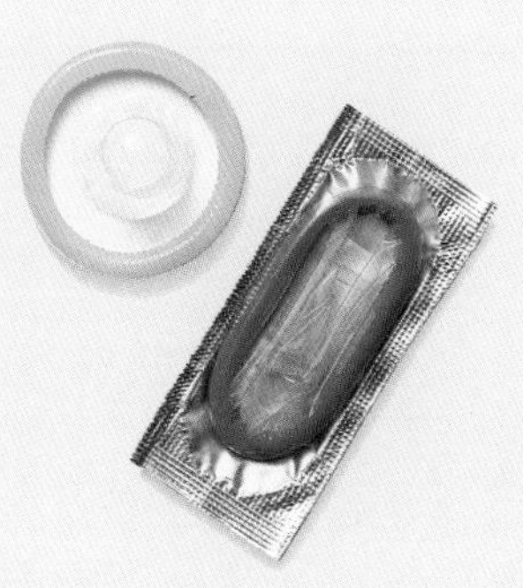

SEXUAL ENERGY

IN CHINESE medicine, sexual energy reflects the most subtle aspect of Qi – namely, the essence or Jing of a person. This form of energy is closely related to the Kidneys, the ultimate source of all Yin and Yang energy in the body. Too much sexual activity is considered to deplete the Kidney Jing and Qi and can lead to premature aging and problems of deficiency in all the Zangfu.

The Chinese view of moderation in sexual activity does not arise from morally defined norms and mores, and certainly does not reflect a sexually repressed culture. Rather, sexual activity is seen in terms of the overall energetic health of the body as a whole. Indeed, certain Daoist Qigong exercises place emphasis on strengthening and maintaining the essential Jing energy in order to promote health and longevity.

ABOVE
Sexual activity is certainly not seen as harmful in itself.

EFFECTS ON QI

While Kidney Qi is detrimentally affected by too much sex, the right amount of sex is beneficial and keeps the body Qi healthy.

FENG SHUI

THE PLACING of buildings in the landscape and the organization of spaces and objects within the building are of crucial importance in Chinese thinking. Feng Shui, the art/science governing this, is literally translated "Wind and Water," two of the most fundamental forms of energy in the universe. Wind represents air, and water the dynamic, flowing nature of the universe. Feng Shui teaches how to take best advantage of these all-pervading forces.

Within Daoist philosophy, eight constituents of the universe were conceived: represented as eight trigrams, which evolved from the dynamic representation of Yin and Yang. These were used to develop the 64 hexagrams that form the archetypes of human consciousness as revealed in the important treatise of Chinese thinking – the *Yi Jing* (often spelled "I Ching" and commonly known as the *Book of Changes*). The *Yi Jing* recognizes the patterns of change within the cosmic order of the universe. An extension of this is used to provide insight into how the energetics of a physical space can be influenced by all the possible interactions of these fundamental energy patterns.

Each of the eight trigrams represents a specific quality of energy, and the experience of the world emerges from the interactions of these energetic qualities. The representations of the eight basic trigrams are shown below.

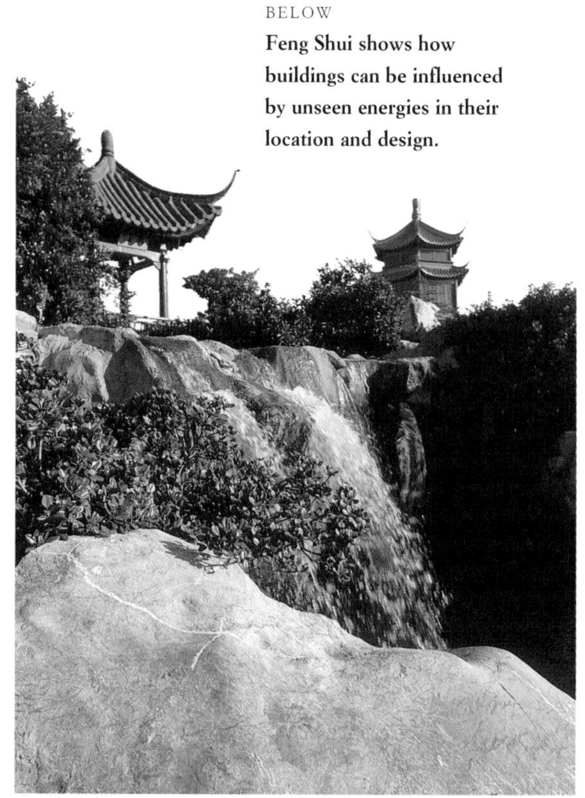

BELOW
Feng Shui shows how buildings can be influenced by unseen energies in their location and design.

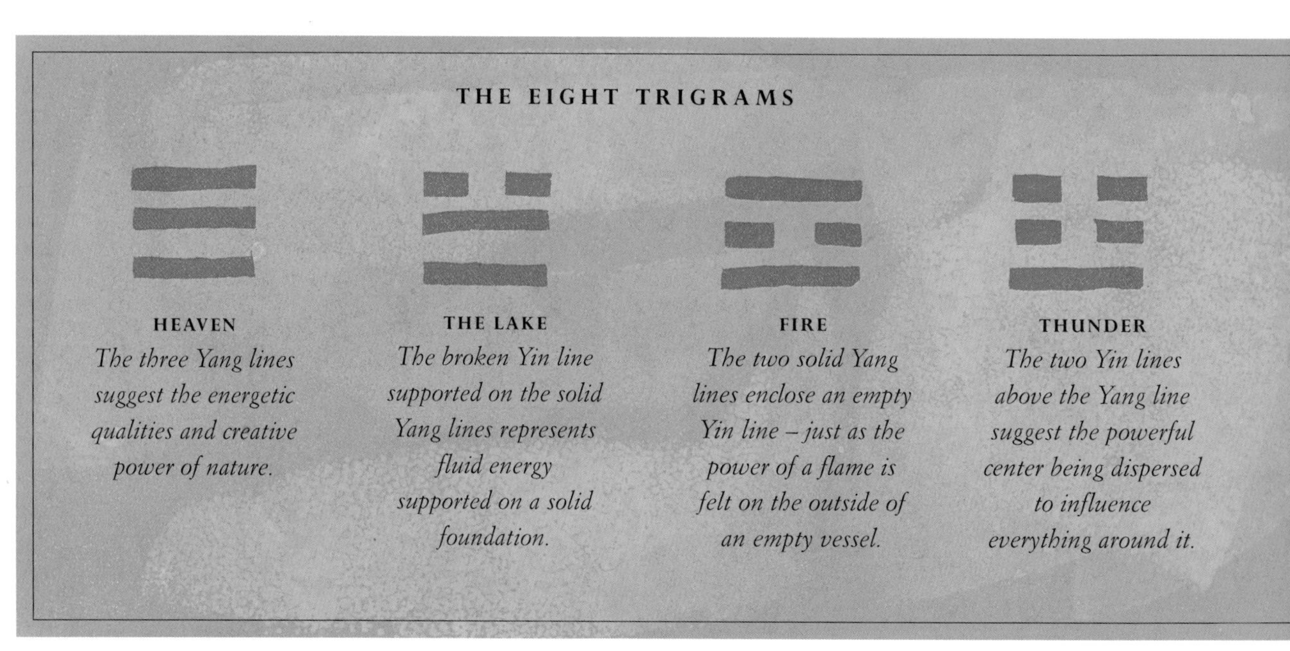

BELOW

The eight trigrams (foot of page) represent the development of the eight possible combinations of Yin and Yang (below).

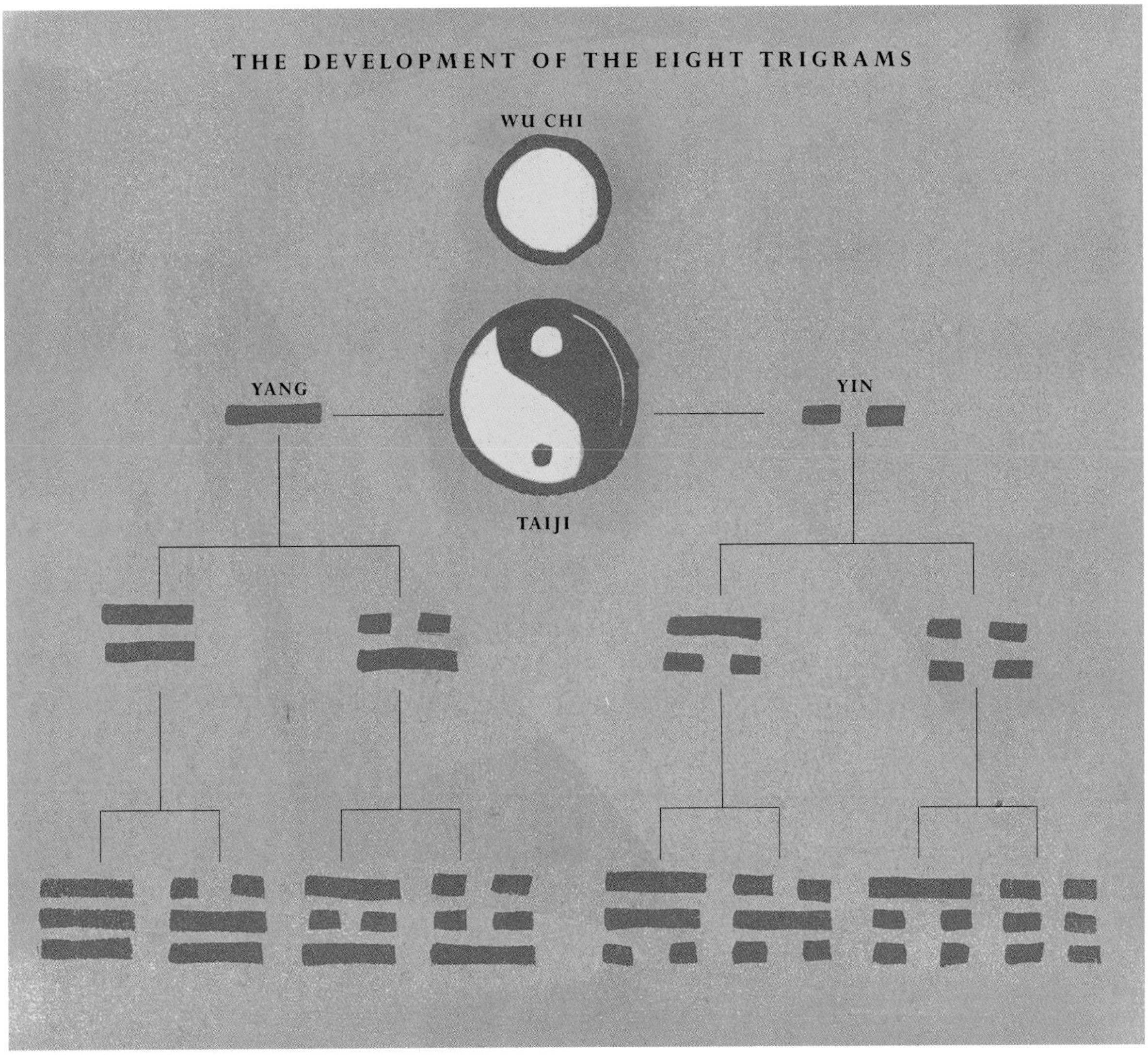

THE DEVELOPMENT OF THE EIGHT TRIGRAMS

WU CHI

YANG

YIN

TAIJI

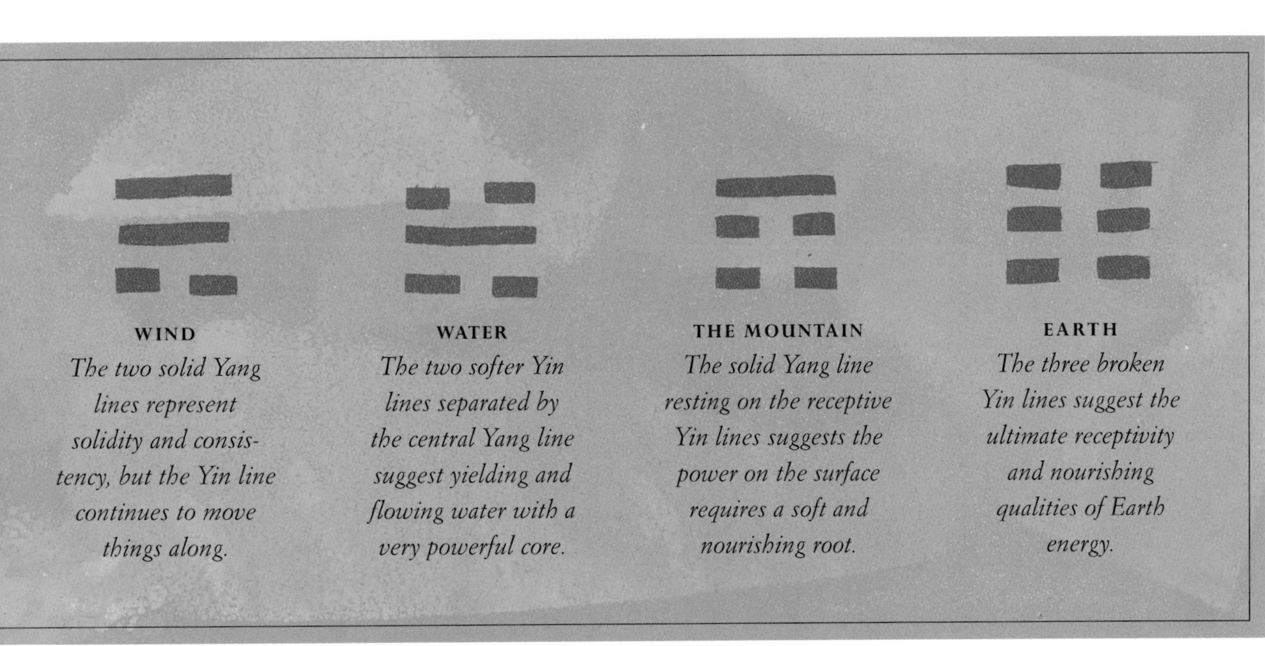

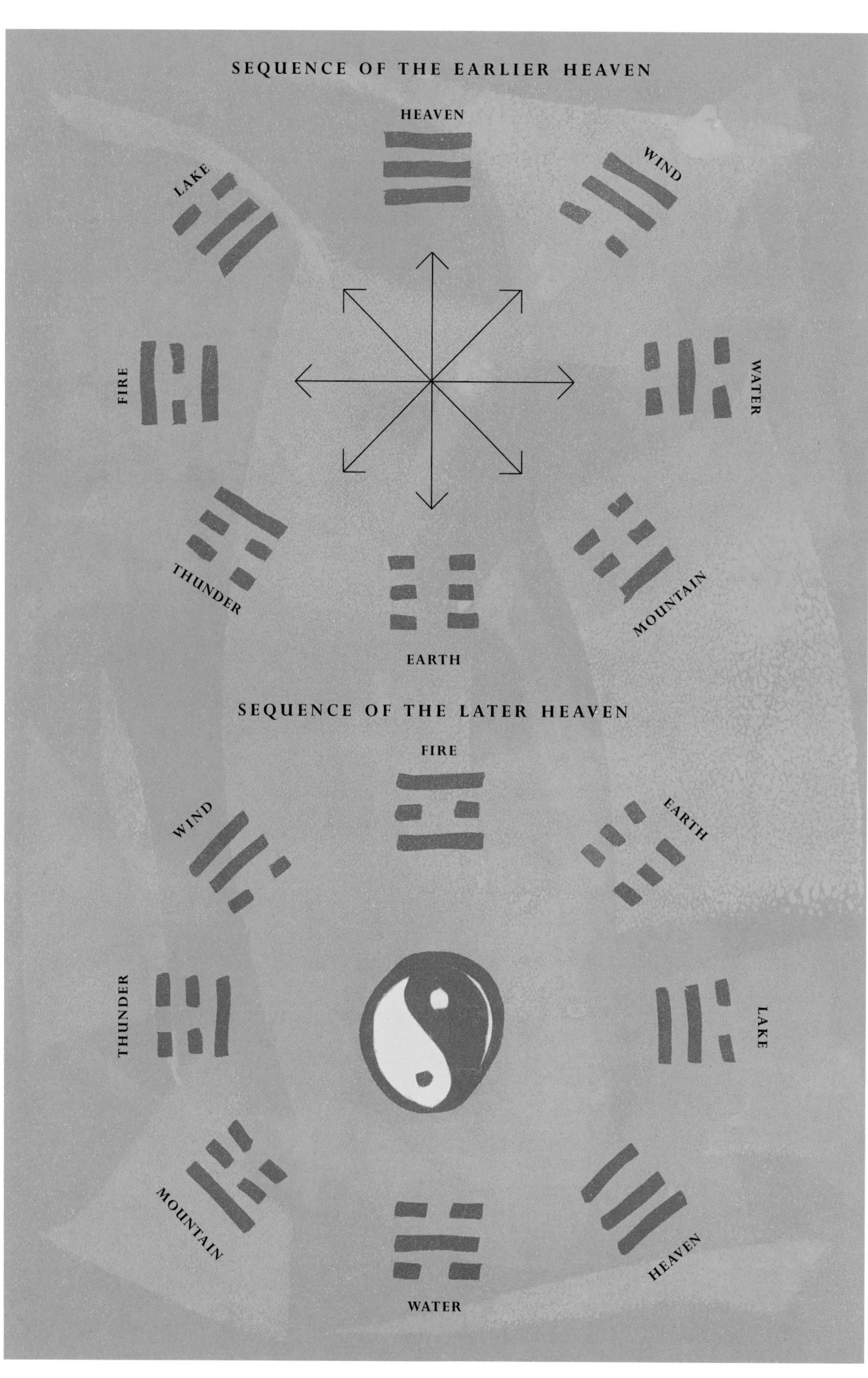
SEQUENCE OF THE EARLIER HEAVEN
HEAVEN
WIND
WATER
MOUNTAIN
EARTH
THUNDER
FIRE
LAKE
SEQUENCE OF THE LATER HEAVEN
FIRE
EARTH
LAKE
HEAVEN
WATER
MOUNTAIN
THUNDER
WIND

Chinese philosophers placed these energetic qualities, in pairs of balancing opposites, in an eight-sided arrangement called the "Sequence of the Earlier Heaven" (the Ba Gua).

While this arrangement seemed to provide a sense of perfect energetic balance, it did not accord with the more dynamic nature of the universe, in which polar opposites are not normally in complete balance. (It is this natural imbalance that gives the universe its sense of dynamic flow.) This observation led to the rearrangement of the energetic qualities into the "Sequence of Later Heaven," which offers a somewhat more dynamic Ba Gua.

This in turn led to a view of the universe as a huge, cascading dynamo of energy – continually in motion, continually and regularly changing and reinventing itself – and suggested that energy dynamics spread out over space and also evolve over time. A development of these ideas is found in the concept of the Five Elements and the "Creative" and "Control" cycles, which is essential to the theory of Chinese medicine.

Ultimately, these ideas were applied to the world of physical form to try to understand how certain places, buildings, room designs and arrangements, objects in space, and so on, are influenced by this huge energetic kaleidoscope, and to ascertain whether these energies are a help or a hindrance with regard to how we experience the world around us. Good Feng Shui can enhance creativity, prosperity, and health; bad Feng Shui can do the exact opposite.

OPPOSITE
The sequences of the Earlier Heaven (above) and of the Later Heaven (below).

BELOW
This mountainous landscape dating from *c.* 970–1050 expresses strongly the Chinese feeling for the natural world.

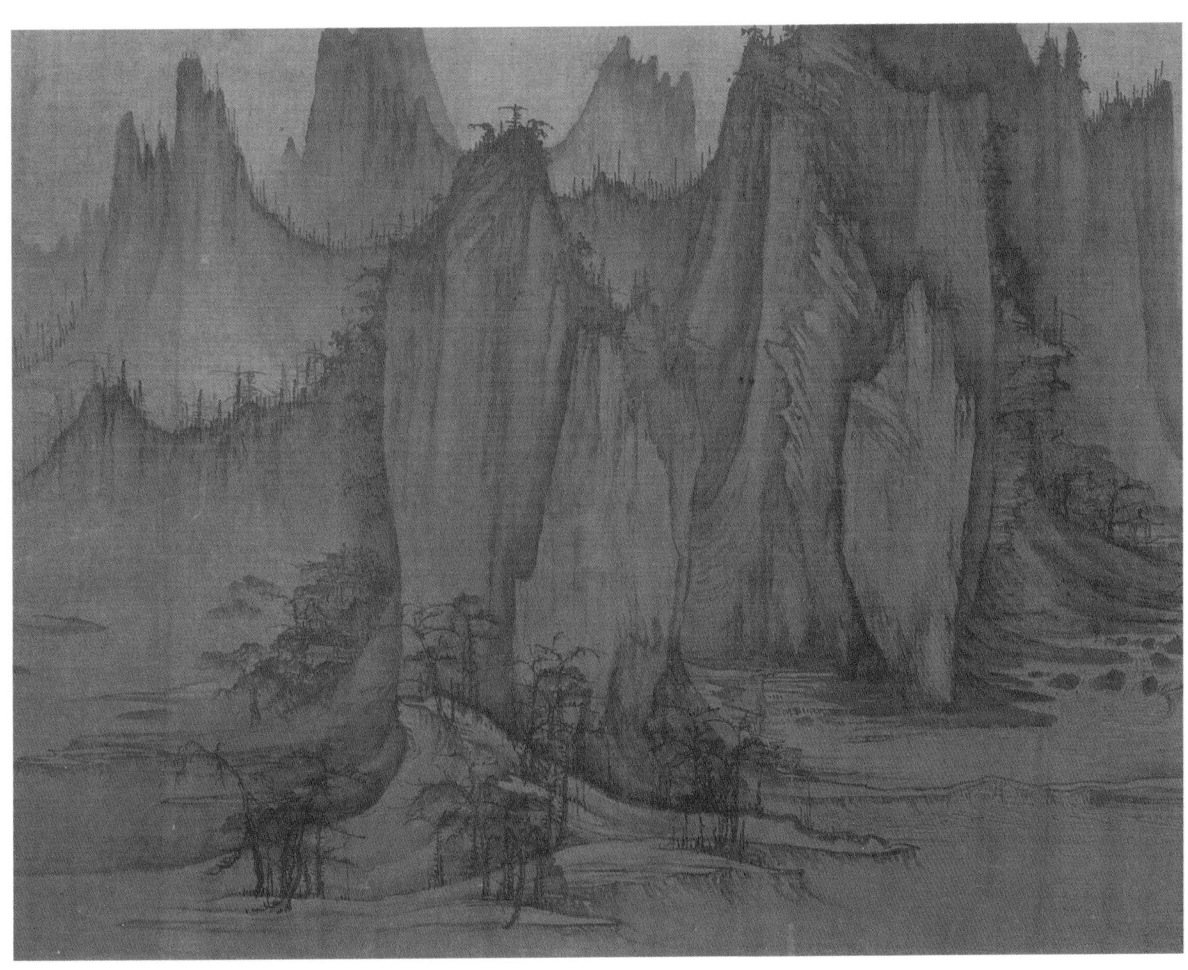

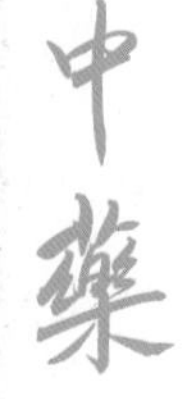

ENERGETICS IN THE NATURAL WORLD

THE PRINCIPLES of Feng Shui suggest that the natural world is alive – energy is moving and changing, Qi is gathering and dispersing. How we experience the world is, for the most part, a function of the interaction between our own Qi and that of the environment around us. This book can but raise an awareness of these ideas. Most readers have probably felt various reactions to different physical environments: some places can uplift the spirit, making us feel alive and vibrant with energy; others smother the spirit, leaving us feeling heavy, lethargic, and depressed. If you can relate to this kind of experience, then you have felt the power of Feng Shui in your life.

An obvious illustration of this experience is the contrast between the beauty of unspoiled areas of nature and the blight of human intervention in rundown urban areas. In the latter, the Qi of the environment has become deficient and stagnated, creating disharmonies – in exactly the same way as deficiency and stagnation cause disharmonies in the body. It is, therefore, hardly surprising that if you live and/or work in an area of "bad" Feng Shui, you will be far more susceptible to both physical and psychological disharmonies. Your own Qi and the Qi of the environment will ultimately vibrate at the same frequency and give out the same energetic signals – unless you take active steps to avoid this.

RIGHT
There are ways in which we can protect ourselves from the disharmonies and stagnations of "bad" Feng Shui.

HOW TO DEAL WITH "BAD" FENG SHUI

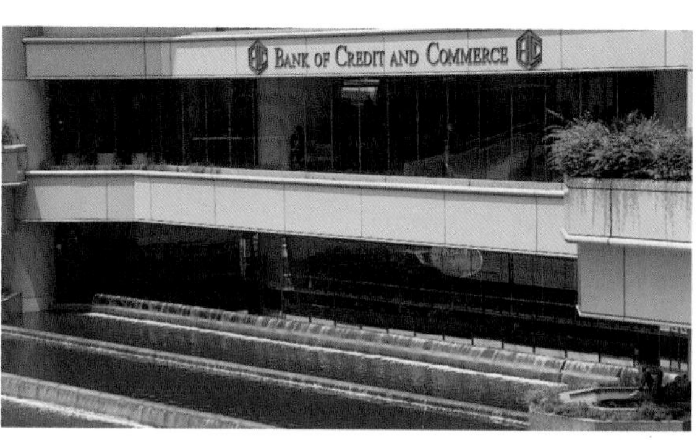

THE FIRST and most obvious solution to this problem is to move to somewhere where you experience "good" Feng Shui. However, this is clearly not a realistic or viable option for most people. Given the realities of life, you need to take active steps to protect yourself in your existing environment. The following approaches may help, but a much more detailed understanding of Feng Shui is necessary in order to gain full benefit. ✦ Follow a healthy and balanced diet, eating at regular times. ✦ Keep physically fit by doing whatever exercise suits you best. ✦ Learn and regularly practice Qigong or Taiji. ✦ Visit the natural world and enjoy its beauty as often as you can. ✦ Spend time every day in a park or "green"area. ✦ Be self-disciplined in your habits and your attitudes to others and the world around you. ✦ Be tidy at all times and do not add to the imbalances of your environment. ✦ Be aware at all times of the effect that the environment is having on you – use your mind intent to send your Qi out into the world in a positive manner.

ABOVE
This bank in Hong Kong blamed its lack of success on the fountain, which was considered to be "bad" Feng Shui.

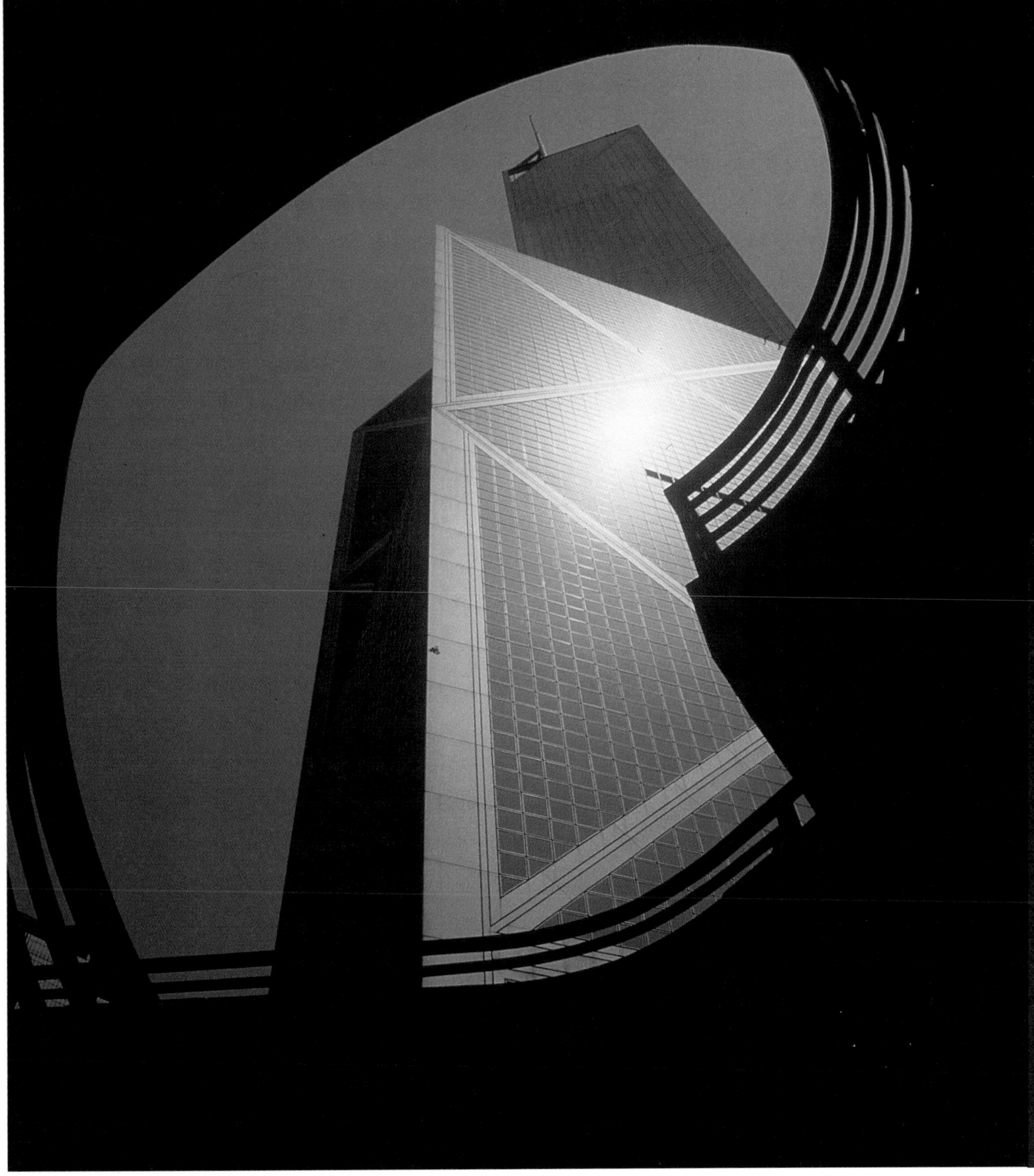

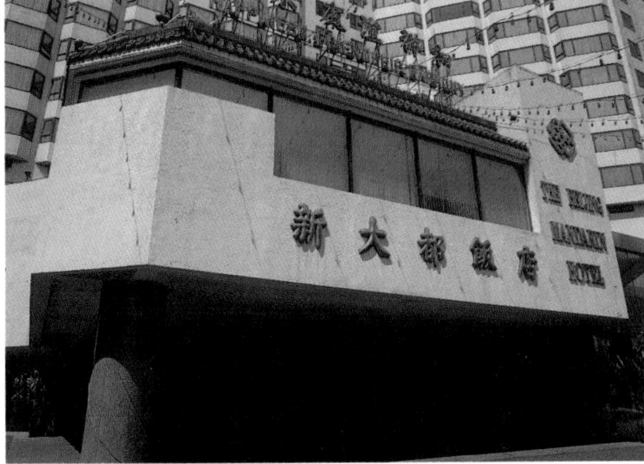

ABOVE
The entrance to the Mandarin Hotel, Beijing is off-set, in accordance with the demands of Feng Shui.

TOP
The Bank of China, Hong Kong, was supposedly designed according to traditional Feng Shui methods.

BALANCE IN THE HOME

There are many ways of making adjustments in your home to create favorable surroundings for yourself. Balance is all important – of hard and soft materials, dark and light colors, areas of light and shade. Mirrors and lights can be used in awkward, dark corners; overlarge windows can be made to seem smaller with curtains that partially cover the frames; small windows can be made to seem larger with simple blinds that reveal their full extent.

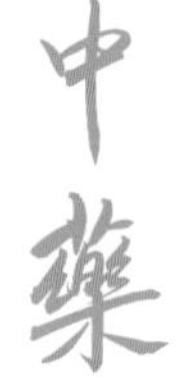

ENERGETICS IN THE HOME AND WORKPLACE

YOU MAY not have much control over the general environment where you live and work, but you do have control over the home you live in and your personal workspace. It is vitally important to consider how Feng Shui principles can work to your benefit in these areas. Again, it is not possible to go into great detail here, but the following general examples illustrate what can be achieved.

QI ENTRY AND EXIT POINTS IN A ROOM

Some door arrangements cause the Qi to rush straight through the room, resulting in a continuous sense of disturbance and unease for anyone sitting in its path. In other circumstances the arrangement of the doors enables the Qi to enter and leave in a smooth, arched motion, giving a more refreshing sense to anyone sitting in its path. This action brings to mind the curve and grace of a Taiji form, which mirrors the natural circulating movement of Qi in a very calming, relaxing, and refreshing manner. This simple example is offered in the hope that you may start to think about the energetics of your rooms. There are many other ways in which the Qi flow can be improved, but this requires, at the very least, reference to a good book on Feng Shui and, ideally, consultation with a Feng Shui practitioner.

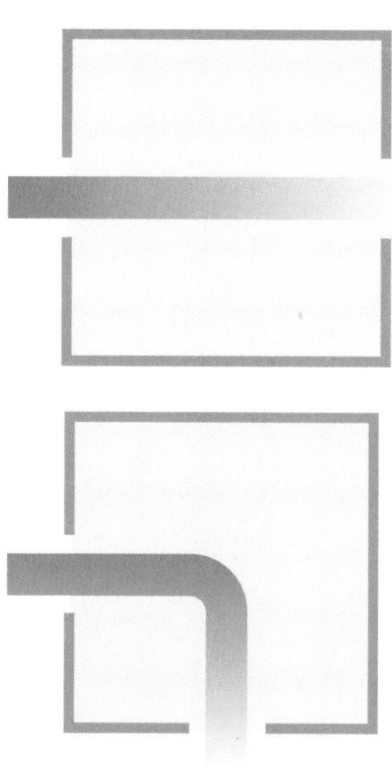

ABOVE
When doors face each other the Qi can rush through the room (top); with other arrangements, (for example as shown above), Qi travels in a curved path.

BLACK TURTLE

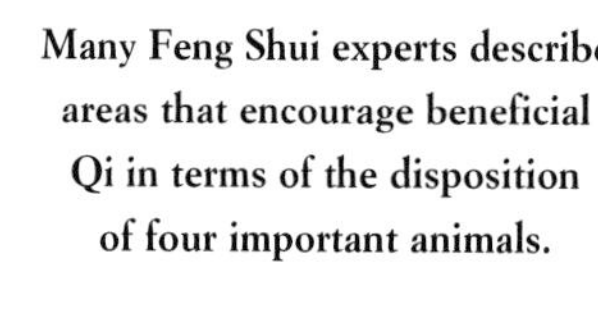

Many Feng Shui experts describe areas that encourage beneficial Qi in terms of the disposition of four important animals.

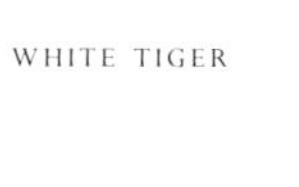

WHITE TIGER

GREEN DRAGON

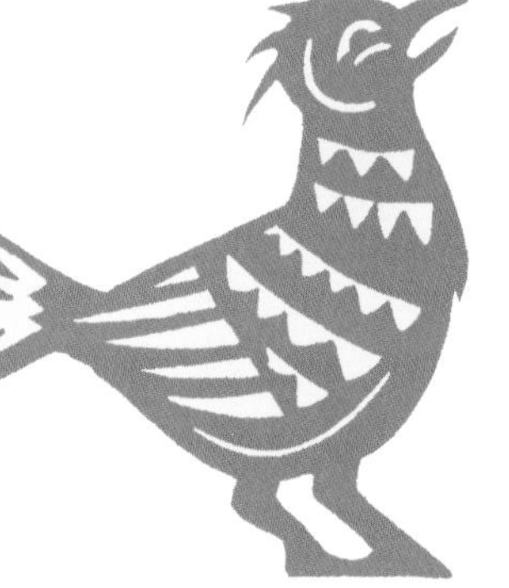

RED PHOENIX

GOOD DESK PLACEMENTS

desk

doorway

The best position is in the corner opposite the door, where the two walls act as protector and make one feel in control.

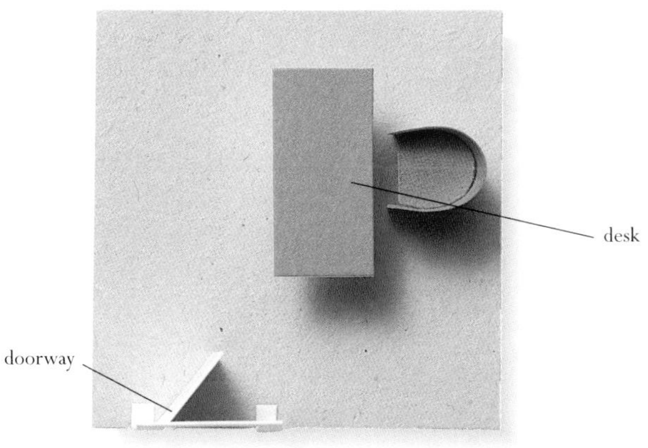

Try to sit facing the door at whatever angle you like, but make sure none of the corners are cutting at you.

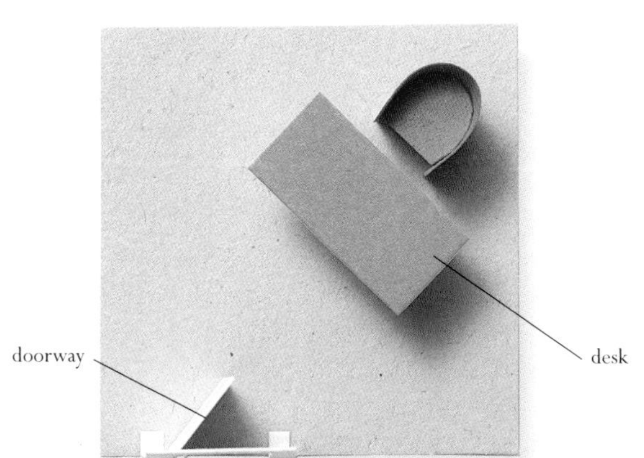

Try not to face the door directly; the incoming Qi could be overpowering.

BAD DESK PLACEMENTS

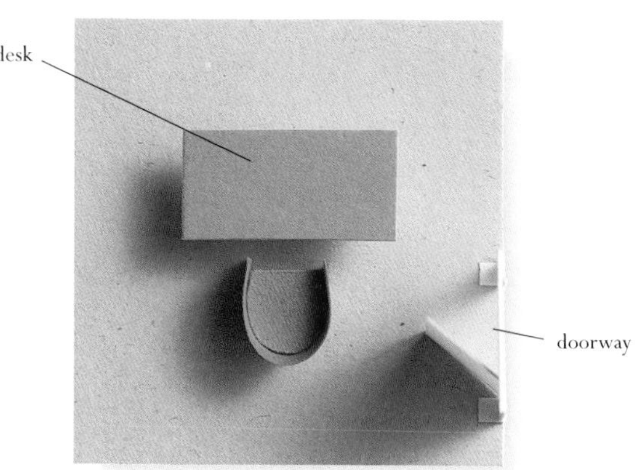

Never sit with your back to the door. You could be betrayed or "stabbed" in the back by a colleague.

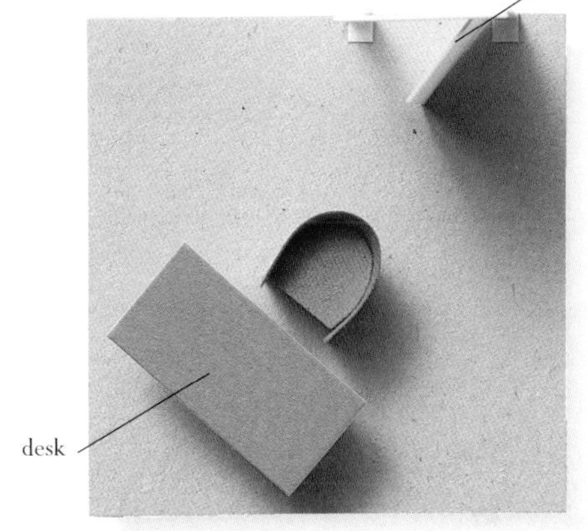

The door at the back of the chair creates a dangerous poison arrow and leaves you vulnerable to attack.

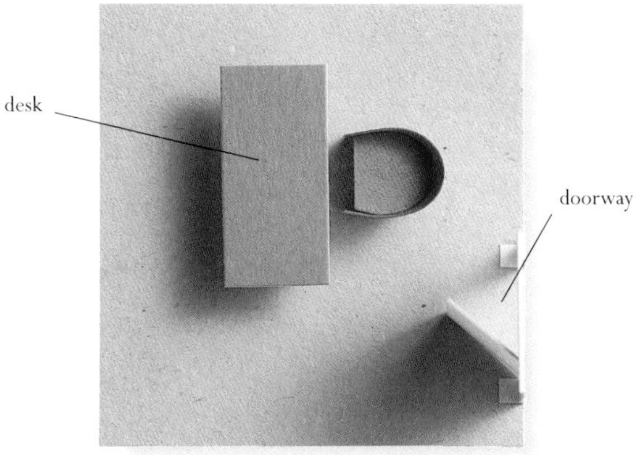

With the door behind or beside you, your concentration and authority could slip out the door.

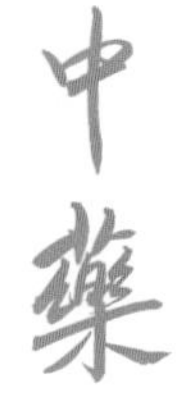

THE BA GUA IN THE HOME

FENG SHUI practitioners use their understanding of the energetics of the Ba Gua *(see pages 226–227)* to analyze the energetics of the home. Each of the eight sections of the Ba Gua is assigned a certain focus in our lives, which is reflected in the energies of that section.

FIRE
This symbolizes the active and abundant energy of summer time. A calm center directs the power around it in a positive and creative manner, representing self-empowerment in everday activity.

TAIJI
(the Supreme Ultimate at the center of the Ba Gua)
This represents the perfection and unity (the Dao) from which everything springs, and which holds everything.

EARTH
This represents the nurturing and supportive energies that can come from our relationships (family, friends, colleagues).

WIND
This represents the energy of good fortune or blessings that are brought into our lives, including good health.

THE LAKE
This represents the energy of creativity. So much potential is hidden in the depths of the lake, and within ourselves.

THUNDER
This represents the most important quality in Chinese culture: respect and honor for our elders (particularly parents), and those above us in the workplace.

HEAVEN
This represents the energy of help and support that comes to us from others and that we must offer freely to others; the natural flow of Yin and Yang.

THE MOUNTAIN
This represents withdrawal and reflection; the energy that requires us to meditate or contemplate on our lives, as did the sages on the mountain.

WATER
This represents the journey of your life, in the way that a river flows from its source to the ocean.

ABOVE
Each area of the home has a special affinity with one of the eight trigrams. For the best energetics, the door will open along the wall, aligning exactly with the water side of the room.

The Feng Shui practitioner overlays this Ba Gua of energetic possibilities and interactions on each room in the home, as in the following example.

Each section of the room is taken to reflect the energetic qualities of the Ba Gua. Thus, for example, if the area of the room covered by the quality of Wind (good fortune and blessings) is messy and unkempt, this would run counter to your desire for good fortune in all aspects of your life, including your health.

Obviously, this is a very simplified example but, ultimately, those individuals who respect the energetic integrity of their home as reflected in the Ba Gua will maintain their health and well-being to a much greater extent than those who ignore these connections.

Much is written in popular Feng Shui literature about the benefits of wind chimes, crystals, house plants, bamboo flutes, correctly positioned mirrors, and so on. But if you are considering Feng Shui as part of your drive for health and well-being, the following advice is probably the most pertinent.

- Focus on and clarify your life's purpose.
- Develop sensible lifestyle habits in all areas of your life.
- Get rid of what is superfluous and unnecessary in your life – both physical and attitudinal.
- When you feel confident that you have done all the above, consult a Feng Shui practitioner for advice on how to improve things further.

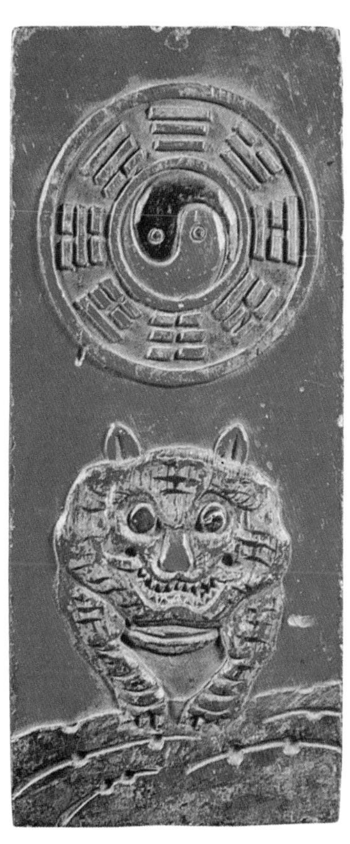

ABOVE
Mirrors and tiger images can both powerfully influence Ba Gua.

Feng Shui is a complex and fascinating branch of Chinese thinking. Although it goes beyond the immediate area of our health, it is none the less intimately tied up with it. Chinese medicine has always seen the individual as a microcosm of the macrocosm and insisted on the energetic interaction of the two. The art and practice of Feng Shui positively make this connection and can be used to support health and well-being in a fundamental way.

With Feng Shui, as with any aspect of Chinese medicine, it is important to consult an experienced and reputable practitioner (who need not be Chinese). Feng Shui is a growing and developing profession in the West. While remaining true to the principles behind this ancient art, Western practictioners are giving a more familiar context to the practice, making it accessible to far more people. Details of how to find a qualified practitioner are given at the end of the book.

This final chapter has sought to place the practice of Chinese medicine in a wider cultural and behavioral context. The theories and principles that underpin Chinese medicine go far beyond acupuncture needles and herbal preparations – they embrace the whole of our lives, and nothing is excluded. When Qi is in harmony, health and well-being are the result. Qi permeates the universe, and our life is defined by this great cosmic dance of energies. Maintaining and improving our health requires us to maintain that universal vision.

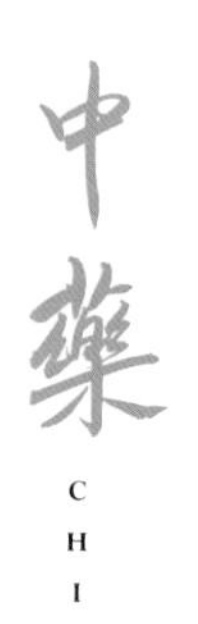

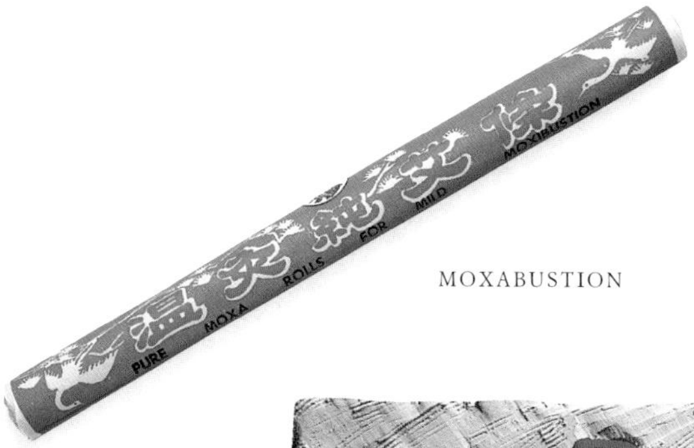

MOXABUSTION

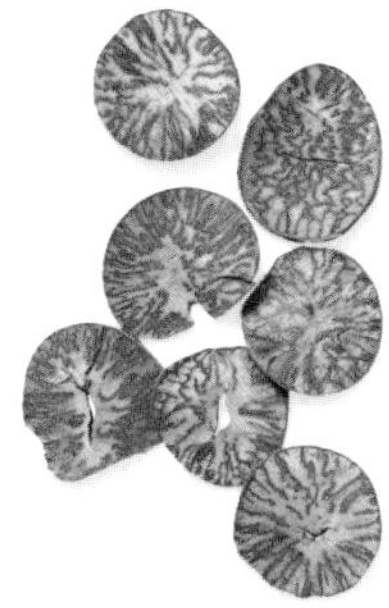

HERBALISM

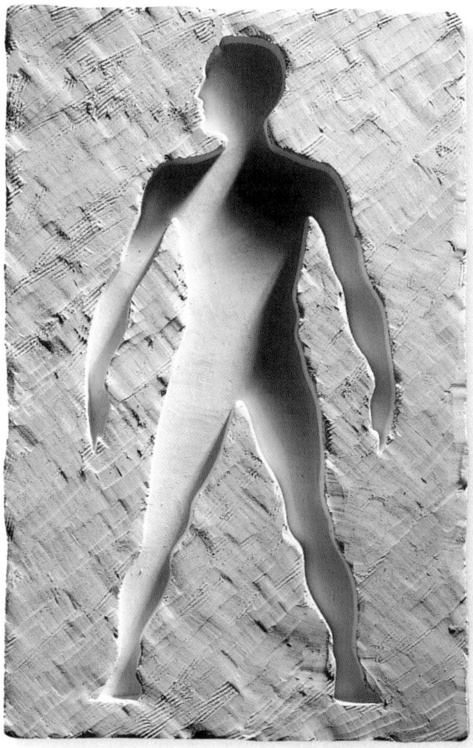

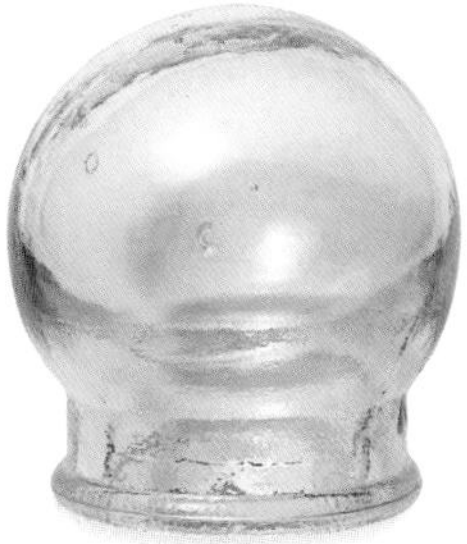

CUPPING

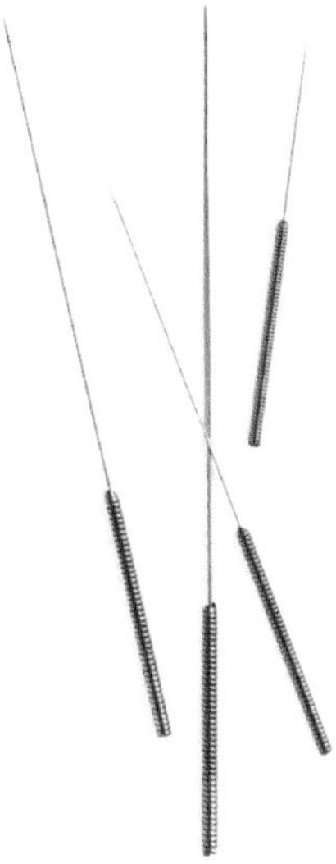

ACUPUNCTURE

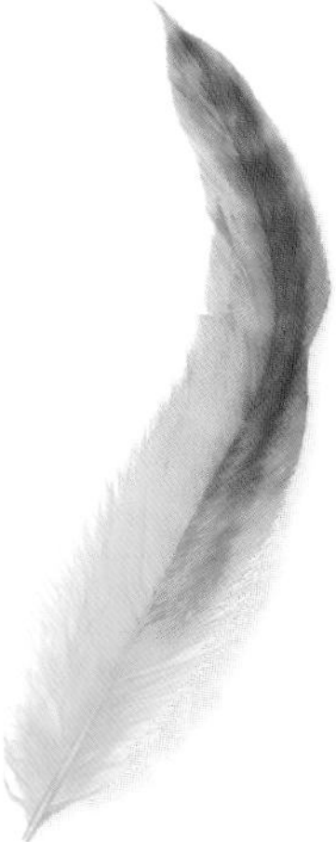

QIGONG

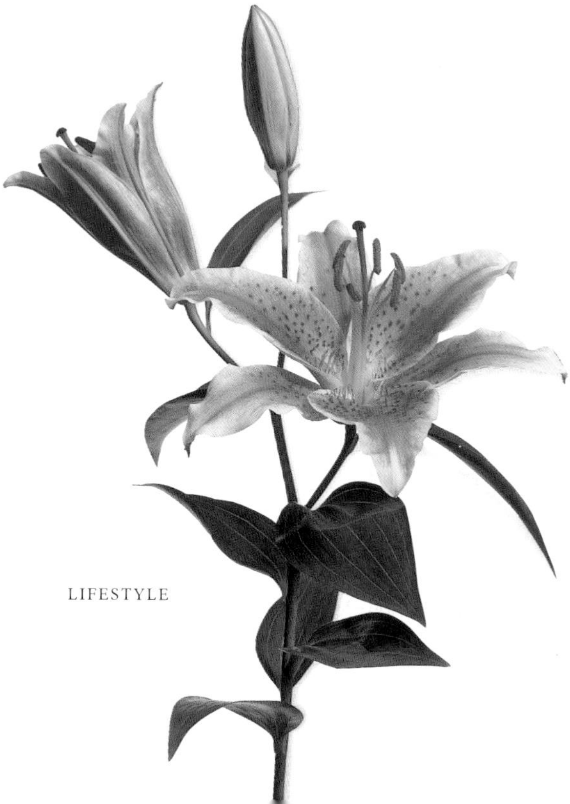

LIFESTYLE

BRINGING IT TOGETHER

THIS BOOK has outlined in some detail both the theories behind and the therapeutic approaches of Chinese medicine. As will be clear, this is a highly developed and sophisticated system of healthcare that has been in existence for thousands of years and that continues to be refined and adjusted even in the present day. No other system offers as clear an articulation of an energy anatomy and physiology. It stands in the forefront of developments that will have massive implications, as we move into the 21st century, for the way in which we understand the workings of our bodies and the manner in which they fail.

In the West, attitudes have shifted dramatically over the last twenty years or so. Acupuncture is no longer treated with the disdain and condescension that was previously the case; the use of herbs is gaining much attention, especially in treating conditions that do not respond well to orthodox approaches; interest in Taiji, Qigong, and meditative practices is no longer confined to marginal groups; and Feng Shui practitioners are increasingly employed to advise in the design of buildings and environmental planning. Despite the fact that many Western-trained practitioners seem intent on trying to shoehorn Chinese medicine into the straitjacket of Western reductionist science – for example, seeking to "isolate" the active chemical ingredient in a herbal remedy – there is no doubt that Chinese practices and ideas are here to stay and will grow and develop in the future.

It is important to get beyond the notion that acupuncture is simply for pain relief, that herbal remedies are nothing but mild tonics, and that Taiji or Qigong are useful adjuncts to "real" physical exercise. Chinese medical practice requires to be contextualized in the illnesses and illness-prevention of everyday people, in terms that they can relate to and in a language that they can understand.

In order to try to give Chinese medicine some real immediacy, the following are examples of real-life problems that have responded well to treatment by Chinese medicine.

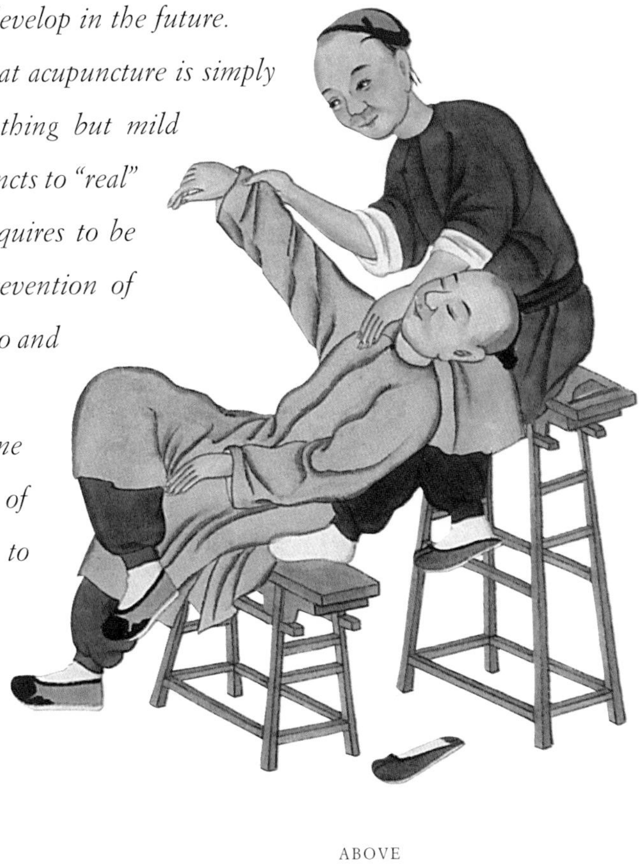

LEFT
Chinese medicine can help us in many ways, and we can help ourselves in our own lifestyle.

ABOVE
The modalities offer treatments for everyday illness.

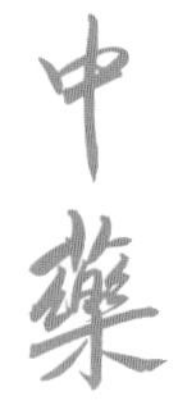

CASE STUDY 1

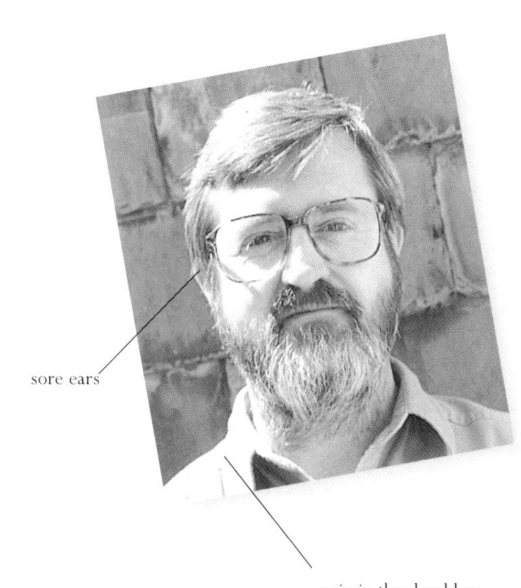

IAN WAS complaining of really sore ears and a general aching that spread over his head and into his shoulders. The focal point of the pain moved around the upper part of the arms, the shoulders, the neck, and the head. The pain around his ears was especially acute. The pain had come on suddenly when he woke up this morning, and he was having to take the day off from his work as an insurance salesman. This was really distressing since he was paid by commission on his sales of policies, and he had turned up at the clinic to see if there was anything that Chinese medicine might be able to do to help. He had taken proprietary analgesics, but these had not really touched the problem.

In a case like this it is sometimes easy to miss the obvious. The information revealed in a full diagnostic interview did not hang together terribly well. Initially, Ian insisted that he had simply got up that morning with these pains, but eventually it turned out that he owns an open-top MG sports car and that the previous evening he had been out for a lengthy country drive with his new girlfriend. He had kept the top down, despite the fact that the warmth of the day was rapidly being lost in the chill of the evening. He estimated that he had driven some thirty to forty miles and they had not arrived home till about 10:30 p.m., by which time it was getting quite cold.

This information provided the key to Ian's problem. He was suffering from Wind and Cold having invaded the channels of the head, neck, and face, causing local Qi stagnation in the relevant channels and collaterals. The type of pain is consistent with a channel disorder, and the fact that the focus seemed to shift shows the influence of the invading Wind.

The treatment of choice was acupuncture, and the principles of treatment were to expel the Wind and Cold and to clear the channels. Appropriate acupuncture points were selected, and the channels around the ears, which were especially painful, were warmed by using a moxa stick in a pecking motion. The condition was very acute but the acupuncture had an immediate effect. After one treatment the pain was markedly reduced. Ian returned the following day for further treatment, and by the end of the week, when he had received a third treatment, he was virtually pain free.

It was suggested to Ian that he keeps the hood up or wears appropriate clothing the next time he wants to impress a new girlfriend with his open-top sports car.

CASE STUDY 2

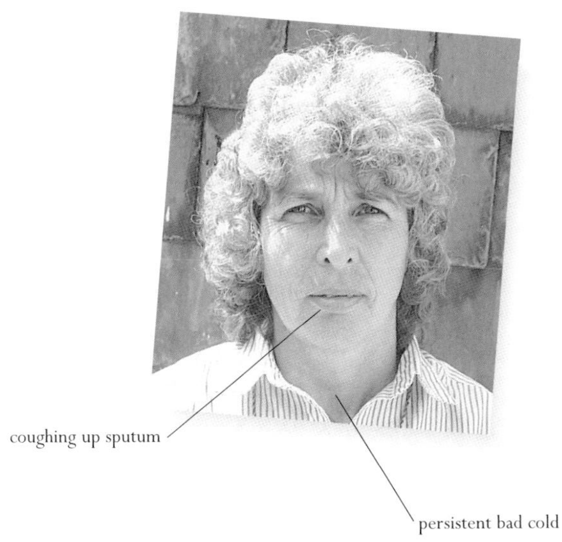

JANET WAS 60 years old and she came to the clinic complaining that she had been diagnosed as having chronic bronchitis but the "pills they give me don't agree with my stomach." The problem had existed for many years but had become particularly bad over this last winter. She had a bad cold in November and since then she had never been right. She was coughing up copious amounts of thick yellow sputum and her coughing was so bad at times that she was almost going into a spasm. Although she no longer smoked, Janet had smoked between thirty and forty a day since she was a teenager. She had eventually stopped about five years ago after she had her first really bad attack of bronchitis. She admitted to still having the odd cigarette, but only very occasionally when "my lungs feel up to it." Janet's tongue was red and dry, with a thick, sticky yellow coating. Her pulses were weak and slippery, especially on the Lung pulse.

The cause and effect here were very obvious: Janet had seriously damaged her Lung function over an extended period of abuse from smoking. Smoking will draw Heat into the Lungs, consuming the Yin fluids and causing Lung function to become impaired. Janet was also somewhat overweight and generally lacking energy. It is therefore likely that Spleen function was impaired, causing Damp to build up. Over time, the Damp had transformed into Phlegm that obstructed the Lungs, which were themselves quite Yin deficient.

The diagnosis was Phlegm Heat in the Lungs with associated Lung Yin deficiency and generalized Spleen Qi deficiency. The treatment principle would be to drain the fire from the Lungs, clear the Phlegm, stop the cough, and tonify the Lungs and the Spleen.

It was felt appropriate to combine acupuncture and herbal treatment: acupuncture to clear the Heat and Phlegm and to tonify the Lungs; herbal treatment to drain Phlegm Heat from the Lungs and, at the same time, stop the cough and moisten the Lungs. One of the benefits of a herbal formula is that the constituent herbs can be selected to address different aspects of the disharmony.

Janet took the herbs in a powdered form. She came weekly for about six weeks, receiving acupuncture treatment each time and reviewing and adjusting the herbal prescription every two weeks. Her cough improved markedly and the Phlegm was much reduced. She felt much better in herself and was now able to get about a little more. She did, however, admit that since she had been feeling better she had smoked the odd cigarette. After eight weeks, acupuncture was discontinued and Janet proceeded with the herbal prescription only. She returned for a follow-up visit every three weeks, and after six months her chest was clearer than it had been for many years.

Fifteen months after her initial visit, Janet is much better and generally feels much more healthy in herself. Her Lung problem is still likely to flare up from time to time, but the use of acupuncture and especially herbs, have made a marked difference to her condition. Provided she avoids smoking, and avoids spending time in places where other people are smoking, she should continue to feel better.

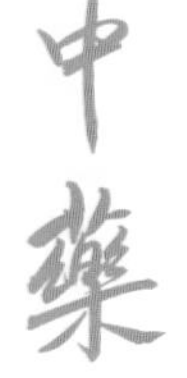

CASE STUDY 3

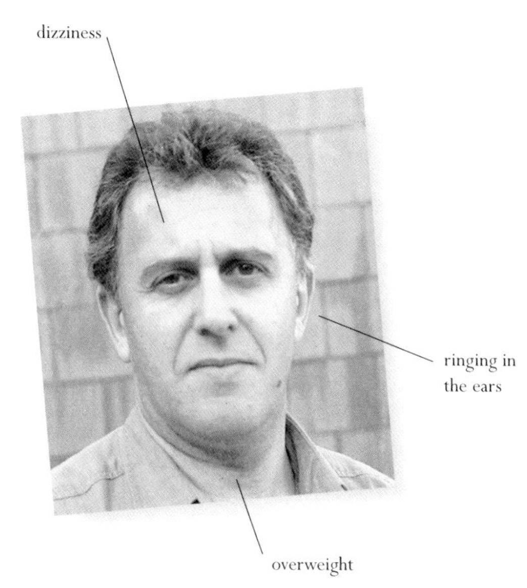

JIM WAS in a high-pressure executive position in a medium-sized engineering firm. The firm was in merger talks with a large multinational company, and Jim felt under inordinate pressure in his efforts to keep his position viable. He believed that if the takeover went ahead, it was likely that he would lose his job.

At the time of his visit Jim was working approximately fifteen hours a day, and most weekends he worked at some time or other. His main complaint was that he was feeling dizzy and at times felt he was going to pass out. He said that he felt that he was losing his place at work and was no longer able to control things the way he used to. He says that he could only come for treatment at 7 a.m. since he was too busy at other times, but he was willing to pay extra for the inconvenience.

He was a bit overweight, with a red face. He complained of ringing in his ears and at times he got headaches. He also said that he had a terrible genital itch that was really annoying him and that he found quite embarrassing at times. His pulse was rapid and slippery and very full. His tongue was red around the edges, with a greasy coating. Throughout the diagnostic interview he was very edgy and at one point he had to suspend the discussion in order to make an urgent phone call on his mobile phone.

It seemed likely from the diagnostic information that the dizziness and other "head" symptoms were caused by Phlegm obstructing the orifices in the head. Also, it seemed likely that there was stagnation in Jim's Liver Qi and that, over time, an imbalance of the Yin and Yang energies had built up, resulting in the Liver Yang energy rising to the head and taking the Phlegm with it.

The main principle of treatment here was to subdue the Liver Yang, promote the smooth flow of Qi and clear the Phlegm from the orifices. In this instance, treatment was begun by giving Jim a relaxing acupressure massage. This was very effective in taking the edginess away and allowing the subsequent treatment to be more effective. This was followed by acupuncture, and a powdered herbal formula was also given to support the main thrust of the treatment.

After several treatments Jim said he was feeling much better – "like a new man." Treatment continued for another three weeks, by which time he felt that he was much better and able to cope on his own. Jim returned about six months later, again feeling under pressure, but by this time the merger in his business life had gone through and his job was secure. His main source of difficulty was the pressures of his new executive position within the enlarged company.

CASE STUDY 4

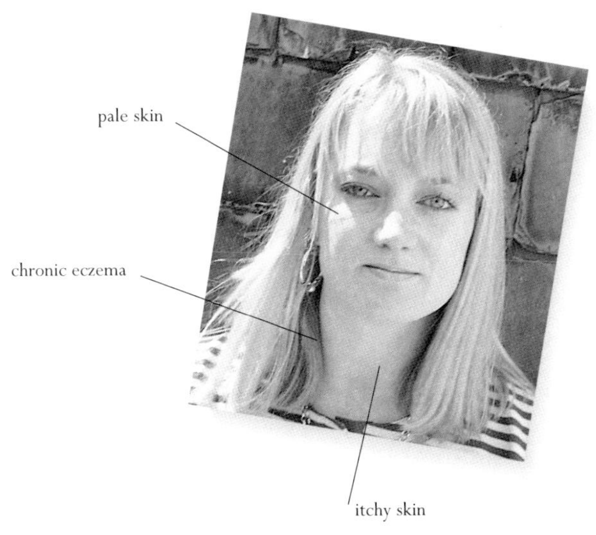

MARIE, AGE 23, was an elementary school teacher. She had suffered from chronic eczema since she was a child. She had been hospitalized and had numerous steroid preparations but nothing had made much impact on the problem.

The eczema was worse on her hands, arms, head, and knees; she also had patches of eczema on her legs and on her trunk. The skin was very dry and flaky; it got very itchy, and when she scratched, it bled. The worst areas were on her hands, where the dryness got so bad that the skin cracked and often became infected. When it was like this, it was extremely painful and she could not write or use her hands at all. She tried to avoid using chalk in the classroom because this sometimes exacerbated the problem. Marie was a thin, somewhat pale young woman. Her tongue was pale and quite dry; her pulse was thin and a bit thready.

In terms of Chinese medicine, a skin condition like this is usually seen as resulting from a deficiency of Blood, allowing Wind to invade the channels. The dry, flaky skin, the pale complexion, and the tongue and pulse all indicated a Blood-deficient condition. The itchiness demonstrated the presence of pathogenic Wind in the channels.

The principle of treatment was to clear the Wind from the channels, tonify the Blood, and nourish the skin. While acupuncture may be of some benefit in such cases, the treatment of choice for skin conditions is herbs. Herbs were selected that clear the Wind, tonify the Yin and Blood, and nourish the skin. There are several classic formulae that would form the basis for a treatment of a condition such as this, and these can be adapted according to the specifics of the presenting signs and symptoms.

Marie initially found that the herbs she was given cleared the itchiness fairly quickly, but the lesions were still very dry and showed no signs of reducing. The formula was adapted and, after a period of about six to eight weeks, there was a significant improvement in the condition. Three months later the skin was healthier than it had been for many years, but there were still lesions, and the ones on the hands were still leading to cracking along the line of the finger joints. After a year of herbs Marie's condition is stable. The skin is much better and her hands are now quite clear. There is the occasional flare-up, and Marie retains a bag of herbs that she takes immediately there is any problem. She will continue to visit on an occasional basis to monitor the condition.

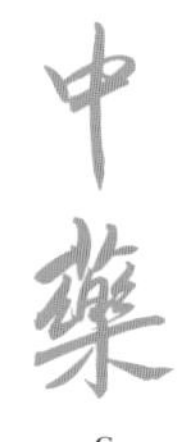

CASE STUDY 5

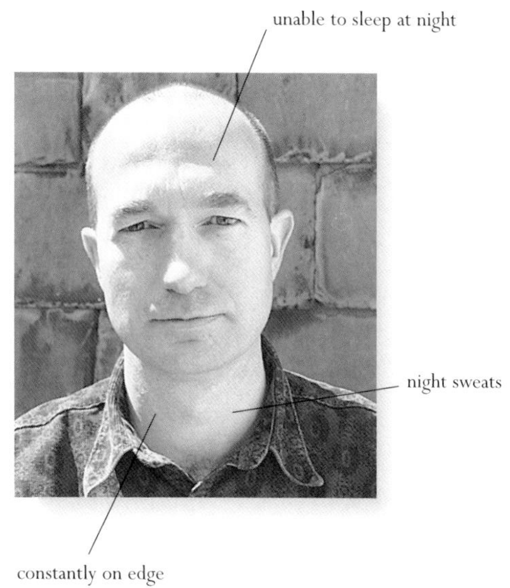

JOHN HAD been diagnosed as HIV positive, and over the last six months this had developed into full-blown AIDS. He was trying to carry on with his life as best he could and was receiving orthodox medical treatment on a regular basis. He came to the clinic to see if it was possible to do anything to help with the worst excesses of the symptoms that he was experiencing. His main complaints were that he had little or no energy, that he could not sleep at night, and that he was burning up with massive night sweats that required him to change his sheets two or three times a night. He was having palpitations and was constantly on edge, even with his partner and other good friends. John looked very thin and almost emaciated. His skin was dry, with lesions on his face and back. His face was red and his tongue was red and peeled, with a bright red tip. His pulse was rapid and thready.

John was presenting the classic signs and symptoms of Empty Heat resulting from an underlying deficiency of Yin energy in the body. The AIDS condition was resulting in the Yin fluids being consumed and the body literally "burning up" from the inside. The Empty Heat was also affecting the Heart Yin and this was resulting in the poor sleep patterns, the edginess, and the palpitations.

It is highly unlikely that Chinese medicine could reverse the AIDS, but there was no reason why the symptoms could not be helped. The principle of treatment would be to clear the Empty Heat, tonify the Yin, and calm the Heart Shen. In John's instance it was decided to use acupuncture. There may be some surprise regarding the choice of acupuncture for a patient with full-blown AIDS, but provided normal common sense and rigorous hygiene procedures are observed, there is absolutely no reason not to use acupuncture in such a case.

John was treated initially twice weekly, and then on a weekly basis. After three months of treatment he was sleeping much better, which naturally helped his general energy level. He was still having night sweats but the intensity was markedly reduced.

John was also encouraged to go along to a Qigong class and learn some simple Qigong postures and exercises that might help him. This he did and, even after he terminated acupuncture treatment, he was continuing to go along to the Qigong class.

After four months John decided to stop his acupuncture treatment. The condition was far from cured, but he had received some significant benefit from the acupuncture and felt that now he was sleeping better he would be more able to continue to fight his condition in his own way, doing Qigong regularly.

CASE STUDY 6

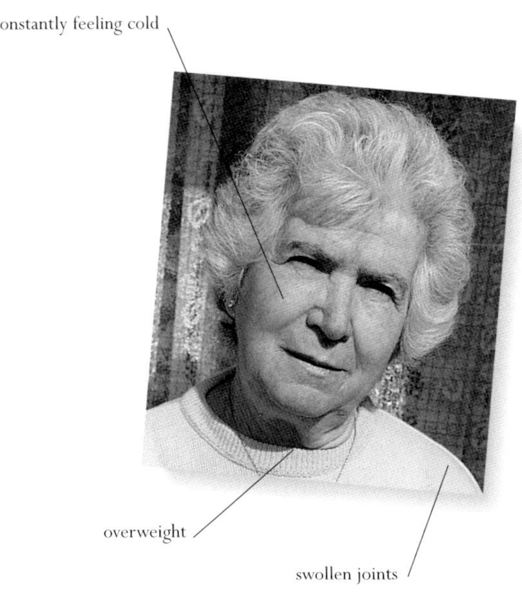

MARTHA WAS 76 and wanted to know if anything could be done to help her arthritis. She was stiff and sore all over, but especially in her knee and ankle joints, which were swollen and painful to the touch. She was overweight and complained that her feet and fingers got quite swollen at times. She found it difficult to keep warm, even when the weather was mild. She also complained of chronic diarrhea, especially first thing in the morning. Martha's tongue was pale and wet and her pulse slow and rather soggy in quality.

Martha's problem suggested the invasion of the channels by Cold and Damp. The invading pathogenic factors tend to lodge in the channels around the joints, causing the pain and swelling of arthritis. There was also evidence of a generalized Yang deficiency, characterized by the cold, chronic diarrhea, and the tongue and pulse indicators. Yang deficiency is a common and natural feature of the aging process.

The principles of treatment are to clear the Damp and Cold from the channels and to tonify the body's underlying Yang energy. Martha was treated with acupuncture, moxabustion, and herbal prescriptions. Cupping was also used to help move the Qi around the worst-affected areas. After twenty weekly sessions Martha's condition was greatly improved. She decided to end the acupuncture and related treatments, but continued to take herbs for the next six months and her condition remained quite stable.

CONCLUSION

THESE CASE studies briefly outline typical conditions that can benefit from the treatments offered in Chinese medicine. There are few, if any, conditions where Chinese medicine cannot be of significant benefit. It is arguable that in many common illness patterns, Chinese medical approaches have a track record which suggests that they ought to be the treatments of first choice.

There is a growing number of practices in which Chinese medical approaches offer a comprehensive healthcare service, ranging from the major modalities of acupuncture and herbalism through to to offering Qigong classes and therapy, and even the services of a Feng Shui practitioner. Ideally, these services would be available alongside other complementary therapies in partnership with the conventional orthodox Western medical approaches.

Chinese medicine is an effective and cost-efficient way of delivering a comprehensive range of medical services, and not only will it open up a range of new treatment possibilities, it will also stand at the front of the growing development in energy medicine as we approach the millennium.

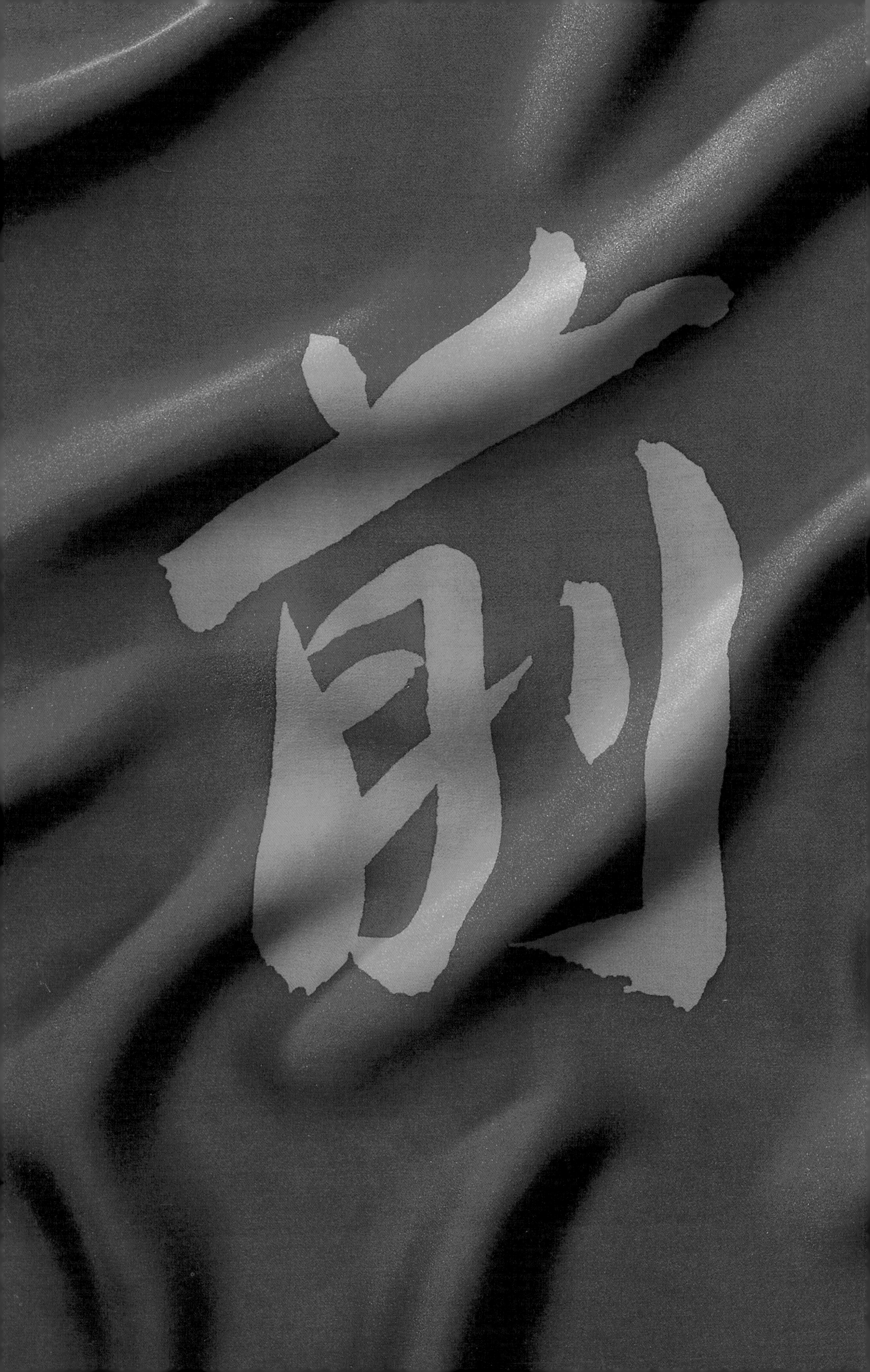
前

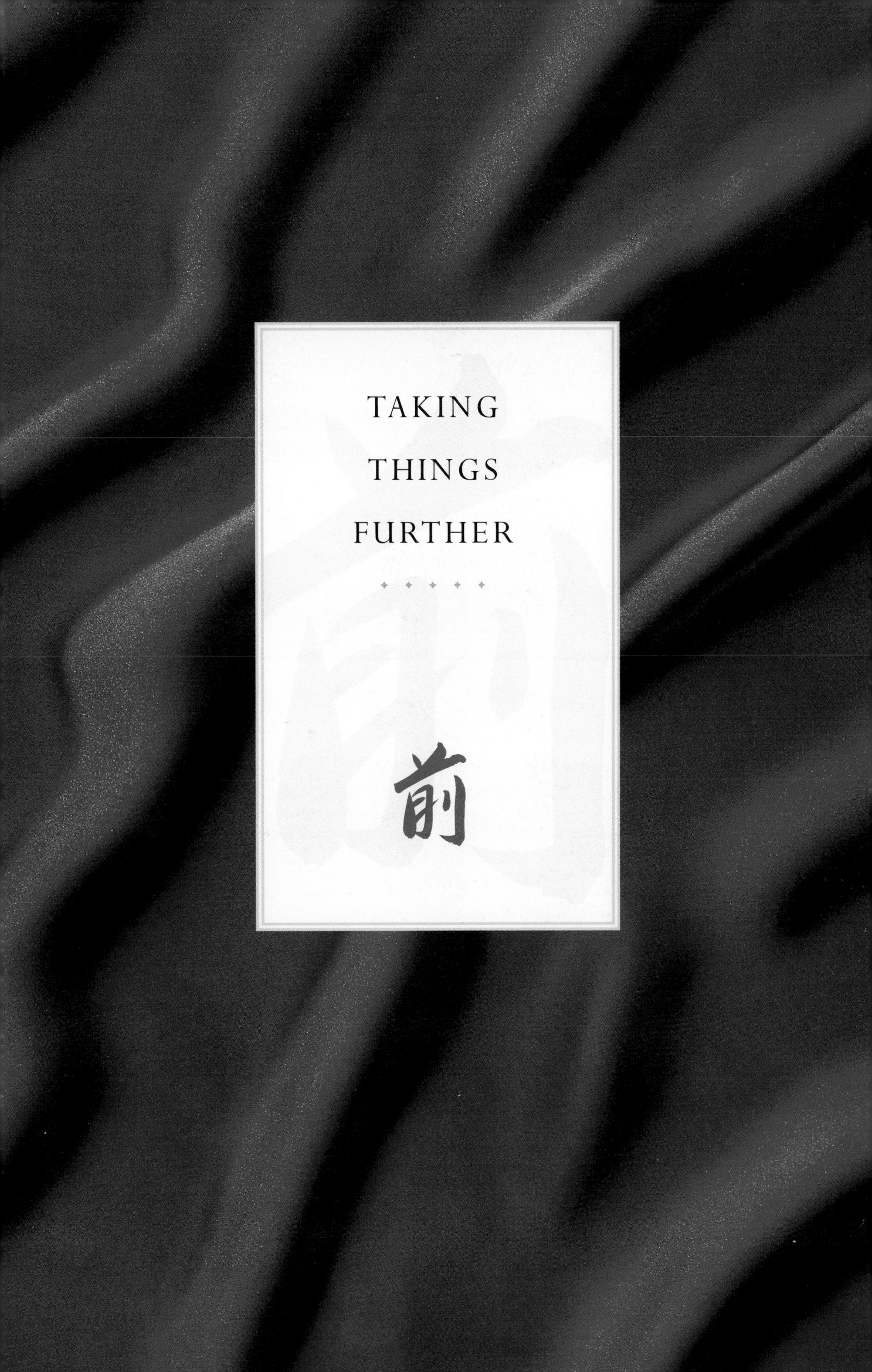
TAKING
THINGS
FURTHER
前

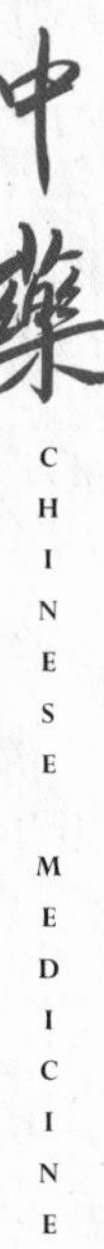

THE NEXT STEPS

THIS BOOK *has offered the background and the practice to Chinese medicine in an easily assimilable format. The interested reader will have a good basic background knowledge as to what this fascinating system is all about, and about what it may have to offer in terms of both treatment for existing health problems and also preventive approaches to health and well-being.*

It will also have been apparent from the almost "mantra-like" insistence on seeking out professional and reputable practitioners that it is absolutely essential for anyone considering using Chinese medicine to know where to go. This section of the book is all about getting further information that you can rely upon and knowing how to access trained practitioners of Chinese medicine.

The section on further reading makes suggestions about books and journals that will deepen and broaden your understanding of the various strands of Chinese medicine, and the section with useful addresses will give information about where you can access practitioners. In each instance every care has been taken to insure that the information is current and accurate.

Chinese medicine is a fascinating and rewarding journey – this is the place to start!

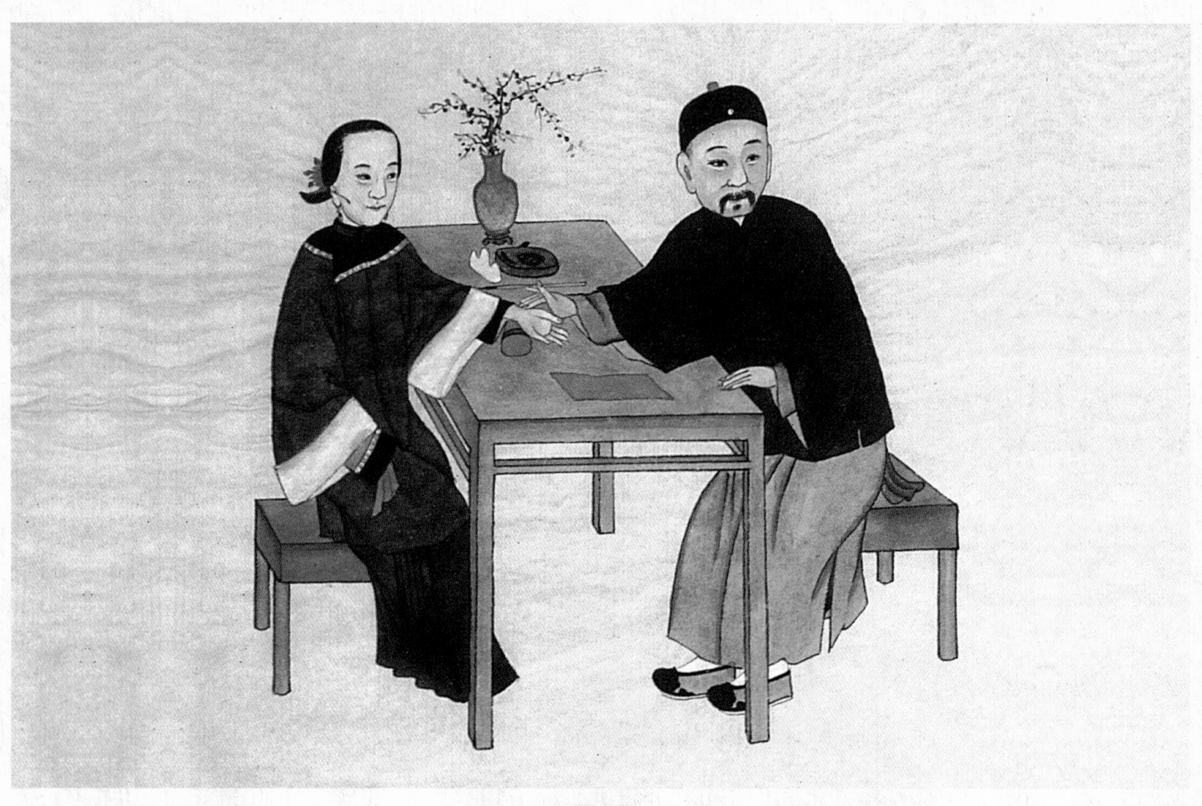

ABOVE
Always seek help from professional practitioners of Chinese Medicine.

FURTHER READING

The following selection of publications is suggested to interested readers in order to offer them the opportunity to expand their understanding of aspects of Chinese medicine. The list is by no means comprehensive, but it does offer a good source guide for further study.

CHINESE MEDICINE – GENERAL

Beinfield, H. and Korngold, E.
Between Heaven & Earth,
Ballantine, New York, 1991

Kaptchuk, Ted
Chinese Medicine, The Web That Has No Weaver,
Rider, London, 1983

Maciocia, Giovanni
The Foundations of Chinese Medicine,
Churchill Livingstone, London, 1989

Maciocia, Giovanni
The Practice of Chinese Medicine,
Churchill Livingstone, London, 1994

Williams, Tom
Chinese Medicine,
Element Books, Shaftesbury, 1995

Wiseman, Ellis, and Zmiewski
The Fundamentals of Chinese Medicine,
Paradigm, Brookline, 1985

ACUPUNCTURE

Connelly, Dianne
Traditional Acupuncture, The Law of Five Elements,
Center for Traditional Acupuncture, Columbia, 1979

Mole, Peter
Acupuncture,
Element Books, Shaftesbury, 1991

O'Connor, J. and Bensky, D.
Acupuncture: A Comprehensive Text,
Eastland Press, Seattle, 1981

CHINESE HERBAL MEDICINE

Bensky, D. and Barolet R.
Chinese Herbal Medicine, Formulas and Strategies,
Eastland Press, Seattle, 1993

Bensky, D. and Gamble, A.
Chinese Herbal Medicine, Materia Medica,
Eastland Press, Seattle, 1993

Fratkin, J.
Chinese Herbal Patent Formulas,
Shya, Boulder, 1986

CHINESE DIETARY THERAPY

Flaws, B.
Arisal of the Clear – a simple guide to eating according to Traditional Chinese Medicine,
Blue Poppy Press, Boulder, 1991

Flaws, B. and Wolfe, H.
Prince Wen Hui's Cook,
Paradigm, Massachusetts, 1983

TAIQI & QIGONG

Chungliang Al Huang
Embrace Tiger, Return to Mountain,
Celestial Arts, Berkeley, CA, 1973

Chungliang Al Huang
Taiji,
Celestial Arts, Berkeley, CA, 1989

Klein, B.
Movements of Magic,
Newcastle, California, 1984

Lam Kam Chuen
The Way of Energy,
Gaia, London, 1991

Liang, T. T.
T'ai Chi Chuan for Health & Self-Defense,
Vintage, New York, 1977

McRitchie, J.
Chi Kung,
Element Books, Shaftesbury, 1993

Reid, H.
The Way of Harmony,
Gaia, London, 1988

Wong Kiew Kit
The Art of Chi Kung,
Element Books, Shaftesbury, 1993

CHINESE PHILOSOPHY

Anthony, C. K.
A Guide to the I Ching,
Anthony, Stow, Massachusetts, 1988

Hua-Ching Ni
I Ching, The Book of Changes,
Eternal Breath of Tao, Santa Monica, 1992

Mitchell, Stephen (Trans.)
Tao Te Ching,
Harper Perennial, New York, 1991

FENG SHUI

Lam Kam Chuen
The Feng Shui Handbook,
Gaia, London, 1995

Rosbach, S.
Feng Shui,
Rider, London, 1984

Rosbach, S.
Interior Design with Feng Shui,
Rider, London, 1987

Spear, W.
Feng Shui Made Easy,
Harper Collins, London, 1995

GENERAL HEALTH CARE

Flaws, B.
Imperial Secrets of Health & Longevity,
Blue Poppy Press, Boulder, Colorado, 1994

Gerber, Richard
Vibrational Medicine,
Bear & Co, Santa Fe, 1988

Myss, Caroline
Anatomy of the Spirit: The seven stages of power in healing,
Crown, Harmony Books, New York, 1996

Myss, C. & Shealy N.
The Creation of Health,
Stillpoint, Walpole NH, 1988

Sheldrake, Rupert
The Presence of the Past,
Collins, London, 1988

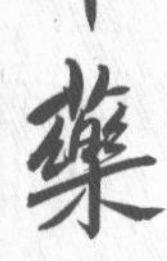

USEFUL ADDRESSES

It is important when considering Chinese medicine as a form of treatment that prospective patients can be sure that they can access a reputable, registered practitioner. This is best done through a professional association or council.

Names and addresses for several countries are given below. Readers in other countries should seek information from appropriate public information offices regarding professional practitioner registers.

AUSTRALIA

Australian Natural Therapists Association
PO Box 308
Melrose Park 5039
South Australia
Tel +61 8 297 9533
Fax +61 8 297 0003

Australian Traditional Medicine Society Limited
(Mailing)
ATMS
PO Box 1027
Meadowbank
NSW 2114
Australia
Tel +61 2 809 6800
(Office)
ATMS
12/27 Bank Street
Meadowbank
NSW 2114
Australia

Qigong Association of Australia
458 White Horse Road
Surrey Hills
Victoria 3127
Australia
Tel +61 3 9836 6961
Fax +61 3 830 5608

CHINA

The World Academic Society of Medical Qigong
No 11 Heping Jie Nei Kou
Beijing 100029
China

FRANCE

Dr. Yves Requena
Institut European de Qi Gong
La Ferme des Vences
13122 Ventabren
France
Tel +33 42 92 56 10
Fax +33 42 92 56 40

NEW ZEALAND

New Zealand Register of Acupuncturists Inc.
PO Box 9950
Wellington 1
New Zealand
Tel/Fax +64 4 476 8578

UNITED KINGDOM

ACUPUNCTURE

The British Acupuncture Council
Park House
206–208 Latimer Road
London
W10 6RE
Tel +44 181 964 0222
Fax +44 181 964 0333

CHINESE HERBALISM

The Register of Chinese Herbal Medicine
PO Box 400
Wembley
Middlesex
HA9 9NZ
Tel +44 181 904 1357

FENG SHUI

Feng Shui Network
PO Box 2133
London
W1A 1RL
Tel +44 171 935 8935
Fax +44 171 935 9295

GENERAL

British Complementary Medicine Association
39 Prestbury Road
Cheltenham
Gloucestershire
GL52 2PT
Tel +44 1242 226770
Fax +44 1242 226778

SHIATSU

Shiatsu Society
31 Pullman Lane
Godalming
Surrey
GU7 1XY
Tel/Fax +44 1483 860771

TAIJI AND QIGONG

British Council for Chinese Martial Arts
Senior Coach (Sp.C. Approved)
28 Linden Farm Drive
Countesthorpe
Leicester
LE8 5SX
Tel/Fax +44 116 2774260

Tai Chi Union for Great Britain
102 Felsham Road
London
SW15 1DQ

ZERO BALANCING

The Zero Balancing Association UK
36 Richmond Road
Cambridge
CB4 3PU
Tel/Fax +44 1223 315480

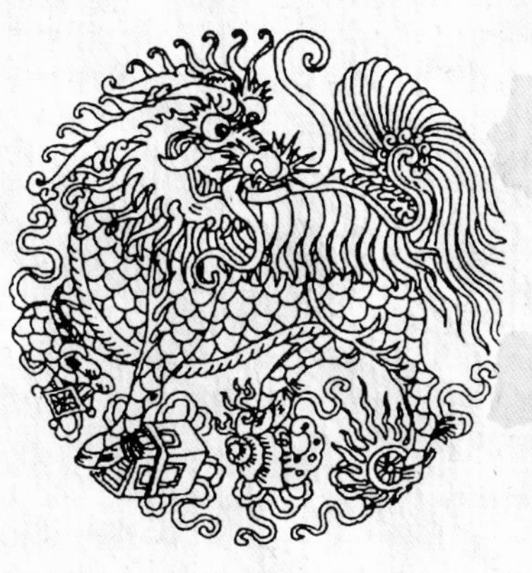

UNITED STATES

American Association of Oriental Medicine (AAOM)
433 Front Street
Catasauqua
PA 18032
Tel +1 610 2661433
Fax +1 610 2642768

American Oriental Bodywork Association
50 Maple Place
Manhasset
NY 19030

The Chi Kung School at The Body-Energy Center
James MacRitchie &
Damaris Jarboux
PO Box 19708
Boulder
CO 80308
Tel +1 303 4422250
Fax +1 303 4423141

The International Chi Kung/ Qi Gong Directory
PO Box 19708
Boulder
CO 80308
Tel +1 303 4423131
Fax +1 303 4423141

National Accreditation Commission for Schools and Colleges of Acupuncture and Oriental Medicine (NACSCAOM)
1010 Wayne Avenue
Suite 1270
Silver Springs
MD 20910
Tel +1 301 6089680
Fax +1 301 6089576

National Acupuncture and Oriental Medicine Alliance (National Alliance)
14637 Starr Road, SE
Olalla
WA 98359
Tel +1 206 8516896
Fax +1 206 8516883

National Commission for the Certification of Acupuncturists (NCCA)
PO Box 97075
Washington DC 20090-7075
Tel +1 202 2321404
Fax +1 202 4626157

Qigong Academy
8103 Marlborough Avenue
Cleveland
OH 44129
Tel/Fax +1 216 8428042

Zero Balancing Association
PO Box 1727
Capitola
CA 95010
Tel/Fax +1 408 4760665

The author would be delighted to hear from any reader who may be interested in obtaining further information regarding Chinese medicine. He can be contacted at:

The Kun Chen Clinic
34 Orchard Drive
Giffnock
Glasgow G46 7NU
Tel/Fax +44 141 638 8801

AT-A-GLANCE DIRECTORY

PRACTITIONERS OF *Chinese therapies generally specialize in one branch or another, but all have the same theoretical framework, and the approach is always to restore or preserve harmony so that the body can maintain energetic equilibrium. Anyone who is interested in Chinese medicine, or the Chinese approach to health, may wonder where to begin, and which approach to try.*

The branches of medicine are known as "modalities," and although they overlap, each has its own essential elements. Each is described separately in the book. Some are forms of treatment and preventive therapy which are relatively passive as far as the "patient" is concerned (acupuncture, moxabustion, cupping, acupressure, herbalism, and qigong healing); the rest are forms of preventive and constitution-building therapy in which the "patient" has to play an active part (qigong, taiji, meditation, and feng shui). Apart from these, the book also gives some advice on diet and social habits from the point of view of Chinese medicine. These two pages give an at-a-glance guide to finding your way about the book when looking for information in these areas.

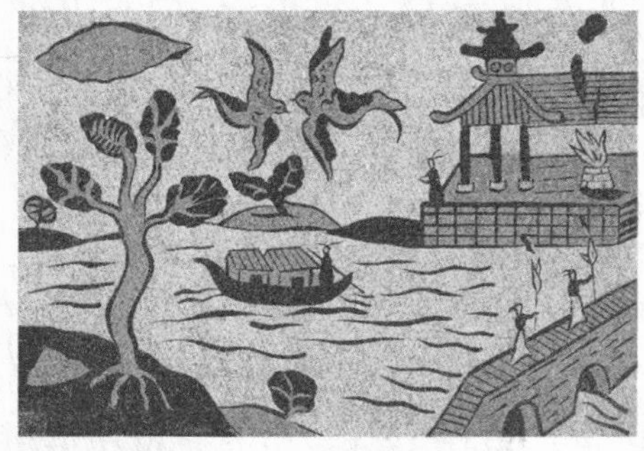

THE THERAPIES

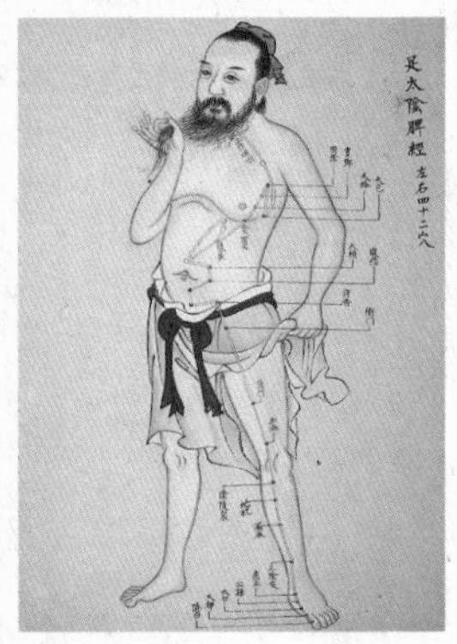

Acupuncture
page 131

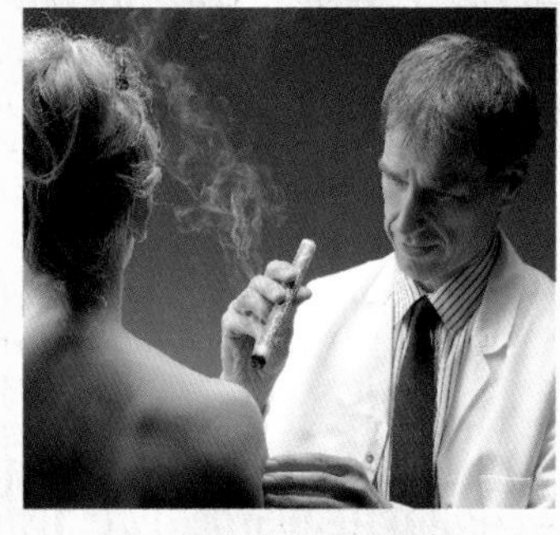

Moxabustion
page 142

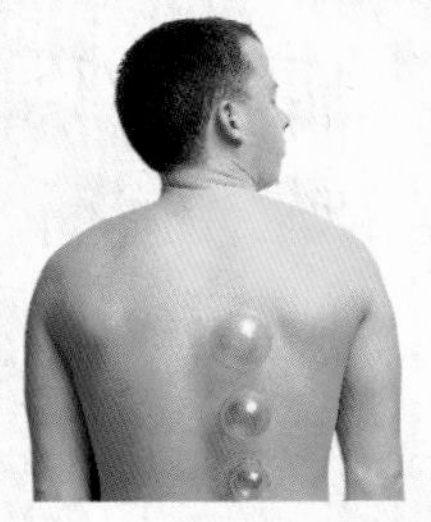

Cupping
page 145

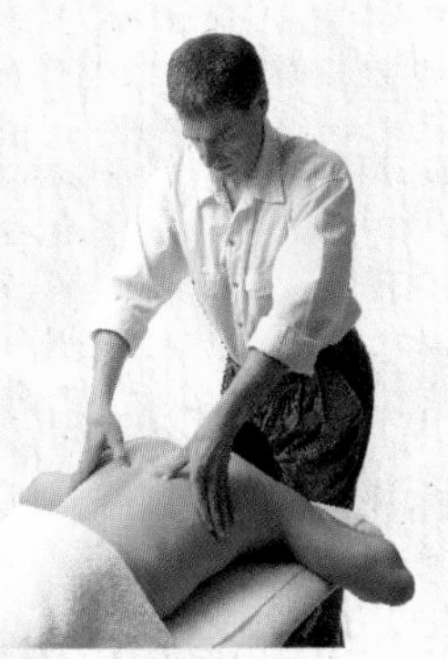

Acupressure
page 150

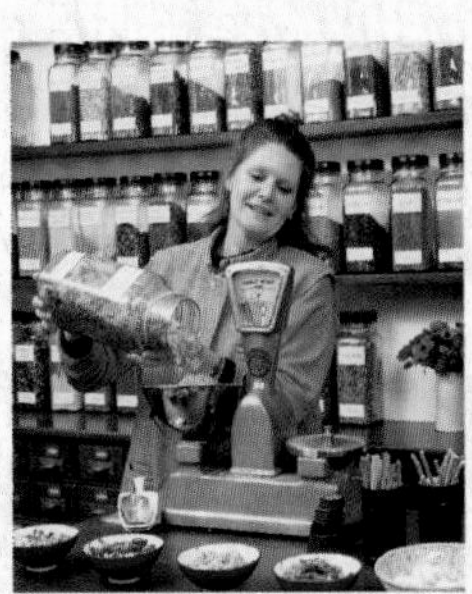

Herbalism
page 163

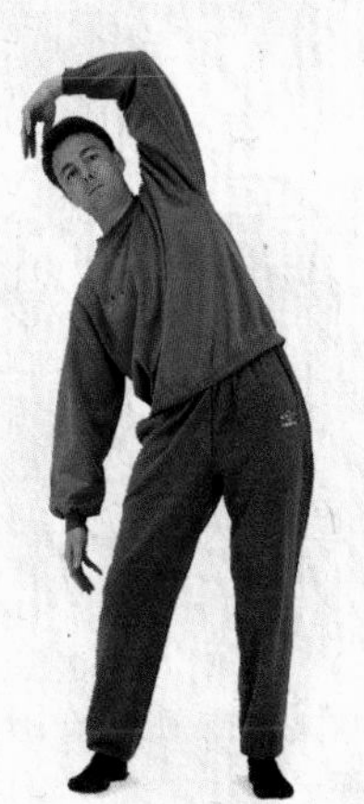

Qigong
page 189

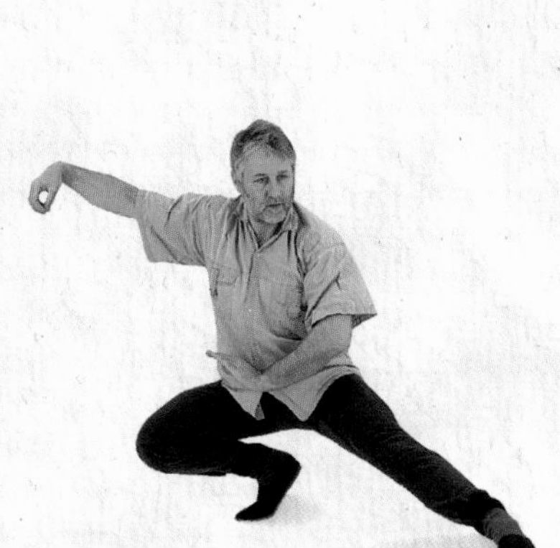

Taiji
page 206

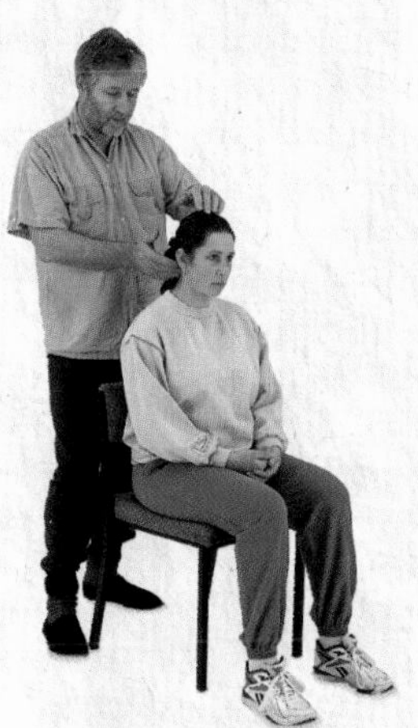

Qigong healing
page 208

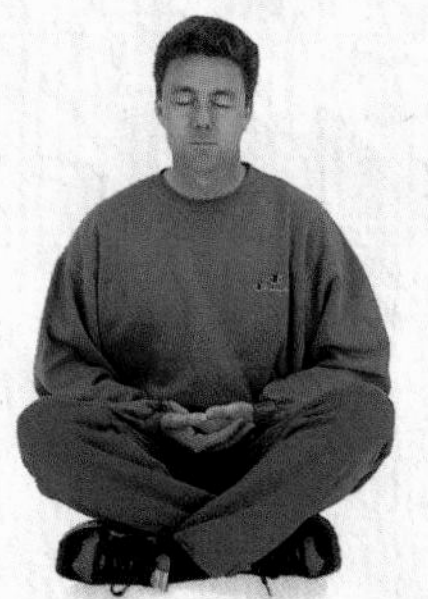

Meditation
page 214

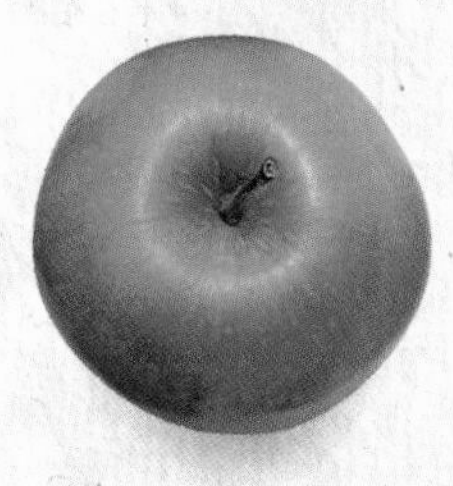

Diet
page 218

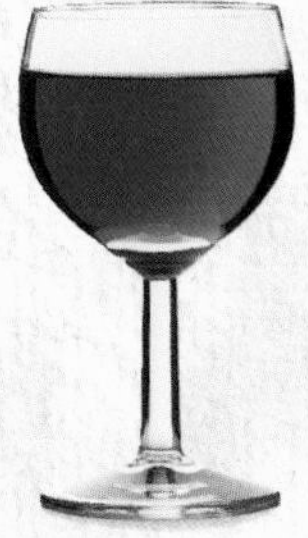

Social habits
page 222

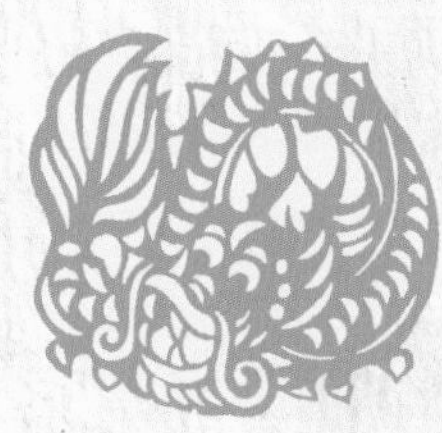

Feng Shui
page 224

GLOSSARY

Abdomen The part of the body lying between chest and pelvis

Acupressure Works on the same basic principle as acupuncture, but the Qi is worked on by pressure and massage instead of needles

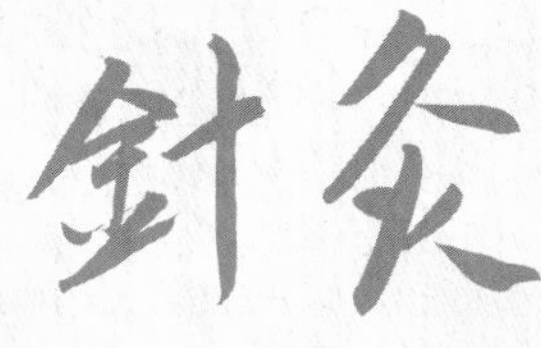

ACUPUNCTURE

Acupuncture Chinese healing therapy designed to rebalance or unblock the flow of energy within the body. Needles are used at certain points on the body, which correspond to points on the meridians along which the energy is thought to flow; see also acupuncture points; meridians.

Acupuncture points Specific points on the body where the energy flow through the body meridians can be adjusted

Analgesic Remedy or agent that deadens pain

Angina pectoris Severe pain in the lower chest, usually on the left side

An Mo The Chinese term for massage, literally "push" and "rub"

Arthritis Painful inflammation of joint tissues

Ashi points Tender spots on the body

Asthma Spasm of the bronchi in the lungs, narrowing the airwaves

Auricular Pertaining to the ear

Blood The Chinese concept of Blood differs from the Western view

Bronchitis Infection of the bronchi, the tubes that take air to the lungs

Chakra One of the energy centers of the body. Based on the Indian understanding of the energy body.

Channels Invisible pathways in which Qi travels; also called meridians. They appear in and on the body.

Chong Mai The penetrating vessel; one of the eight extraordinary meridians

Chronic Persisting for a long time, a state showing no change or very slow change

Constipation Condition where evacuating the bowels is infrequent and difficult

Contraindication Any factor in a patient's condition that indicates that treatment would involve a greater than normal degree of risk and is therefore not recommended

Cupping A treatment technique involving drawing the Qi and blood to the surface of the skin using a vacuum created inside a glass or bamboo cup

Dai Mai The girdle vessel; one of the eight extraordinary meridians

Damp In Chinese medicine, Damp is considered a Yin pathogenic influence, leading to sluggishness, tired, and heavy limbs and general lethargy

Dan Tien Energy centers in the body. In Chinese medicine there are considered to be three; an upper (between the eyebrows); a middle (in the center of the trunk); and a lower (in the lower abdomen). Qi is considered as being stored there.

Dao/Daoism Chinese philosophical and spiritual system. Dao literally means "the way." Sometimes spelt "Tao."

Dayan Qigong Wild goose Qigong form. A sequence of moving exercises based on the movements of wild geese.

Decoction A herbal preparation, where the plant material (usually hard or woody) is boiled in water and reduced to make a concentration extract

Deficient condition In Chinese medicine, any disorder that is caused by the body's inability to maintain balance, through inadequate function of the Zangfu

Deqi Literally, "acquiring the Qi" – the sensation of accessing the Qi with the needle, which the patient may experience as a tingling or numb sensation

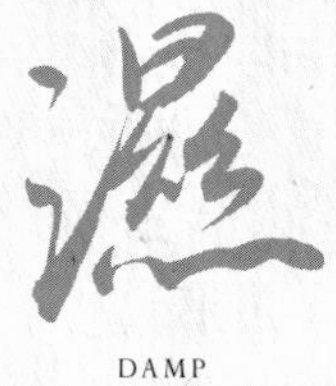

DAMP

Diagnostic process The identification of a disease by means of its symptoms

Diarrhea Frequent evacuation of loose (watery) stools

Disharmony Lack of harmony and balance in the body

Du Mai The governing vessel; one of the eight extraordinary meridians

Dysfunction Abnormal functioning of a system or organ within the body

Eczema Term for a wide range of skin conditions

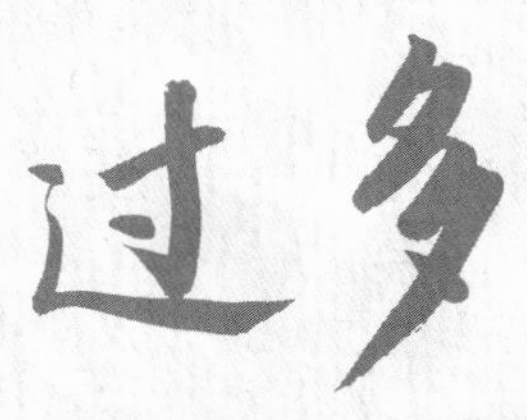

EXCESS

Edema A painless swelling caused by fluid retention beneath the skin's surface

Eight Principle patterns The system of organizing diagnostic information in Chinese medicine according to the principles of Yin, Yang; Interior, Exterior; Hot, Cold; Excess, Deficiency

Empty Heat Internal Heat in the body resulting from a deficiency of Yin

Energy bodies The energy "sheaths" that are considered to surround the physical body

Enuresis Involuntary bedwetting while asleep

Epigastrium The part of the abdomen extending from the sternum toward the navel

Epilepsy Abnormality of brain function causing seizures

Equilibrium A state of even balance

Excess condition A condition in which Qi, Blood, or Body Fluids are imbalanced, accumulating in parts of the body

External In Chinese medicine, any factors influencing the body from outside

Extra Fu Less important "minor" organs in Chinese medicine

Feng Shui The Chinese system of analyzing the energy patterns of the physical environment

Five Elements/Phases The system in Chinese medicine based on observations of the natural world. The system is built around the elements of water, wood, fire, metal, and earth.

Five Palm Sweat Characteristic sweat associated with Yin deficiency appearing on the palms, the soles of the feet, and the chest

Four Levels System for diagnosis in Chinese medicine

Fu The hollow Yang organs of the body

Gan Sweet; used to assign taste to Chinese herbs

Gu Qi The Qi extracted in the Stomach through the digestion of food and drink

Hegu The acupuncture point Large Intestine 4; translates as "Tiger's Mouth"

Hemophiliac Someone suffering from hemophilia, a hereditary disease causing excessive bleeding when any blood vessel is even slightly injured

Holistic Aiming to treat the individual as an entity, incorporating body, mind, and spirit, from the Greek word *holos*, meaning whole

Homeostasis Tendency for the internal environment of the body to remain constant in spite of varying external conditions

Hypertension Raised blood pressure

Hypochondrium The region of the abdomen on either side, under the costal cartilages and short ribs

Hypothermia Subnormal body temperature, caused by exposure to cold, or induced

Insomnia Condition where falling asleep is difficult or impossible

Internal In Chinese medicine, refers to aspects of disharmonies that arise within the body

Jiao Refers to the areas of the body; "Heater" or "Burner"

Jin Ye Body Fluids; Jin refers to the lighter fluids, Ye to the denser fluids

Jing A Chinese term for the vital essence that is the source of life and individual development

Jing Luo Zhi Qi Qi flowing through the meridians

Jue Yin Arm and leg channels of the Pericardium and the Liver

Ke Cycle The cycle of mutual control in the Five Elements system

Kong Qi Qi derived in the Lungs from the air

Ku Bitter; used to assign taste to Chinese herbs

Laogong Acupuncture point in the center of the palm – Pericardium 8. Literally translates as "Labor Palace"

Lesion A term used to explain an abnormality or damage to the body

Lethargy Heavy unnatural slumber or torpor

Leucorrhea Vaginal discharge, often indicating infection

Luo The system of connecting channels between the major channels

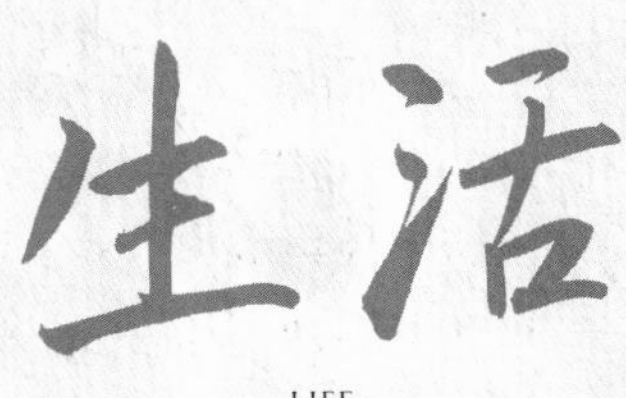

LIFE

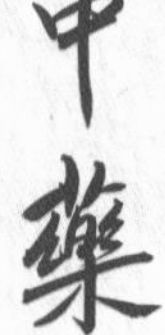

Marrow The substance that makes up the brain and the spinal column in Chinese medicine
Materia medica A branch of science dealing with the origins and properties of remedies; the complete description of all Chinese herbs
Meditation Serious continuous contemplation, especially on a religious or spiritual theme

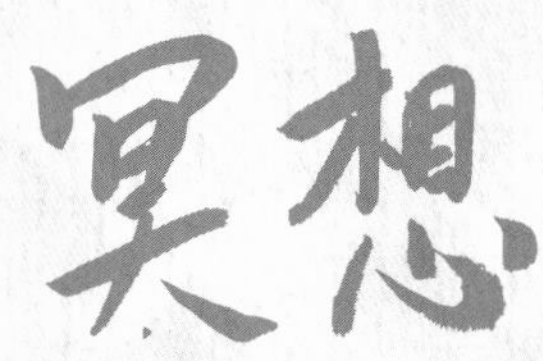

MEDITATION

Meridians The channels through which vital energy flows in the body. In Chinese acupuncture, there are 59 meridians in all; Indian medicine recognizes several hundred.
Mingmen Fire The nature of the essential warming energy of Kidney Yang. Considered to be vital in maintaining the heat in the body.
Modality Factor that makes symptoms better or worse
Morphology The science of form, especially of living organisms and their parts
Moxa Dried mugwort, which is burned on the end of needles, or rolled into a stick, and then heated in moxabustion. It is said to warm the Qi in the body, in order to increase its flow. It is made from the species of mugwort *Artemisia vulgaris.*
Moxabustion The treatment approach involving the burning of the Chinese herb moxa.
Mucus Slimy fluid secreted by various membranes in the body
Myocardial infarction Destruction of the muscular substance of the heart due to interruption of the blood supply
Nadis Subtle energetic channels that connect the chakras and link them through the body
Obese Abnormally fat
Palpation Examination with the hands
Palpitation Erratic/fast beating or abnormal rhythm of the heart
Parkinson's Disease A progressive disease of the nervous system
Pathogenic Causing or producing disease
Pediatric Relating to the medical treatment of children
Phlegm In Chinese medicine, a disharmony of the Body Fluids produces either external or visible Phlegm, or internal or invisible Phlegm.

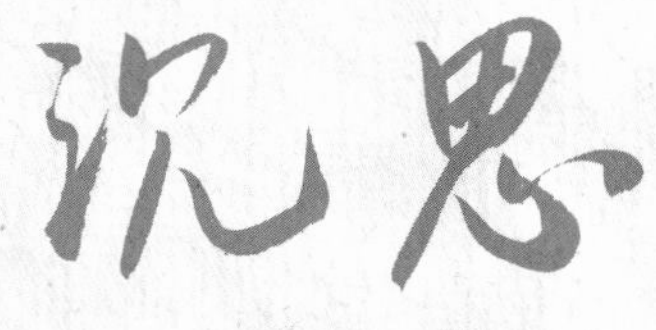

PENSIVENESS

Postnatal/After Heaven Qi/Jing Qi or Jing manufactured from air or food
Prenatal/Before Heaven Qi/Jing Qi or Jing passed on from our parents
Psoriasis Skin disorder causing skin to become dry or itchy
Psychotic Person suffering from a serious mental disorder

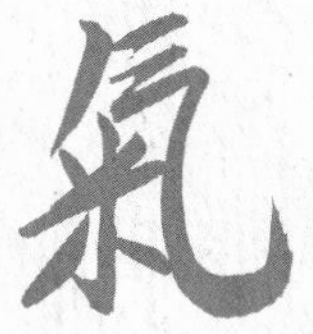

QI

Qi (chi) The Chinese term for the life force or vital energy of the universe, which is fundamental to all aspects of life. It permeates the whole body and concentrates in the channels.
Qigong (Chi Kung) Literally translates as "energy cultivation." A series of moving and static exercises designed for this function.
Qihai The "Sea of Qi" in the lower Dantian. The acupuncture point Ren 6.
Qi Ni Rebellious Qi; Qi that moves in the "wrong" direction
Qi Xian Sinking Qi; Qi sinks when it is too deficient to perform its holding function
Qi Xu Deficient Qi
Qi Zhi Stagnant Qi; Qi that has become sluggish and that ceases to move correctly
Quchi Acupuncture point Large Intestine 11. Literally translates as "crooked pool."
Radial Near the radius of the arm
Reductionist Breaking down something into its constituent parts
Ren Mai The conception vessel, one of the eight extraordinary meridians
Ren Shen Ginseng root
San Jiao The Triple Warmer/Heater/Burner. A process organ in the Chinese Zangfu system

Sciatica Pain in the lower back, usually a sign of some other problem, like a slipped disk

Sea of Marrow The Chinese believe the brain is composed of Marrow, which is then called the "sea"

Semen Palace The male source of sexual energy in the Lower Dantian

Shao Yang San Jiao and Gall Bladder channels

Shao Yin Heart and Kidney channels

Shen An important aspect of mind or spirit in Chinese medicine

Sheng Cycle The cycle of mutual production or promotion in the Five Element system of Chinese medicine

Shiatsu A therapy derived from acupuncture in which pressure is applied to more than 600 acupuncture points by finger, thumb, or palm; from the Japanese word *shiatsu*, meaning "finger pressure"

Six Stage patterns A diagnostic system in Chinese medicine

Stool Feces

Suan Sour; a description of taste for Chinese herbs

Taiji Literally translates as "the supreme ultimate." Usually refers to the martial form of moving practice, which should correctly be termed Taijiquan – Supreme Ultimate Fist or Boxing Art (sometimes written as T'ai Chi Chaun).

Tai Yang The Small Intestine and Bladder channels

Tai Yin The Lung and Spleen channels

Three Treasures The collective term used to describe Qi, Jing, and Shen

Tincture A herbal remedy or perfumery material prepared in an alcohol base

Tinnitus A condition where sounds (ringing) appear in the ear for no apparent reason

Tonification A process in Chinese medicine that involves strengthening and supporting the Blood and Qi

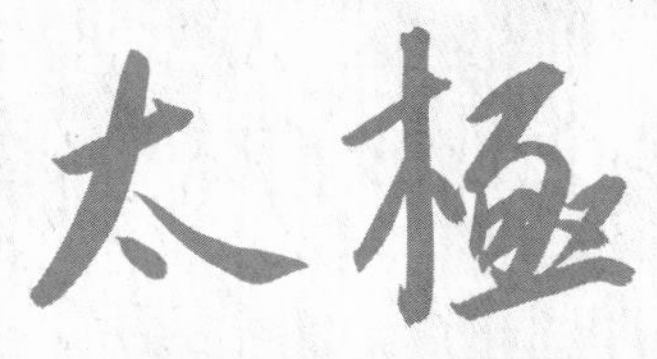

TAIJI

Toxic Poisonous to the body

Trigram An inscription of three letters or figure of three lines

Triple Warmer See San Jiao

Tumor Abnormal growth of the cells anywhere in the body

Varicose veins A condition in which veins become distended and twisted, particularly in the leg

Wei Qi Defensive Qi, which protects the body from invasion by external pathogenic factors. It flows just beneath the skin.

Xian Salty; a description of taste for Chinese herbs

Xin Acrid; a description of taste for Chinese herbs

Xu Deficiency; a common disharmony in Chinese medicine

Xue The Chinese term for Blood

Yang One aspect of the complementary opposites in Chinese philosophy. Reflects the more active, moving, warmer aspects; see also Yin.

Yang Ming Large Intestine and Stomach channels

Yin One aspect of the complementary opposites in Chinese philosophy. Reflects the more passive, still, reflective aspects; see also Yang.

Ying Qi Nutritive aspects of Qi that nourish the body

Yuan Qi Original or source Qi. That aspect of Qi passed on from our parents.

Zang The solid Yin organs of the body

Zangfu The term used in traditional Chinese medicine for the complete Yin and Yang organs of the body (different from those of Western medical science)

Zangfu Zhi Qi Qi of the organs; the Qi that nourishes the organs of the body

Zheng Qi Normal or upright Qi; Qi that circulates through the channels and the organs of the body

Zong Qi Gathering Qi; the Qi that gathers in the chest area through the coming together of Gu Qi and Kong Qi

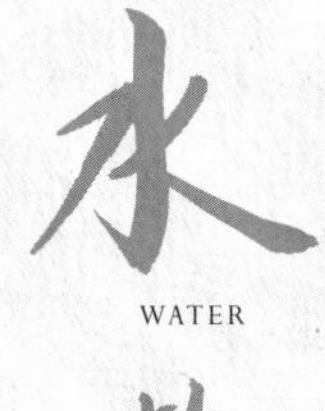

WATER

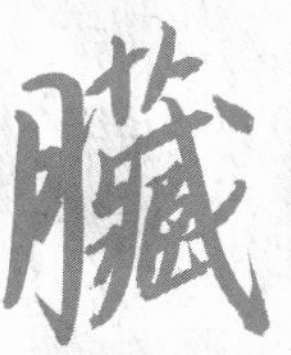

ZANG

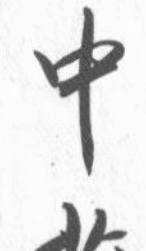

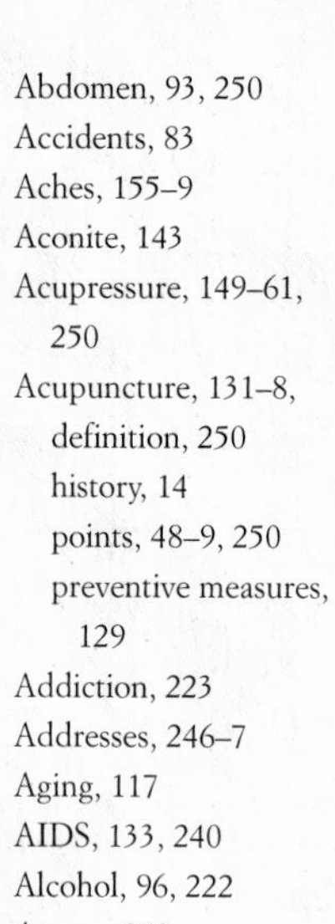

INDEX

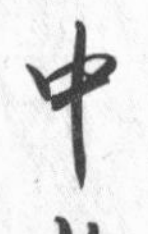

C H I N E S E M E D I C I N E